Manual of Cancer Chemotherapy

Manual of Cancer Chemotherapy

Edited by
Roland T. Skeel, M.D.

Professor of Medicine and Chief, Section
of Hematology and Oncology, Medical
College of Ohio, Toledo

Little, Brown and Company
Boston

Library of Congress Catalog Card No. 82-81884

ISBN 0-316-79572-0

Printed in the United States of America

HAL

Preface

Cancer chemotherapy is an area of medicine that often appears to non-oncologists as an irrational discipline. Numerous drugs, everchanging drug combinations, and endless acronyms seem at best confusing and may lead the nononcologist to give up attempting to understand the oncologist's treatment plan for patients whose care they share. The result is that the primary care physician, on whom the patient continues to rely for guidance and care, is ill-equipped to help the patient with very critical health, and even life or death, decisions.

There is a certain degree of validity to the complaints leveled against the oncologist—and especially the chemotherapist—regarding the rapidity with which one treatment program gives way to another and another. Nonetheless, it is quite possible for the nononcologist to readily learn and understand the principles underlying rational chemotherapy, the categories of antineoplastic chemotherapeutic agents, the goals and strategies of treating various cancers, and the major supportive care problems arising in the patient with cancer. Once these principles and strategies are well understood, the individual treatment programs are more easily understood, and the changes that evolve can be seen as less arbitrary or capricious.

This is not to claim that *every* chemotherapy regimen in each disease has a sound pharmacologic, biologic, or even clinical basis or that we understand why each effective treatment works as well as it does. Ten or twenty years from now, we surely will look back with disbelief at how unrefined our methods are today, perhaps wondering how we managed to do as well as we have. But just as surely, we can look upon our knowledge now with great respect and pride at what has been learned and accomplished over the past twenty years through a rapid incorporation of tumor biology and pharmacology into clinical application.

The purpose of this book is to provide physicians who are not oncologists with a manual that will help them care for their patients who have cancer, particularly those who are receiving chemotherapy. For some cancers—in some stages—the chemotherapy program will be sufficiently straightforward so that the physician who is not an oncologist will feel comfortable directing and administering the chemotherapy. At times, the treatment will be so complex, the toxicity so severe, or dosage modification so critical that an oncologist should both direct and administer the drugs. More often, the care will be best accomplished through a joint management program carved out by the oncologist and the primary care physician. Whatever the circumstance, this manual is designed to help the nononcologist understand the basis for, and participate in, the safe and effective administration of cancer chemotherapy.

R.T.S.

Acknowledgments

I thank my friend, Gordon Reid, M.D., who many years ago planted the idea for this manual in my head, and my chief, Patrick J. Mulrow, M.D., who encouraged me to get the task off the ground. Many people helped prepare the manuscript, checking everything from sentence structure to drug doses, making phone calls, and cheerfully typing and retyping. Among those to whom I am particularly indebted are Georgiann Monhollen, Mary Kesling, Donna Freshour, Gloria Gluntz, and Kristi Skeel. To my mentors, Edward S. Henderson, M.D., and Joseph R. Bertino, M.D., I owe a special thanks for their expert guidance during my training and development in oncology. Most of all, I am grateful to the patients who have allowed me to enter their lives to learn about them, their diseases, and their care.

Contents

Contributing Authors

Robert S. Benjamin, M.D.

Associate Professor of Medicine, University of Texas System Cancer Center; Chief, Melanoma-Sarcoma Section, M. D. Anderson Hospital and Tumor Institute, Houston, Texas

Ronald C. DeConti, M.D.

Associate Clinical Professor of Medicine, Tufts University School of Medicine, Boston; Acting Chief, Hematology and Oncology Unit, Baystate Medical Center, Springfield, Massachusetts

William D. DeWys, M.D.

Chief, Clinical Investigations Branch, Cancer Therapy Evaluation Program, Division of Cancer Treatment, National Cancer Institute, National Institutes of Health, Bethesda, Maryland

Roberto Franco-Saenz, M.D.

Professor of Medicine and Chief, Division of Endocrinology and Metabolism, Medical College of Ohio, Toledo

Robert B. Livingston, M.D.

Chairman, Department of Hematology and Medical Oncology, Cleveland Clinic Foundation, Cleveland, Ohio

Gerald W. Marsa, M.D.

Clinical Associate Professor of Radiology, Medical College of Ohio, Toledo; Director, Radiation Oncology, Flower Hospital Oncology Center, Sylvania, Ohio

John C. Marsh, M.D.

Professor of Medicine and Lecturer in Pharmacology, Yale University School of Medicine, Section of Medical Oncology, Department of Medicine, Yale-New Haven Hospital, New Haven, Connecticut

Larry Nathanson, M.D.

Professor of Medicine, State University of New York at Stony Brook School of Medicine; Director, Division of Oncology/ Hematology, Department of Medicine, Nassau Hospital, Mineola, New York

Martin M. Oken, M.D.

Assistant Professor of Medicine, University of Minnesota Medical School; Staff Physician, Veterans Administration Hospital, Minneapolis, Minnesota

Roland T. Skeel, M.D.	Professor of Medicine and Chief, Section of Hematology and Oncology, Medical College of Ohio, Toledo
Mary R. Smith, M.D.	Associate Professor of Medicine and Assistant Professor of Pathology, Medical College of Ohio, Toledo
Richard S. Stein, M.D.	Associate Professor of Medicine, Vanderbilt University School of Medicine, Nashville, Tennessee
Steven E. Vogl, M.D.	Associate Professor of Medicine, Albert Einstein College of Medicine, Bronx, New York
Michael Weintraub, M.D.	Associate Professor of Pharmacology and Medicine, University of Rochester School of Medicine, Rochester, New York

Manual of Cancer
Chemotherapy

Basic Principles and Considerations of Rational Chemotherapy

It is often difficult to deliver the best treatment for a patient with cancer for no two persons are exactly alike with respect to the biologic behavior and therapeutic responsiveness of their cancer, or to the toxic effects of the chemotherapy (or other modality). Therefore, therapeutic decisions must always take individual factors into account. Individualization of therapy does not mean that therapy for each patient must be selected de novo or be substantially different from the therapy of other patients with the same disease. On the contrary, similarities among patients and their cancers are common and can be exploited in the selection of therapy most likely to result in a beneficial response.

Several principles underlie the selection of optimal therapy for each patient. While the chemotherapist does not systematically review each principle nor the laboratory and clinical data that form their basis every time a patient is treated, each principle is critical at some point in developing treatment and applying these programs to individual patients. These principles that form the basis of rational chemotherapy relate to the drugs, to the patient, and to other modalities of treatment.

1. Rational chemotherapy has a biologic and pharmacologic basis.
2. Systematic assessment of the patient is critical for selection and administration of effective chemotherapy.
3. Chemotherapy is only one part of good cancer treatment.

In the three chapters of Part I, each of these principles will be considered in some detail in order to provide a background for the following parts of the manual, in which the individual agents and cancers are discussed.

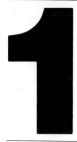

The Biologic and Pharmacologic Basis of Cancer Chemotherapy

Roland T. Skeel

I. General mechanisms by which chemotherapeutic agents control cancer. The purpose of treating cancer with chemotherapeutic agents is to prevent cancer cells from multiplying, invading, metastasizing, and ultimately killing the host (patient). Most agents currently in use appear to have their effect primarily on cell multiplication and tumor growth. Because cell multiplication is a characteristic of many normal cells as well as cancer cells, most cancer chemotherapeutic agents also have toxic effects on normal cells, particularly those with a rapid rate of turnover, such as bone marrow and mucous membrane cells. The goal in selecting an effective drug, therefore, is to find an agent that has marked growth inhibitory or controlling effect on the cancer cell with minimal toxic effect on the host. In the most effective chemotherapeutic regimens, the drugs are capable not only of inhibiting but of completely eradicating all neoplastic cells while sufficiently preserving normal marrow and other target organs to allow a return to normal, or at least satisfactory, function.

Ideally, the pharmacologist or medicinal chemist would like to look at the cancer cell, discover how it differs from the normal host cell, and then design a chemotherapeutic agent to capitalize on that difference. In practice, more often, less rational means are used. The effectiveness of agents is discovered by treating either animal or human neoplasms, and then the pharmacologist attempts to discover why they work as well as they do. With few exceptions, the reasons why chemotherapeutic agents are more effective against cancer cells than normal cells are poorly understood.

Inhibition of cell multiplication and tumor growth can take place at several levels within the cell, including

1. Macromolecular synthesis and function
2. Cytoplasmic organization
3. Cell membrane synthesis function

Nearly all agents currently in use or under investigation, with the exception of immunotherapeutic agents and other biologic response modifiers, appear to have their primary effect on either macromolecular synthesis or function. This effect means that they interfere with either the synthesis of DNA, RNA, or proteins, or with the appropriate functioning of the preformed molecule. When interference in the macromolecular synthesis or function of the neoplastic cell population is sufficiently great, a proportion of the cells die. (Cell death may or may not take place at the time of exposure to the drug. Often a cell must undergo several divisions before the lethal event that took place earlier finally results in the death of the cell.) Because only a proportion of the cells die with a given treatment, repeated doses of

3

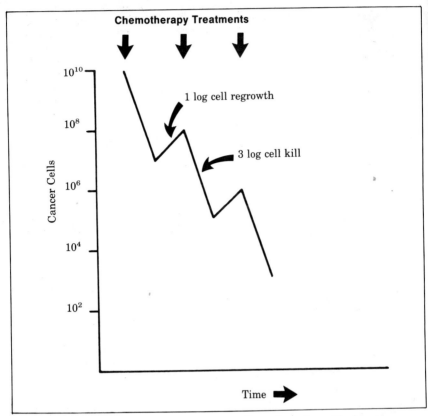

Fig. 1-1. The effect of chemotherapy on cancer cell numbers. In an ideal system, chemotherapy kills a constant proportion of the remaining cancer cells with each dose. Between doses, cell regrowth occurs. When therapy is successful, cell killing is greater than cell growth.

chemotherapy must be used to continue to reduce the cell number (Fig. 1-1). Each time the dose is repeated, the same *proportion* of cells—not the same absolute number—is killed. In the example shown in Figure 1-1, 99.9 percent (3 logs) of the cancer cells are killed with each treatment, and there is a tenfold (1 log) growth between treatments for a net reduction of 2 logs with each treatment. Starting at 10^{10} cells (about 10 g or 10 cm^3), it would take five treatments to reach less than 10^0, or one, cell. Such a model makes certain assumptions that rarely are strictly true in clinical practice:

1. All cells in a tumor population are equally sensitive to a drug.
2. Cell sensitivity is independent of the location of the cells within the host and independent of local host factors, such as blood supply or surrounding fibrosis.
3. Cell sensitivity does not change during the course of therapy.

The lack of curability of most initially sensitive tumors is probably a reflection of the degree to which these assumptions do not hold true.

II. Tumor cell kinetics and chemotherapy. Cancer cells, unlike other body cells, are characterized by a growth process whereby their sensitivity to normal controlling factors has been completely or partially lost. As a result of this uncontrolled growth, it was once thought that cancer cells grew or multiplied faster than normal cells, and that this growth rate was responsible for their sensitivity to chemotherapy. It now is known that most cancer cells grow less rapidly than the more active normal cells, such as bone marrow. Thus, growth rate alone cannot explain the greater sensitivity of cancer cells to chemotherapy.

  A. Tumor growth. The growth of a tumor is dependent on several interrelated factors.

    1. Cell cycle time, or the average time for a cell that has just completed mitosis to grow and again divide and pass through mitosis, determines the maximum growth rate for a tumor but probably does not determine drug sensitivity. As is explained in section **B,** the relative proportion of cell cycle time taken up by the DNA synthetic phase may relate to drug sensitivity.

    2. Growth fraction, or the fraction of cells undergoing cell division, represents the portion of cells that will be sensitive to drugs whose major effect is exerted on cells that are actively dividing. If the growth fraction approaches one and the cell death rate is low, then the tumor doubling time will approximate the cell cycle time.

    3. Total number of cells in the population (determined at some arbitrary time at which the growth measurement is started) is clinically important because it is an index of how advanced the cancer is and frequently correlates with normal organ dysfunction.

    4. Intrinsic cell death rate of tumors is difficult to measure in patients but probably makes a major contribution to slow the growth rate of many solid tumors.

  B. Cell cycle. The cell cycle of cancer cells is qualitatively the same as that of normal cells (Fig. 1-2). Each cell begins its growth during a postmitotic period or phase called G_1 during which enzymes necessary for DNA

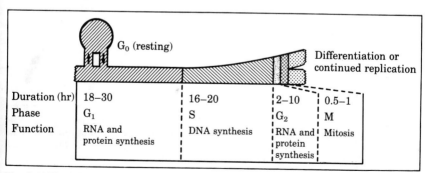

Duration (hr)	18–30	16–20	2–10	0.5–1
Phase	G_1	S	G_2	M
Function	RNA and protein synthesis	DNA synthesis	RNA and protein synthesis	Mitosis

G_0 (resting)

Differentiation or continued replication

Fig. 1-2. The cell cycle time for human tissues has a wide range (16–260 hr) with marked differences among normal and tumor tissues. Normal marrow and gastrointestinal-lining cells have cell cycle times of 24 to 48 hours. Representative durations and the kinetic or synthetic activity are indicated for each phase.

Table 1-1. Cell Cycle Phase-Specific Chemotherapeutic Agents

Phase of Greatest Activity	Class	Type	Agent
Gap 1 (G_1)	Natural product	Enzyme	Asparaginase
	Hormone	Corticosteroid	Prednisone
DNA synthesis (S)	Antimetabolite	Pyrimidine analog	Cytarabine, fluorouracil
	Antimetabolite	Folic acid analog	Methotrexate
	Antimetabolite	Purine analog	Thioguanine
	Miscellaneous	Substituted urea	Hydroxyurea
Gap 2 (G_2)	Natural product	Antibiotic	Bleomycin, etoposide
Mitosis (M)	Natural product	Mitotic inhibitor	Vinblastine, vincristine, vindesine

production, other proteins, and RNA are produced. G_1 is followed by a period of *DNA synthesis (S)* in which essentially all DNA synthesis for a given cycle takes place. When DNA synthesis is complete, the cell enters a *premitotic period (G_2)* during which further protein and RNA synthesis occur. This gap is followed immediately by *mitosis (M)* at the end of which actual physical division takes place, two daughter cells are formed, and each again enters G_1. The G_1 phase is in equilibrium with a resting state called G_0. Cells in G_0 are relatively inactive with respect to macromolecular synthesis and are consequently insensitive to many chemotherapeutic agents, particularly those that affect macromolecular synthesis.

C. Phase and cell cycle specificity. Most chemotherapeutic agents can be grouped according to whether they depend on cells being in cycle (i.e., not in G_0) and, if they depend on the cell being in cycle, whether their activity is greater when the cell is in a specific phase of the cycle.

   1. Phase-specific drugs. Those agents that are most active against cells that are in a specific phase of the cell cycle are called *cell cycle phase-specific* drugs (Table 1-1).

   a. Implications of phase-specific drugs. Phase specificity has important implications for cancer chemotherapy.

   (1) Limitation to single-exposure cell kill. With a phase-specific agent, there is a limit to the number of cells that can be killed with a single instantaneous (or very short) drug exposure, because only those cells in the sensitive phase will be killed. A higher dose will kill no more cells.

   (2) Increasing cell kill by prolonged exposure. For more cells to be killed requires either a prolonged exposure to the drug or repeated doses of the drug to allow more cells to enter the sensitive phase of the cycle. Theoretically, all cells could be killed if the blood level, or more importantly the intracellular concentration, of the drug remains sufficiently high while all cells in the target population pass through one complete cell cycle. This theory assumes that the drug does not prevent the passage of cells from one (insensitive) phase to another (sensitive).

(3) **Recruitment.** A higher number of cells could be killed by a phase-specific drug if the proportion of cells in the sensitive phase could be increased (recruited).

b. **Cytarabine.** One of the best examples of a phase-specific agent is cytarabine (ara-C), which is an inhibitor of DNA synthesis and thus is active in only the S phase (at standard doses). Ara-C is rapidly deaminated in vivo to an inactive compound, ara-U, and rapid injections result in very short, effective levels of ara-C. As a result, single doses of ara-C are quite nontoxic to the normal hematopoietic system and are generally ineffective in treating leukemia. If the drug is given as a daily rapid injection, some patients with leukemia will respond well but not nearly as well as when ara-C is given on an every 12-hour schedule. The apparent reason for the greater effectiveness of the 12-hour schedule is that the S phase (DNA synthesis) of human acute nonlymphocytic leukemia cells lasts about 18 to 20 hours. If the drug is given every 24 hours, some cells that have not entered the S phase when the drug is first administered would not be sensitive to its effect. Therefore, these cells could pass all the way through the S phase before the next dose is administered and would completely escape any cytotoxic effect. However, when the drug is given every 12 hours, no cell that was "in cycle" would be able to escape exposure to ara-C, since none would be able to get through one complete S phase without the drug being present.

If all cells were in active cycle, that is, if none were resting in a prolonged G_1 or G_0, it would be theoretically possible to kill all cells in a population by a continuous or scheduled exposure equivalent to one complete cell cycle. Experiments with patients with acute leukemia have shown that if tritiated thymidine is used to label cells as they enter DNA synthesis, it may be 7 to 10 days before the maximum number of leukemia cells have all passed through the S phase. This factor means that for ara-C to have a maximum effect on the leukemia, the repeated exposure must be continued for a 7- to 10-day period. Clinically, this type of schedule for ara-C administration appears to be most effective in treating newly diagnosed patients with acute nonlymphocytic leukemia. Even with such prolonged exposure, however, a few of the cells appear not to have passed through the S phase.

2. **Cell cycle-specific drugs.** Agents that are effective while cells are actively in cycle, but are not dependent on the cell being in a particular phase, are called *cell cycle-specific drugs (phase-nonspecific)*. This group includes most of the alkylating agents, antitumor antibiotics, and some miscellaneous agents (Table 1-2). Some agents in this group are not totally phase-nonspecific; they may have greater activity in one phase than in another, but not to the degree of the phase-specific agents. Many of the agents in this group also appear to have some activity in cells that are not in cycle, although not as much as when the cells are rapidly dividing.

3. **Cell cycle-nonspecific drugs.** A third group of drugs appears to be effective whether cancer cells are in cycle or are resting. In this respect, these agents are similar to photon irradiation. Drugs in this

Table 1-2. Cell Cycle-Specific Chemotherapeutic Agents

Class	Type	Agent
Alkylating agent	Nitrogen mustard	Chlorambucil, cyclophosphamide, melphalan
	Alkyl sulfonate	Busulfan
	Triazine	Dacarbazine
	Metal salt	Cisplatin
Natural product	Antibiotic	Dactinomycin, daunorubicin, doxorubicin

Table 1-3. Cell Cycle-Nonspecific Chemotherapeutic Agents

Class	Type	Agent
Alkylating agent	Nitrogen mustard	Mechlorethamine
	Nitrosourea	Carmustine, lomustine, semustine

category are called *cell cycle-nonspecific,* and include mechlorethamine (nitrogen mustard) and the nitrosoureas (Table 1-3).

D. Changes in tumor cell kinetics and therapy implications. As cancer cells grow from a few cells to a lethal tumor burden, certain changes occur in the growth rate of the population that affect the strategies of chemotherapy. These changes have been determined by observing the characteristics of experimental tumors in animals and neoplastic cells growing in tissue culture. These model systems readily permit accurate cell number determinations to be made and growth rates to be determined. (Since tumor cells cannot be injected or implanted into humans and permitted to grow, studies of growth rates of intact tumors in humans must largely be limited to observing the growth rate of macroscopic tumors.)

1. **Stages of tumor growth.** Immediately after inoculating a tissue culture or an experimental animal with tumor cells, there is a *lag phase* during which there is little tumor growth. Presumably the cells in this phase are becoming accustomed to the new environment and are preparing to enter into cycle. The lag phase is followed by a period of rapid growth called *log phase,* during which there are repeated doublings of the cell number. In those populations in which the growth fraction approaches 100 percent and the cell death rate is low, the population doubles within a period approximating the cell cycle time. As the cell number or tumor size becomes macroscopic, the doubling time of the tumor cell population becomes prolonged and levels off (*plateau phase*). The prolongation in tumor doubling time may be due to a smaller growth fraction, a change in the cell cycle time, an increased intrinsic death rate, alone or in combination. Factors responsible for these changes include decrease of nutrients, increase of inhibitory metabolites, and inhibition of growth by cell-cell interaction.

2. **Growth rate and effectiveness of chemotherapy.** Chemotherapeutic agents are most effective during the period of logarithmic growth. As might be expected, this result is particularly true for the antimetabo-

lites, which are largely S-phase-specific. As a result, when human tumors become macroscopic, the effectiveness of many chemotherapeutic agents is reduced because only part of the cell population is actively dividing. Theoretically, if the cell population could be reduced sufficiently by other means, such as surgery or radiotherapy, chemotherapy would be more effective because a higher fraction of the remaining cells would be in logarithmic growth. The validity of this theoretical premise is supported by the considerable success of combined surgery and chemotherapy or of radiotherapy and chemotherapy in breast cancer, Wilms' tumor, ovarian cancer, and oat-cell carcinoma of the lung.

III. **Combination chemotherapy.** Combinations of drugs are frequently more effective in producing responses and prolonging life than the same drugs used sequentially. There are several reasons that combinations are likely to be more effective than single agents.

A. **Reasons for effectiveness of combinations**

1. **Prevention of resistant clones.** If one in 10^5 cells is resistant to drug A and one in 10^5 resistant to drug B, it is likely that treating a macroscopic tumor (10^6 cells/cm^3) with either agent alone will result in several clones of cells that are resistant to that drug. Once a resistant clone has grown to macroscopic size and if the same mutant frequency persists for drug B, resistance to that agent will also emerge. If both drugs are used at the outset of therapy or in close sequence, however, the likelihood of a cell being resistant to both drugs will be only one in 10^{10}. Thus the combination confers considerable advantage against the emergence of resistant clones.

2. **Cytotoxicity to resting and dividing cells.** The combination of a drug that is cell cycle-specific (phase-nonspecific) or cell cycle-nonspecific with a drug that is cell cycle phase-specific can kill cells that are slowly dividing as well as cells that are actively dividing. The use of cell cycle-nonspecific drugs can also help recruit cells into a more actively dividing state, which results in their being more sensitive to the cell cycle phase-specific agents.

3. **Biochemical enhancement of effect.** Combinations of drugs that affect different biochemical pathways or steps in a single pathway can enhance each other.

4. **Drug interactions.** Combinations can result in beneficial effects of one drug on the other, including

   a. An intracellular increase in the drug or its active metabolites

   b. Reduced metabolic inactivation of the drug

   c. Cooperative inhibition of a single enzyme or reaction

5. **Sanctuary access.** Combinations can be used to provide access to sanctuary sites for reasons such as drug solubility or affinity of specific tissues for a particular drug type.

6. **Rescue.** Combinations can be used in which one agent rescues the host from the toxic effects of another drug.

B. **Principles of selection of agents.** In selecting appropriate agents for use in a combination, the following principles should be observed:

1. Choose individually active drugs. Do not use a combination in which one agent is inactive when used alone unless there is a clear, specific biochemical or pharmacologic reason to do so, such as high-dose methotrexate followed by leucovorin rescue.

2. When possible, choose drugs in which the dose-limiting toxicities differ qualitatively or in time of occurrence. Often, however, two or more agents that have marrow toxicity will have to be used, and the selection of a safe dose of each is critical. As a starting point, two drugs in combination can usually be given at two thirds of the dose used when the drugs are given alone. Whenever a new drug combination is tried, a careful evaluation for both expected and unanticipated toxicities must be carried out.

3. Select agents for a combination for which there is a biochemical or pharmacologic rationale. Preferably this rationale will have been tested in an animal tumor system and in the appropriate model system and will have been found to be better than either agent alone.

4. Be cautious when attempting to improve on a successful two-drug combination by adding a third, fourth, and fifth drug. Although this approach may be beneficial, two undesirable results may be seen:

   a. An intolerable level of toxicity that leads to excessive morbidity and mortality.

   b. Unchanged or reduced antitumor effect because of the necessity to reduce the dose of the most effective drugs to a level below which antitumor responses will not be seen, despite the theoretical advantages of the combination. Therefore, the addition of each new agent to a combination must be carefully considered, the principles of combination therapy closely followed, and controlled clinical trials carried out to compare the efficacy of any new regimen with a more established (standard) treatment program.

C. **Clinical effectiveness of combinations.** Combinations of drugs have been clearly demonstrated to be better than single agents in many, but not all, human cancers. The benefit of combinations of drugs compared with the same drugs used sequentially has been quite marked in diseases such as acute lymphocytic leukemia, Hodgkin's lymphoma, breast carcinoma, oat-cell carcinoma of the lung, and testicular carcinoma. The benefit is less clear in cancers such as non-oat-cell carcinoma of the lung, non-Hodgkin's lymphomas with favorable prognoses, ovarian carcinoma, head and neck carcinomas, melanoma, and colorectal carcinomas, although reports exist for each of these in which combinations are better in one respect or another than single agents.

IV. **Resistance to antineoplastic agents.** Resistance to antineoplastic chemotherapy is a combined characteristic of a specific drug, a specific tumor, and a specific host whereby the drug is ineffective in controlling the tumor without excessive toxicity. Resistance of a tumor to a drug is the reciprocal of selectivity of that drug for the tumor. The problem for the chemotherapist or pharmacologist is not simply to find an agent that is cytotoxic, but to find an agent that can selectively kill neoplastic cells while preserving the essential host cells and their function. Were it not for the problem of resistance of human cancer to antineoplastic agents, or conversely, the lack of selectivity of those agents, cancer chemotherapy would be similar to antibacterial chemotherapy in which complete eradication of infection is regularly observed. Such a utopian state of cancer chemotherapy has not yet been achieved for the majority of human cancers. Thus the problem of resistance and ways to overcome or even exploit it remains an area of major interest for the chemotherapist.

Resistance to antineoplastic chemotherapeutic agents may be either natural or acquired. *Natural resistance* refers to the initial unresponsiveness of a tumor to a given drug, while *acquired resistance* refers to the unresponsiveness that emerges after initially successful treatment. There are four basic categories of resistance to chemotherapy: kinetic, biochemical, pharmacologic, and nonselectivity.

A. Cell kinetics and resistance. Resistance based on cell population kinetics relates to cycle and phase specificity, growth fractions, and the implications of these factors for responsiveness to specific agents and schedules of drug administration. A particular problem with many human tumors is that they are in a plateau growth phase with a small growth fraction. This factor renders many of the cells insensitive to the antimetabolites and relatively unresponsive to many of the other chemotherapeutic agents. Strategies to overcome resistance due to cell kinetics include

1. Reducing tumor bulk with surgery or radiotherapy

2. Using combinations to include drugs that affect resting populations (with many G_0 cells)

3. Scheduling of drugs to prevent phase escape or to synchronize cell populations and increase cell kill

B. Biochemical causes of resistance. Resistance can occur for biochemical reasons. These include the inability of a tumor to convert a drug to its active form, the ability of a tumor to inactivate a drug, or the location of a tumor in a site where substrates are present that bypass an otherwise lethal blockade. Combination chemotherapy can overcome biochemical resistance by increasing the amount of active drug intracellularly as a result of biochemical interactions or effects on drug transport across the cell membrane. The use of a second agent to rescue normal cells may also permit the use of very high doses of the first agent, which can overcome the resistance caused by a low rate of conversion to the active metabolite or a high rate of inactivation.

C. Pharmacologic causes of resistance. Apparent resistance to cancer chemotherapy can result from poor absorption, increased excretion or catabolism, and drug interactions leading to inadequate blood levels of the drug. Strictly speaking, this result is not true resistance, but, to the degree that the insufficient blood levels are not appreciated by the clinician, resistance appears to be present. The variation from patient to patient in the highest tolerated dose has led to dose-modification schemes that permit dose escalation when the toxicities of the chemotherapy regimen are minimal or nonexistent, as well as dose reduction when toxicities are great. This regulation is particularly important for some chemotherapeutic agents for which the dose-response curve is quite steep.

True pharmacologic resistance is caused by the poor transport of agents into certain body tissues and tumor cells. For example, the central nervous system (CNS) is a site that many drugs do not reach well. Several drug characteristics favor transport into the CNS, including high lipid solubility and low molecular weight. For tumors that originate in the CNS or metastasize there, drugs of choice should be those that achieve effective antitumor concentration in brain tissue and are effective against the tumor cell type being treated.

D. Nonselectivity and resistance. Nonselectivity is not really a mechanism for resistance, but rather an acknowledgment that for most cancers and most drugs, the reasons for resistance and selectivity are poorly understood.

Given a rather limited understanding of the biochemical differences between normal and malignant cells, it is gratifying that chemotherapy is successful as frequently as it is. It is to be hoped that in 20 years we will view current chemotherapy as a very crude beginning, and that many more tumor target-directed agents will be found that will have a high potential for curing the majority of human cancers that now defy successful treatment.

Selected Reading

Baserga, R. The relationship of the cell cycle to tumor growth and control of cell division. A review. *Cancer Res.* 25:581, 1965.

Baserga, R. The cell cycle. *N. Engl. J. Med.* 304:453, 1981.

Bender, R. A., and Dedrick, R. L. Cytokinetic aspects of clinical drug resistance. *Cancer Chemotherapy Rep.* 59:805, 1975.

Clarkson, B., et al. Studies of cellular proliferation in human leukemia. *Cancer* 25:1237, 1970.

DeVita, V. T., and Schein, P. S. The use of drugs in combination for the treatment of cancer. Rationale and results. *N. Engl. J. Med.* 288:998, 1973.

Schabel, F. M., Jr. The use of tumor growth kinetics in planning "curative" chemotherapy of advanced solid tumors. *Cancer Res.* 29:2384, 1969.

Skeel, R. T., and Lindquist, C. A. Clinical Aspects of Resistance to Antineoplastic Agents. In F. F. Becker (Ed.), *Cancer, A Comprehensive Treatise,* Vol. 5. New York: Plenum Pr., 1977.

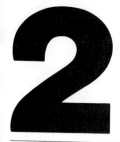

Systematic Assessment of the Patient with Cancer

Roland T. Skeel

I. Establishing the diagnosis

A. A pathologic diagnosis is critical.
Although it is a truism to state that the diagnosis of cancer must be firmly established before chemotherapy or any other treatment is administered, the critical nature of accurate diagnosis warrants a reminder. As a rule, there must be cytologic or histologic evidence of neoplastic cells, together with a clinical picture consistent with the diagnosis of the cancer under consideration.

Most commonly, patients will present to their physician with a complaint such as a cough or a lump; through a logical sequence of evaluation, the presence of cancer is revealed on a cytologic or histologic specimen. Less frequently, lesions will be discovered fortuitously during routine examination, in systematic screening for cancer, or during evaluation of an unrelated disorder. With some types of cancer, pathologists can establish the diagnosis on very small amounts of material obtained from needle biopsies, aspirations, or tissue scrapings. Other cancers may require larger pieces of tissue for special staining or examination under the electron microscope. It is often helpful to confer with the pathologist prior to obtaining a specimen in order to determine what kind and size of specimen will be adequate to establish the complete diagnosis. When a tissue diagnosis of cancer is made by the pathologist, it is incumbent on the clinician to review the material with the pathologist. This is not only good medicine (and good learning), but it helps to be able to tell the patient you have seen the cancer with your own eyes when you give the diagnosis. It also prevents the physician from administering chemotherapy without a pathologic diagnosis. The pathologist will often give a better consultation—not just a tissue diagnosis—if the clinician shows a personal interest.

B. Pathologic and clinical diagnosis must be consistent.
Once the tissue diagnosis is established, the clinician must be certain that the pathologic diagnosis is consistent with the clinical findings. If the two are not consistent, then a search must be made for additional information, either clinical or pathologic, which will allow the clinician to make a unified diagnosis. (On rare occasions, two simultaneous diagnoses of cancer may be made.)

C. Treatment without a pathologic diagnosis.
There are rare circumstances in which treatment is undertaken before a pathologic diagnosis is established. Such circumstances are clearly exceptions, however, and constitute less than 1 percent of all patients with cancer. Therapy is begun without a pathologic diagnosis only when

   1. Withholding prompt treatment or carrying out the procedures required to establish the diagnosis would greatly increase a patient's morbidity or mortality.

   2. The likelihood of a benign diagnosis is remote.

   Two examples of such circumstances would be (1) a primary tumor of the midbrain and (2) superior vena cava syndrome.

II. Staging. Once the diagnosis of cancer is firmly established, it is important to determine the anatomic extent or stage of the disease. The steps taken in staging vary considerably among cancers because of their differing natural histories.

   A. Staging system criteria. For most cancers, a system of staging has been established based on the following:

   1. The natural history and mode of spread of the cancer

   2. The prognostic import for the staging parameters used

   3. The value of the criteria used for decisions about therapy

   B. Staging and therapy decisions. In the past, surgery and radiotherapy were used to treat patients with cancer in "early" stages, and chemotherapy was used when surgery and radiotherapy were no longer effective or when the disease was in an advanced stage at presentation. In such circumstances, chemotherapy was only palliative (except for gestational choriocarcinoma) and in the absence of exquisitely sensitive tumors or strikingly potent drugs, the likelihood of increasing survival was low. As we have learned more about cancer growth and tumor cell kinetics, the value of early intervention with chemotherapy has been transposed from animal models to human cancers. To plan this intervention and evaluate its effectiveness, careful staging has become increasingly important. Only when the exact extent of disease has been established can the most rational plan of treatment for the individual patient be devised, whether it be surgery, radiotherapy, or chemotherapy, alone or in combination. No single staging system is universally used for all cancers, and none of the several systems will be presented here in detail. When relevant to the specific cancers whose chemotherapy is discussed in Part III, the staging system most commonly used for that cancer will be discussed.

III. Performance status. The performance status refers to the level of activity of which a patient is capable. It is an independent measurement (independent from the anatomic extent or histologic characteristics of the cancer) of how much the cancer has affected the patient and a prognostic indication of how well the patient is likely to do with treatment.

   A. Types of performance status scales. Two performance status scales are in wide use.

   1. The Karnofsky Performance Status Scale (Table 2-1) has 10 levels of activity. It has the advantage of allowing discrimination over a wide scale, but it has the disadvantage of being difficult to remember easily and perhaps makes discriminations that are not clinically useful.

Table 2-1. Karnofsky Performance Status Scale

Functional Capability	Level of Activity
Able to carry on normal activity; no special care is needed	100% Normal; no complaints, no evidence of disease 90% Able to carry on normal activity; minor signs or symptoms of disease 80% Normal activity with effort, some signs or symptoms of disease
Unable to work; able to live at home; cares for most personal needs; a varying amount of assistance is needed	70% Cares for self; unable to carry on normal activity or to do active work 60% Requires occasional assistance but is able to care for most of own needs 50% Requires considerable assistance and frequent medical care
Unable to care for self; requires equivalent of institutional or hospital care	40% Disabled; requires special medical care and assistance 30% Severely disabled; hospitalization is indicated, although death not imminent 20% Very sick; hospitalization necessary; active supportive treatment necessary 10% Moribund; fatal processes progressing rapidly 0% Dead

Table 2-2. ECOG Performance Status Scale

Grade	Level of Activity
0	Fully active, able to carry on all pre-disease performance without restriction (Karnofsky 90–100)
1	Restricted in physically strenuous activity but ambulatory and able to carry out work of a light or sedentary nature, e.g., light house work, office work (Karnofsky 70–80)
2	Ambulatory and capable of all self-care but unable to carry out any work activities; up and about more than 50% of waking hours (Karnofsky 50–60)
3	Capable of only limited self-care, confined to bed or chair more than 50% of waking hours (Karnofsky 30–40)
4	Completely disabled. Cannot carry on any self-care; totally confined to bed or chair (Karnofsky 10–20)

2. **The Eastern Cooperative Oncology Group (ECOG) Performance Status Scale** (Table 2-2) has the advantages of being easy to remember and use for making discriminations that are clinically useful.

Using the criteria of each scale, patients who are fully active or mildly symptomatic respond more frequently to treatment than do patients who are less active or severely symptomatic. A clear designation of the performance status distribution of patients in therapeutic clinical trials is thus critical in determining comparability of trials and effectiveness of the treatments used.

B. **Use of performance status in choosing treatment.** In the individualization of therapy, the performance status is often a useful parameter in helping the clinician decide whether the patient will benefit from treatment or will be made worse. For example, unless there is some reason to expect a dramatic response of a cancer to chemotherapy, treatment is often withheld from patients with an ECOG performance status of four, since responses to therapy are infrequent and toxic effects of the treatment are likely to be great.

IV. **Response to Therapy.** Response to therapy may be measured by (1) survival, (2) objective change in tumor size or in tumor product (e.g., antibody in myeloma), and (3) subjective change.

A. **Survival.** One goal of all cancer therapy modalities is to allow patients to live as long as they would have had they not had the cancer. If this is achieved, it can be said that the patient is cured of the cancer. From a practical standpoint, we do not wait to see whether patients live a normal life span before saying that a given treatment is capable of achieving a cure, but we follow a cohort of patients to see whether their survival in a given time span is different from a comparable cohort without the cancer. It is, of course, possible that a patient may be cured of the cancer but die earlier from complications associated with the treatment. Unless the complications are acute, such as bleeding or infection, survival is likely to be longer than if the treatment had not been given, but shorter than if the patient never had the cancer.

If cure is not possible then the reduced goal is to allow the patient to live longer than if the therapy under consideration were not given. It is important for physicians to know whether, and with what likelihood, any given treatment will result in a longer life. Such information is important to the physician in choosing whether to recommend treatment and may be important to the patient in deciding whether to undertake the recommended treatment program.

B. **Objective response.** Although survival is important to the individual patient, it is not easy to predict how long a patient is going to live; thus survival does not give an early measurement of treatment effectiveness. Tumor regression, on the other hand, frequently occurs early in the course of effective treatment and is therefore a readily used measurement of treatment benefit. Tumor regression can be determined by the reduction in size of a tumor or the reduction of tumor products, such as hormones or antibodies.

1. **Tumor size.** When tumor size is measured, responses are usually classified as follows:

    a. **Complete response** is the complete disappearance of all evidence of the cancer for at least 2 measurement periods separated by at least 4 weeks.

    b. **Partial response** is a decrease of 50 percent or greater in the product of the largest diameter and the diameter perpendicular to the largest (diameter product) of all measurable lesions with no appearance of any new lesions for at least 4 weeks.

c. **Stable disease** is a decrease of less than 50 percent to an increase of less than 25 percent in the diameter product of any measurable lesions.

d. **Progression** is an increase of more than 25 percent in the diameter product or the appearance of any new lesions.

If survival curves of populations of patients having different categories of response are compared, those patients with complete response frequently survive longer than those with lesser response. If a sizable number of complete responses occur within a treatment program, the survival rate of patients treated with that program is likely to be significantly greater than that of patients who are untreated. When the number of complete responders in a population rises above 50 percent, the possibility of cure for a small number of patients begins to appear. With increasing percentages of complete responders, the frequency of cures is likely to increase correspondingly.

Although those patients who have partial response to a treatment usually survive longer than those patients who have stable disease or progression, it is often not easy to demonstrate that the overall survival of the treated population is better than a comparable untreated group. In part, this difficulty may be due to a phenomenon of small numbers. If only 15 to 20 percent of a population responds to therapy, the median survival rate may not change at all, and there may not be enough numbers to demonstrate a significant difference in the 5 or 10 percent survival duration for treated and untreated populations. It is also possible that those patients who achieve a partial response to therapy are those who have less aggressive disease at the outset of treatment and thus will survive longer than the nonresponders regardless of therapy. These caveats notwithstanding, most clinicians and patients welcome a partial response and are little concerned at that point with the vagaries of survival statistics.

2. **Tumor products.** For many cancers, objective tumor size changes are difficult or impossible to document. For some of these neoplasms, tumor products (hormones, antigens, or antibodies) may be measurable and may provide a good objective way to evaluate tumor response.

Two examples of such markers are the abnormal immunoglobulins produced in multiple myeloma and the human chorionic gonadotropin (HCG) produced in choriocarcinoma, both of which closely reflect tumor cell mass.

3. **Evaluable disease.** Other kinds of objective changes may occur but are not easily quantifiable. When these changes are not easily measurable they may be termed *evaluable*. For example, neurologic changes secondary to primary brain tumors cannot be measured with a caliper, but they can be evaluated using neurologic testing. An arbitrary system of grading the degree of severity of the neurologic deficit can be devised that will permit an objective evaluation of tumor response.

4. **Performance status** changes may also be used as a measure of objective change, although in many respects the performance status is

more representative of subjective rather than objective status of the disease.

C. Subjective change. A subjective change is one that is perceived by the patient, but not necessarily by the physician or others around the patient. Subjective improvement is often of far greater importance to the patient than objective improvement, for if the cancer shrinks, but the patient feels worse than before treatment, he is not likely to believe that the treatment was worthwhile. It is not valid to look at subjective change in isolation, however, because temporary worsening in the perceived state of well-being may be necessary to achieve subsequent long-term improvement.

This is particularly well illustrated in combined modality treatment in which chemotherapy is used to treat micrometastases after surgical removal of the macroscopic tumor. In such a circumstance, the patient is likely to feel entirely well after the primary surgical procedure, but the side effects of chemotherapy will increase the symptoms and make the patient feel subjectively worse, *for the period of treatment.* The winner's stakes are quite valuable, however, for if the chemotherapy treatment of the micrometastases is successful, the patient will be cured of the cancer and can be expected to have a normal or near-normal life expectancy rather than dying from recurrent disease. Most patients will agree that the temporary subjective worsening is not only tolerable but well worth the price if cure of the cancer is a distinct possibility.

When chemotherapy is given with a palliative intent, patients (and less often physicians) may be unwilling to tolerate significant side effects or subjective worsening. Fortunately, subjective improvement often accompanies objective improvement so that patients who have measurable improvement of their cancer will also feel better as a result of the treatment. The degree of subjective worsening that each patient is willing to tolerate varies, and the patient and physician together must discuss and evaluate whether the chemotherapy treatment program is worth continuing. Such discussions should include a clear presentation of the scientific facts and a sensitive consideration of the expressed desires and the social, economic, psychological, and spiritual situation of the patient and his or her family.

V. Toxicity

A. Factors affecting toxicity. One of the characteristics that separates cancer chemotherapeutic agents from most other drugs is the frequency and severity of anticipated side effects at usual therapeutic doses. Because of the severity of the side effects, it is critical to carefully monitor the patient for adverse reactions so that therapy can be modified before the toxicity becomes life threatening. Most toxicities are dependent on

1. Specific agent

2. Dose

3. Schedule of administration

4. Route of administration

5. Predisposing factors in the patient, which may be known and predictive for toxicity, or unknown and result in unexpected toxic effects

B. Clinical testing of new drugs for toxicity. Before the introduction of any agent into wide clinical use, the agent must undergo testing in carefully controlled clinical trials. The first set of clinical trials are called *phase I* clinical trials. Phase I clinical trials are carried out with the express purpose of determining toxicity in humans and establishing the maximum tolerated dose although they are done only in patients who potentially might benefit from the drug. Such trials are only undertaken after extensive tests in animals have been completed. Many human toxicities are predicted by animal studies, but because of significant species' differences, initial doses used in human studies are several times lower than doses at which toxicity is first seen in animals. Phase I trials are carried out using several schedules, and the dose is escalated in successive groups of patients once the toxicity of the prior dose has been established.

At the completion of phase I trials, there is usually a great deal of information about the spectrum and anticipated severity of acute drug effects (toxicity). However, because patients on phase I trials often do not live long enough to receive many months of treatment, chronic or cumulative effects may not be discovered. Discovery of these toxicities may occur only after widespread use of the drug in *phase II* trials (to establish the spectrum of effectiveness of the drug) or *phase III* trials (to compare the new drug with standard agents).

C. Common toxicities. Some toxicities are relatively common among cancer chemotherapeutic agents. Common toxicities include the following:

1. Myelosuppression with leukopenia, thrombocytopenia, and anemia
2. Nausea and vomiting
3. Mucous membrane ulceration
4. Alopecia

Aside from nausea and vomiting, these toxicities occur because of the cytotoxic effects of chemotherapy on rapidly dividing normal cells of the bone marrow and epithelium (mucous membranes, skin, and hair follicles).

D. Selective toxicities. Other toxicities are less common and are specific to individual drugs or classes of drugs. Examples of these toxicities include the following:

1. Vinca alkaloids: neurotoxicity
2. Cyclophosphamide: hemorrhagic cystitis
3. Anthracyclines: cardiomyopathy
4. Bleomycin: pulmonary fibrosis
5. Asparaginase: anaphylaxis (allergic reaction)

E. Recognition and evaluation of toxicity. Anyone who administers chemotherapeutic agents *must be* familiar with the expected and the unusual toxicities of the agent the patient is receiving, prepared to avert severe toxicity when that is possible, and able to manage toxic complications when they cannot be avoided.

For the purpose of reporting toxicity in a uniform manner, criteria are often established to grade the severity of the toxicity. Figure 2-1 shows

ECOG Toxicity Criteria

		0	1	2	3	4
Leuko-penia	WBC × 10³ Neut × 10³	≥4.5 ≥1.9	3.0–<4.5 1.5–<1.9	2.0–<3.0 1.0–<1.5	1.0–<2.0 0.5–<1.0	<1.0 <0.5
Thrombo-cytopenia	Plt × 10³	≥130	90–<130	50–<90	25–<50	<25
Anemia	Hgb gm% Hct % Clinical	≥11 ≥32	9.5–10.9 28–31.9	<9.5 <28 Sx of anemia	Req transfusions	
Hemorrhage		None	Minimal	Mod—Not debilitating	Debilitating	Life threatening
Infection		None	No active Rx	Requires active Rx	Debilitating	Life threatening
GU	BUN mg% Creatinine Proteinuria Hematuria	≤20 ≤1.2 Neg Neg	21–40 1.3–2.0 1+ Micro-Cult–positive	41–60 2.1–4.0 2+–3+ Gross-Cult–positive	>60 >4.0 4+ Gross+Clots	Symptomatic uremia c̄ obst uropathy

Urinary tract infection should be graded under infection, not GU.
Hematuria resulting from thrombocytopenia is graded under hemorrhage.

		0	1	2	3	4
Hepatic	SGOT Alk Phos Bilirubin Clinical	<1.5 × nl <1.5 × nl <1.5 × nl	1.5–2 × normal 1.5–2 × normal 1.5–2 × normal	2.1–5 × normal 2.1–5 × normal 2.1–5 × normal	>5 × normal >5 × normal >5 × normal Precoma	 Hepatic coma

Viral hepatitis should be recorded as infection rather than liver toxicity.

		0	1	2	3	4
N & V		None	Nausea	N & V controllable	Vomiting intractable	
Diarrhea		None	No dehydration	Dehydration	Grossly bloody	
Pulm	PFT Clinical	Nl	25–50% decrease in Dco or VC Mild Sx	>50% decrease in Dco or VC Moderate Sx	 Severe Sx–Intermittent O₂	 Assisted vent or continuous O₂

Pneumonia is considered infection and not graded as pulmonary toxicity unless felt to be resultant from pulmonary changes directly induced by treatment.

		0	1	2	3	4
Cardiac		Nl Nl	ST–T changes Sinus tachy >110 at rest	Atrial arrhythmias Unifocal PVC's	Mild CHF Multifocal PVC's Pericarditis	Severe or refract CHF Ventric tachy Tamponade
Neuro	PN	None	Decr DTR's Mild paresthesias Mild constipation	Absent DTR's Severe paresthesias Severe constipation Mild weakness	Disabling sens loss Severe PN pain Obstipation Severe weakness Bladder dysfunct	Resp dysfunction 2° to weakness Obstipation req surg Paralysis—confining pt to bed wheelchair
	CNS	None	Mild anxiety Mild depression Mild headache Lethargy	Severe anxiety Mod depression Mod headache Somnolence Tremor Mild hyperactivity	Confused or manic Severe depression Severe headache Cord dysfunction Confined to bed due to CNS dysfunct	Seizures Suicidal Coma
Skin & Mucosa		Nl	Transient erythema Pigmentation, atrophy	Vesiculation Subepidermal fibrosis	Ulceration Necrosis	
	Stomatitis	None	Soreness	Ulcers—can eat	Ulcers—cannot eat	
Alopecia		None	Alopecia—mild	Alopecia—severe		
Allergy		None	Transient rash Drug fever ≤38°C (≤100.4°F)	Urticaria Drug fever >38°C (>100.4°F) Mild bronchospasm	Serum sickness Bronchospasm–req parenteral meds	Anaphylaxis
Fever		≤37.5°C	≤38°C (≤100.4°F)	>38°C (>100.4°F)	Severe c̄ chills (>40°C)	Fever c̄ hypotension

Fever felt to be caused by drug allergy should be graded as allergy.
Fever due to infection is graded under infection only.

		0	1	2	3	4
Local Tox		None	Pain	Pain + Phlebitis	Ulceration	

1. The toxicity grade should reflect the most severe degree occurring during the evaluated period, not an average.
2. When two criteria are available for similar toxicities, e.g., leukopenia, neutropenia, the one resulting in the more severe toxicity grade should be used.
3. Toxicity grade = 5 if that toxicity caused the death of the patient.
4. Refer to detailed toxicity guidelines or to study chairman for toxicity not covered on this table.

Fig. 2-1. The ECOG toxicity criteria are an example of a systematic scheme for evaluating toxicity from chemotherapy. This kind of scoring of toxicity helps in assessing the severity of adverse effects both for individual patients and for groups of patients undergoing similar or diverse treatments.

the criteria used by the Eastern Cooperative Oncology Group (ECOG) for the most common toxic manifestations. The specific toxicities of the most commonly used individual chemotherapeutic agents are detailed in Chapter 4.

Selected Reading

Cadman, E. Toxicity of Chemotherapeutic Agents. In F. F. Becker (Ed.), *Cancer, A Comprehensive Treatise,* Vol. 5. New York: Plenum Pr., 1977.

Kennealley, G. T., and Mitchell, M. S. Factors that Influence the Therapeutic Response. In F. F. Becker (Ed.), *Cancer, A Comprehensive Treatise,* Vol. 5. New York: Plenum Pr., 1977.

Rubin, P. Statement of the Clinical Oncologic Problem. In P. Rubin and R. F. Bakemeier (Eds.), *Clinical Oncology for Medical Students and Physicians* (5th ed.). Rochester: American Cancer Society, 1978.

Terry, R. Pathology of Cancer. In P. Rubin and R. F. Bakemeier (Eds.), *Clinical Oncology for Medical Students and Physicians* (5th ed.). Rochester: American Cancer Society, 1978.

Selection of Treatment for the Patient with Cancer

Roland T. Skeel

I. **Treatment objective.** Before deciding on a course of treatment for a patient with cancer, the objective of treatment must be clearly defined. If the objective is to cure the patient of cancer, then the strategy of therapy is likely to be very different from the strategy chosen if the objective is to prolong useful life or to relieve symptoms. Several considerations may help determine the treatment objective. Those factors discussed in Chapter 2—the type of cancer, the stage of the disease, and the performance status of the patient—must be assessed to determine the possible responses and the likelihood with which they may be expected to occur.

Armed with this information, the physician can plan a course of treatment and make a recommendation to the patient. Although most often this will be accepted, some patients may reject the recommendation as inappropriate for them for a variety of reasons. Some may ask the physician for another recommendation, while others may seek the opinion of a second physician. The physician must clearly present the reasons for the treatment recommendations and why they seem to be the best way to achieve the treatment objective. At the same time, it is important for the physician to allow the patient to share in the setting of objectives and treatment decisions, since it is the patient who must undergo the treatment and be willing to abide its consequences.

II. **Choice of treatment modality**

A. **Surgery.** The oldest, most established, and still most effective way to cure most cancers is surgery. Surgery is selected as the treatment if the cancer is limited to one area and if it is anticipated that all cancer cells can be removed without unduly compromising vital structures. If it is believed that the patient can survive the surgery and return to a worthwhile life then surgery is recommended. If the risk of surgery is greater than the risk of the cancer, if metastasis always occurs despite complete removal of the primary tumor, or if the patient will be left so debilitated that, although cured of cancer, the patient feels life is not worthwhile, then surgery will not be recommended.

Most commonly, surgery is reserved for treatment of the primary neoplasm, although at times it may be used effectively to remove isolated metastases (e.g., in lung, brain, or liver) with curative intent. Surgery is also used palliatively, as in decompression of the brain for gliomas or decompression, with biliary bypass procedures, for carcinoma of the pancreas. In nearly all nonhematologic cancers, a surgeon should be consulted to determine the role of surgery in the optimal treatment of the patient.

B. Radiotherapy. Radiotherapy is used for the treatment of local or regional disease when surgery cannot completely remove the cancer or when surgery would unduly disrupt normal structures or functions. In the treatment of some cancers, radiotherapy is as effective as surgery in eradicating the cancer. In this circumstance, factors such as the anticipated side effects of the treatment, the expertise and experience of local oncologists, or the preference of the patient may influence the choice of treatment.

One of the factors used to determine the appropriateness of radiotherapy is the inherent sensitivity of the cancer to ionizing radiation. Some kinds of cancers, such as the lymphomas and seminomas, are quite sensitive to radiotherapy. Other kinds, such as melanomas and sarcomas, tend to be less sensitive. Such considerations do not preclude the use of radiotherapy, however, and it is helpful to obtain the evaluation of the radiotherapist prior to initiating treatment, so that treatment planning can take into consideration the possible contribution of this modality.

Although radiotherapy is frequently used as the primary curative mode of therapy, it is also well suited to palliative management of problems such as bony metastases, superior vena cava syndrome, or local nodal metastases. The use of radiotherapy in the management of bony metastases and superior vena cava syndrome is discussed in Chapters 21 and 22.

C. Chemotherapy. Chemotherapy has as its primary role the treatment of disease that is no longer confined to one site or region and has spread systemically. In the earliest days of chemotherapy, this interpretation directed its use in diseases that regularly presented in a disseminated form, such as leukemia, or after disease recurred following primary management with surgery or radiotherapy. It is now understood that widespread systemic micrometastases commonly occur early in cancer. These metastases are associated with certain predictive factors such as axillary node metastases in carcinoma of the breast, and large tumor size and poorly differentiated histologic features in sarcomas. Therefore, chemotherapy is now applied earlier to treat systemic disease. When this treatment is used for micrometastases, the response of an individual patient cannot be measured. Rather, the effectiveness of therapy must be determined by comparing the survival of high-risk patients who receive therapy with similar (control) patients who do not receive therapy for the micrometastases.

Chemotherapy also has a role in the treatment of localized or regional disease. These specialized uses are discussed in **III.B** and **C** and also in Part III (see pages 69–192).

D. Biologic response modifiers. It has long intrigued cancer biologists that cancer does not occur randomly, but preferentially selects specific populations: the young, the elderly, the immunosuppressed (certain types of cancer only), and those with a strong family history of cancer. These observations have led cancer biologists to postulate that some kind of biologic control over the emergence of cancer exists, which some people have and others do not, at least at the time the cancer becomes established. One prime candidate for the mechanism of biologic control of cancer has been immunity. That immunity plays some role in controlling the development of cancer has been clearly demonstrated in animal models and a few, though not most, human neoplasms. Other biologic factors, although less well defined at the present, may be equally or more important than immunity in the development of cancer.

In an attempt to exploit and enhance the biologic control that is presumed to exist to some degree in everyone, a variety of agents called *biologic response modifiers* have been used in the treatment of cancer. Although the most widely used group of biologic response modifiers— included broadly under the term *immunotherapy*—has been used extensively for many years, none has yet demonstrated substantial benefit in the treatment of human cancer. This is an area of intensive research and, in the future, may provide an important component of effective cancer therapy.

E. **Combined modality therapy.** Neither surgery, radiotherapy, nor chemotherapy alone is appropriate for the treatment of all cancers. Frequently, patients present with cancer in which there is a bulky primary, macroscopically evident regional disease, and presumed microscopic or submicroscopic systemic disease. For this reason, oncologists have turned to a multidisciplinary approach to the treatment of cancer, selecting two or more modalities of therapy for sequential or simultaneous use. This approach requires close cooperation between the surgical oncologist, radiation oncologist, and medical oncologist to provide the patient with the best overall treatment plan. Although combined modality therapy is not effective or desirable for all kinds or stages of cancers, the regular practice of a multidisciplinary approach provides the best opportunity to exploit the advantages of each mode of treatment.

III. Modes of chemotherapy administration

A. **Systemic treatment.** Chemotherapeutic agents are most often administered systemically by one of the following routes: intravenous, intramuscular, subcutaneous, or oral. Which of these routes is chosen will depend primarily on chemical and pharmacologic factors, such as solubility, effects of stomach acid and digestive enzymes, absorption, local irritation at the site of injection, and rapidity of metabolism of the drug once it has entered the blood stream. Occasionally, the oral route has been used for systemic administration of a drug (e.g., fluorouracil) with the secondary intention of achieving high concentrations in the liver as the drug passes through the portal circulation. (Unfortunately, this does not appear to have any advantage in patients who have liver metastases from gastrointestinal carcinomas, perhaps because hepatic metastases are fed more by the hepatic artery than by the portal vein.)

Regardless of the route of administration, the goal of systemic therapy is to achieve a sufficient drug concentration multiplied by time product to result in a therapeutic cytotoxic effect on cancer cells wherever they may be in the body. This goal is realistic and achievable for some cancers if the cells are sufficiently sensitive and if they are located in accessible sites. It is unachievable if the cancer cells are resistant or are located in sanctuary sites that are inaccessible to the drug, or drugs, being used.

B. **Intraarterial infusion.** At times cancer may be localized to a region that is unresectable or that cannot receive sufficient radiotherapy to effect a cure or palliation. In such circumstances it is desirable to administer chemotherapy in such a way that the cancer is exposed to a much higher concentration of drug than the rest of the body.

1. **Conditions for effective treatment.** For this kind of treatment to be effective, at least three conditions must exist:

   a. The region (frequently an organ or limb) must have an accessible artery for infusion of the drug.

   b. The drug must be rapidly bound or inactivated after one pass through the region, so that the systemic concentration does not build up to essentially the same level as the regional level. (If this occurs, the advantage of regional administration will be obviated.)

   c. The drug must be active in its administered form (or activated by tumor cells) without requiring passage through a systemic organ such as the liver.

2. **Clinical use.** Intraarterial infusion appears to benefit some patients with primary or metastatic liver tumors. Hepatic artery catheterization may be performed intraoperatively or percutaneously through the femoral or brachial arteries. Treatment regimens are outlined in Chapter 7. Beneficial results in extremity cancers (melanoma, sarcoma), head and neck cancer, and primary brain tumors have been less common and at present intraarterial infusion for these sites remains experimental.

3. **Complications** unique to intraarterial infusion require that special precautions be taken. Common problems include thrombosis of the artery with distal or retrograde arterial occlusion, bleeding, infection, catheter cracking and leaking, and catheter dislodgement. Careful technique and care of the catheter will help minimize these problems, but even in the best of hands, some complications may occur and occasional deaths may result.

C. **Intracavitary instillation.** Pleural, peritoneal, and less commonly, pericardial and subarachnoid spaces may be treated by instillation of a chemotherapeutic agent directly into the space. In all of the spaces, this instillation has the result of achieving a higher concentration of drug than would be achieved if the drug were given systemically, providing three criteria are met.

1. **The dilution volume is small.** To prevent dilution or inactivation, pleural, peritoneal, and pericardial spaces are drained prior to instillation of the drug.

2. **There is open communication within the space.** Open communication cannot be assumed, and loculations may prevent successful treatment, particularly of pleural effusions.

3. **Adequate mixing is assured.** Adequate mixing usually can be achieved in the peritoneal, pleural, and pericardial spaces, but it is a major problem in treating meningeal carcinomatosis, leukemia, or lymphoma: cases in which the drug is injected into the lumbar space. Strategies to overcome this latter problem have included injecting the drug into the cerebrospinal fluid through an implanted subcutaneous

reservoir that communicates with one of the lateral ventricles. The specific treatment of effusions are discussed in Chapter 23.

Selected Reading

Lundberg, W. B. Intraarterial Chemotherapy. In F. F. Becker (Ed.), *Cancer, A Comprehensive Treatise,* Vol. 5. New York: Plenum Pr., 1977.

Nealon, T. F., Jr., and Russo, E. P. Surgical Principles. In J. Horton and G. J. Hill, II (Eds.), *Clinical Oncology.* Philadelphia: Saunders, 1977.

Papac, R. J. Treatment of Malignant Disease in Closed Spaces. In F. F. Becker (Ed.), *Cancer, A Comprehensive Treatise,* Vol. 5. New York: Plenum Pr., 1977.

Perez, C. A. Principles of Radiation Therapy. In J. Horton and G. J. Hill, II (Eds.), *Clinical Oncology.* Philadelphia: Saunders, 1977.

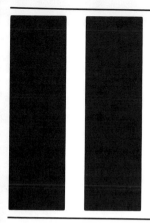

Chemotherapeutic Agents

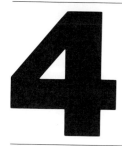

Antineoplastic Drugs: Classification and Clinically Useful Agents

Roland T. Skeel

I. Classes of drugs. Chemotherapeutic agents are customarily divided into several classes. For two of the classes, the *alkylating agents* and the *antimetabolites*, the names indicate the mechanism of cytotoxic action of the drugs in their class. For *hormonal agents*, the name designates the physiologic type of drug; and for the *natural products*, the name reflects the source of the agents. Finally, for those drugs that do not easily fit into any other category, there is a *miscellaneous* category. Although some would include an additional category, the *biologic response modifiers*, these agents fit more into the realm of immunotherapy than chemotherapy and will not be included in this description of the chemotherapeutic agents.

Within each class are several types of agents (Table 4-1). As with the criteria for separating into class, the types are also grouped according to the mechanism of action, the biochemical structure or derivation, or a physiologic action. In some instances, these groupings into classes and types are rather arbitrary, and some drugs may seem to fit into either more than one category or none. However, the classification of chemotherapeutic agents in this fashion is helpful in several respects. For example, because the antimetabolites interfere with purine and pyrimidine metabolism and the formation of DNA and RNA, they are all at least cell cycle-specific and in some instances primarily cell cycle phase-specific. The nitrosourea group of alkylating agents, on the other hand, contains drugs that are predominantly or entirely cell cycle-nonspecific. Such knowledge can be helpful in planning therapy for tumors when sufficient kinetic information permits a rational selection of agents and when drugs are selected for use in combination.

The classification scheme also may help to predict cross-resistance between drugs. Tumors that are resistant to one of the nitrogen-mustard types of alkylating agents thus would be likely to be resistant to another of that same type, but not necessarily to one of the other types of alkylating agents, such as the nitrosoureas or the metal salts (cisplatin).

A. Alkylating agents

1. General description. The alkylating agents are a diverse group of chemical compounds that are capable of forming molecular bonds with nucleic acids, proteins, and many molecules of low molecular weight. Either the compounds are electrophiles or they generate electrophiles in vivo to produce polarized molecules with positively charged regions. These polarized molecules then can interact with electron-rich regions of most cellular molecules. The cytotoxic effect of the alkylating agents appears to relate primarily to the interaction between the electrophiles and DNA. This interaction may result in

Table 4-1. Useful Chemotherapeutic Agents

Class	Type	Agent
Alkylating agent	Nitrogen mustard	Chlorambucil, cyclophosphamide, estramustine, mechlorethamine, melphalan
	Ethylenimine derivative	Thiotepa (triethylenethiophosphoramide)
	Alkyl sulfonate	Busulfan
	Nitrosourea	Carmustine, chlorozotocin,* lomustine, semustine,* streptozocin*
	Triazine	Dacarbazine
	Metal salt	Cisplatin
Antimetabolite	Folic acid analog	Methotrexate
	Pyrimidine analog	Azacytidine,* cytarabine, fluorouracil floxuridine
	Purine analog	Mercaptopurine, thioguanine
Natural product	Mitotic inhibitor	Vinblastine, vincristine, vindesine*
	Podophyllum derivative	Etoposide*
	Antibiotic	Bleomycin, dactinomycin, daunorubicin, doxorubicin (Adriamycin™), mithramycin, mitomycin
	Enzyme	Asparaginase
Hormone and hormone antagonist	Androgen	
	Corticosteroid	
	Estrogen	
	Progestin	
	Estrogen antagonist	Tamoxifen
Miscellaneous agent	Substituted urea	Hydroxyurea
	Methyl hydrazine derivative	Procarbazine
	Adrenal cortical suppressant	Mitotane
	Steroid synthesis inhibitor	Aminoglutethimide
	Substituted melamine	Hexamethylmelamine*
	Halogenated hexitol	Dibromodulcitol*

*Investigational agents, not yet approved by the FDA for general use.

substitution reactions, cross-linking reactions, or strand-breaking reactions. The most sensitive part of the DNA is the 7 position of guanosine, although other sites may have equal biologic significance. The net effect of the alkylating agent's interaction with DNA is to alter the information coded in the DNA molecule. This alteration results in inhibition of or inaccurate DNA replication with resultant mutation or cell death. One implication of the mutagenic capability of alkylating agents is the possibility that they are teratogenic and carcinogenic. Because they interact with preformed DNA, RNA, and protein, the alkylating agents are not phase specific, and at least some are cell cycle-nonspecific.

2. Types of alkylating agents

a. Nitrogen mustards.
This group of compounds all produce highly reactive carbonium ions that react with the electron-rich areas of

susceptible molecules. They vary in reactivity from mechloreth-amine, which is highly unstable in aqueous form, to cyclophos-phamide, which must be biochemically activated in the liver.

b. Ethylenimine derivatives. Triethylenethiophosphoramide (thio-tepa) is the only compound in this group that has much clinical use. Ethylenimine derivatives are capable of the same kinds of re-actions as the nitrogen mustards.

c. Alkyl sulfonates. Busulfan is the only clinically active compound in this group. It appears to interact more with cellular thiol groups than with nucleic acids.

d. Triazine. Dacarbazine, the only agent of this type, was originally thought to be an antimetabolite because of its resemblance to 5-aminoimidazole-4-carboxamide (AIC). Dacarbazine is now known to act as an alkylator after AIC is cleaved from active diazometh-ane.

e. Nitrosoureas. The nitrosoureas undergo rapid spontaneous acti-vation in aqueous solution to form products capable of alkylation and carbamoylation. They are unique among the alkylating agents with respect to being non-cross-resistant with other alkylating agents, highly lipid soluble, and having delayed myelosuppressive effects (6–8 weeks).

f. Metal salts. Cisplatin inhibits DNA synthesis probably through the formation of intrastrand crosslinks in DNA. It may also react with DNA through chelation or through binding to the cell mem-brane.

B. Antimetabolites

1. General description. The antimetabolites are a group of low molecu-lar-weight compounds that exert their effect by virtue of their struc-tural or functional similarity to naturally occurring metabolites in-volved in nucleic acid synthesis. Because they are mistaken by the cell for the normal metabolite, they either inhibit critical enzymes involved in nucleic acid synthesis or become incorporated into the nucleic acid and produce incorrect codes. Both types of mechanisms result in an inhibition of DNA synthesis and ultimate cell death. Because of their primary effect on DNA synthesis, the antimetabo-lites are most active in cells that are in active growth and are largely cell cycle phase-specific.

2. Types of antimetabolites

a. Folic acid analogs. These drugs, of which methotrexate is the only member in wide clinical use, inhibit the enzyme dihydrofolate re-ductase. This inhibition blocks the production of the reduced N^5-, N^{10}-methylenetetrahydrofolate, the coenzyme in the synthesis of thymidylic acid. Other metabolic processes in which there is a one carbon unit transfer are also affected, but are probably of less importance in the cytotoxic action of methotrexate.

b. Pyrimidine analogs. These compounds inhibit critical enzymes necessary for nucleic acid synthesis and may become incorporated into DNA and RNA.

c. Purine analogs. The specific site of action for the purine analogs is less well defined than for pyrimidine analogs, although it is well demonstrated that they interfere with normal purine interconversions and thus with DNA and RNA synthesis. Some of the analogs also are incorporated into the nucleic acids.

C. Natural products

1. **General description.** The natural products are grouped together not on the basis of activity, but because they are all derived from natural sources. The clinically useful drugs are (1) plant products, (2) fermentation products of various species of the soil fungus *Streptomyces,* and (3) bacterial products.

2. **Types of natural products**

   a. **Mitotic inhibitors.** Vincristine, vinblastine, and its semisynthetic derivative vindesine are derived from the periwinkle plant (*Catharanthus roseus*), a species of myrtle. They appear to act primarily through their effect on microtubular protein with a resultant metaphase arrest and inhibition of mitosis.

   b. **Podophyllum derivative.** Etoposide, a semisynthetic podophyllotoxin derived from the root of the mayapple plant (*Podophyllum peltatum*), arrests cells in the G_2 phase. It also has some effects on DNA, RNA, and protein synthesis.

   c. **Antibiotics.** The antitumor antibiotics are a group of related antimicrobial compounds produced by *Streptomyces* species in culture. Their cytotoxicity, which limits their antimicrobial usefulness, has proved to be of great value in treating a wide range of cancers. All of the clinically useful antibiotics affect the function and synthesis of nucleic acids.

      (1) Dactinomycin and the anthracylines, doxorubicin and daunorubicin, intercalate between base pairs of DNA to interfere with the template function of DNA. This interference results in an inhibition of DNA-dependent DNA and RNA synthesis.

      (2) Bleomycins cause DNA-strand scission; the resulting fragmentation is believed to underlie the drug's cytotoxic activity.

      (3) Mitomycin causes cross links between complementary strands of DNA that impair replication.

      (4) Mithramycin complexes with Mg^{2+} to DNA and blocks RNA synthesis.

   d. **Enzymes.** Asparaginase, the one example of this type of agent, catalyzes the hydrolysis of asparagine to aspartic acid and ammonia, and deprives selected malignant cells of an amino acid essential to their survival.

D. Hormones and hormone antagonists

1. **General description.** The hormones and hormone antagonists that are clinically active against cancer include steroidal estrogens, progestins, androgens, corticoids and their synthetic derivatives, and nonsteroidal synthetic compounds with steroid or steroid-antagonist

activity. Each agent has diverse effects: some effects are mediated directly at the cellular level by the binding of the drug to specific cytoplasmic receptors, and other effects are mediated through indirect effects on the hypothalamus and its anterior pituitary regulating hormones. The final common pathway in most circumstances appears to lead to the malignant cell, which has retained some sensitivity to hormonal control of its growth. An exception to this mechanism is the effect of corticosteroids on leukemias and lymphomas in which the steroids appear to have direct lytic effects on abnormal lymphoid cells that have high numbers of glucocorticoid receptors.

2. Types of hormones and hormone antagonists

a. Androgens may exert their antineoplastic effect by altering pituitary function or directly affecting the neoplastic cell.

b. Corticosteroids cause lysis of lymphoid tumors that are rich in specific cytoplasmic receptors, but may have other indirect effects as well.

c. Estrogens suppress testosterone production (through the hypothalamus) in males and alter breast cancer cell response to prolactin.

d. Progestins appear to act directly at the level of the malignant cell receptor to promote differentiation.

e. Estrogen antagonists compete with estrogen for binding on the cytosol estrogen receptor protein in cancer cells, although the sites of binding may not be identical.

E. Miscellaneous agents are listed in Table 4-1. Descriptions of specific agents are found in section **III**.

II. Clinically useful chemotherapeutic agents. Section III of this chapter contains an alphabetically arranged description of the chemotherapeutic agents that are recognized to be clinically useful. Each drug is listed by its generic name with other common or trade names included. A brief description is given of the probable mechanism of action, the clinical uses, recommended doses and schedules, precautions, and side effects.

A. Recommended doses: caution. Although every effort has been made to ensure that the drug dosages and schedules herein are accurate and in accord with published standards, readers are advised to check the product information sheet included in the package of each Food and Drug Administration approved drug and to read FDA/NCI (National Cancer Institute) guidelines for drugs not yet approved for general use to verify recommended dosages, contraindications, and precautions.

B. Drug toxicity: frequency designation. The doses are listed using body surface area (m^2) as the base. Doses from the adult literature, which are expressed using a weight base, have been converted by multiplying the mg/kg dose by 37 to give the mg/m^2 dose. Doses using a weight base, which have been taken from pediatric literature, have been converted using a factor of 25. As many of the drugs are given in combination with other agents, doses most commonly used in popular combinations may also be indicated. The data sheets should not be used as the sole source of information for any of the drugs, but rather used as a guide to confirm and compare dose ranges and schedules and to identify potential problems. The designation of the frequency of toxic side effects is indicated as follows (probability of occurrence equals percent of patients):

1. Universal (90%–100%).

2. Common (15%–90%).

3. Occasional (5%–15%).

4. Uncommon (1%–5%).

5. Rare (<1%).

These designations are only meant to be guides and the likelihood of a side effect in each patient will depend on their physical and psychological status, previous treatment, the dose and schedule of drug administration, and other concurrent treatment.

C. Dose modification

  1. Philosophy. The optimal dose and schedule of a drug is one that gives maximum benefit with minimal toxicity. Because most chemotherapeutic agents have a steep dose-response curve, if no toxicity is seen, as a rule a higher dose should be given to get the best possible therapeutic benefit. If toxicity is too great, however, the patient's life may be threatened or the patient may decide that the treatment is worse than the disease and refuse further therapy. How much toxicity the patient and the physician are willing to tolerate depends both on the likelihood that more intensive treatment will make a major therapeutic difference (e.g., cure versus no cure) and on the patient's physical and psychological tolerance for adverse effects.

  2. Guidelines

    a. Nonhematologic toxicity

      (1) Acute effects. Acute drug toxicity that is limited to 1 or 2 days and is not cumulative is not usually a cause for dose modification unless it is of grade 3 or 4 (see Fig. 2-1). Occasionally repeating a dose that caused intractable nausea and vomiting or temperature greater than 40C (104F) is warranted, but for any other grade 3 or 4 toxicity, the subsequent doses should be reduced by 50 percent. If the acute drug effects last longer than 48 hours, for example, severe paresthesias or abnormalities of renal or liver function, then the subsequent doses should be reduced by 35 to 50 percent.

      A recurrence of the side effects at the reduced doses would be an indication to either reduce by another 50 percent or discontinue the drug altogether. Non-dose-related toxicity, such as anaphylaxis, is an indication to discontinue the offending drug.

      (2) Chronic effects. Chronic or cumulative toxicity, such as pulmonary function changes with bleomycin or decrease in cardiac function with doxorubicin, is nearly always an indication to discontinue the responsible agent.

    b. Hematologic toxicity. The degree of myelosuppression and attendant risk of infection and bleeding that are acceptable depend on

Table 4-2. Dose Modification for Myelosuppressive Drugs with Nadir*
Less than 3 Weeks (Blood Count on Day of Scheduled Treatment)

WBC/μl		Platelets/μl	Dose (%)
$\geqslant$4000	*and*	$\geqslant$125,000	100
3500–4000	*or*	100,000–125,000	75
2500–3500	*or*	75,000–100,000	50
<2500	*or*	< 75,000	0†

*If nadir WBC is <1500/μl or platelets are <40,000/μl, decrease dose by 25% in subsequent cycles.
†If WBC is <2500/μl or platelets are <75,000/μl, obtain blood count weekly and resume treatment when they are above this level.

Table 4-3. Dose Modification for Myelosuppressive Drugs
with Nadir Greater than 3 Weeks*

WBC/μl		Platelets/μl	Dose (%)
BLOOD COUNT AT NADIR			
>3500	*and*	>100,000	125
2000–3500	*and*	> 75,000	100
2000–3500	*and*	< 75,000	50
<2000	*and*	> 75,000	75
<2000	*and*	< 75,000	50
BLOOD COUNT ON DAY OF SCHEDULED TREATMENT			
<4000	*or*	<100,000	0†

*The nitrosoureas or other agents if the observed nadir is prolonged.
†Obtain weekly blood counts and withhold treatment until counts are normal; then treat with dosage adjustment based on above table.

the cancer, the duration of the myelosuppression, and the general health of the patient. For example, in acute nonlymphocytic leukemia remission is unlikely unless sufficient therapy is given to cause profound pancytopenia for at least 1 week. Since there is little benefit with lesser treatment, grade 4 leukopenia and thrombocytopenia are acceptable toxicities in this circumstance. In breast cancer, on the other hand, responses are seen with less aggressive treatment, and prolonged pancytopenia is not acceptable, which is particularly true if chemotherapy is being used in an adjuvant setting in which a portion of the patients would not have recurrence even without chemotherapy, and excessive toxicity would pose an unacceptable risk.

With these caveats in mind, the dose modification schemes shown in Tables 4-2 and 4-3 can serve as a guide to reasonable dose changes for drugs that have myelosuppression as a major toxicity. Separate schemes are given for the nitrosoureas and for drugs that have less prolonged myelosuppression. Lesser dose reductions are justifiable for drugs for which myelosuppression is not a major effect.

III. Data for clinically useful chemotherapeutic agents

> **Note:** Although every effort has been made to ensure that the drug dosage and schedules herein are accurate and in accord with published standards, users are advised to check the product-information sheet included in the package of each FDA-approved drug and FDA/NCI guidelines for drugs that are not yet approved for general use (see Table 4-1) to verify recommended dosages, contraindications, and precautions.
>
> Agents that have not yet been approved by the FDA are included, either because they have some demonstrated usefulness or are widely used in investigational studies. As their efficacy and toxicity are more firmly established, it is expected that some will become FDA approved for general use while others will remain investigational or be dropped from further study.

Aminoglutethimide

Other names. Cytadren®, Elipten®

Mechanism of action. Interferes with conversion of cholesterol to Δ^5-pregnenolone, thereby blocking the biosynthesis of all steroid hormones. This drug causes, in effect, a reversible chemical adrenalectomy.

Primary indications. Breast carcinoma (investigational) and adrenocortical carcinoma.

Usual dosage and schedule. 1000 mg daily in 4 divided doses.

Special precautions. Hydrocortisone must be given concomitantly to prevent adrenal insufficiency. Suggested dose is 100 mg daily in divided doses for 2 weeks, then 40 mg daily in divided doses.

Toxicity
1. **Myelosuppression.** Leukopenia and thrombocytopenia are rare, and if they occur they resolve rapidly when the drug is stopped.
2. **Nausea and vomiting** are occasional and usually mild.
3. **Mucocutaneous.** A morbilliform rash is commonly seen in the first week of treatment, but it usually disappears within 1 week.
4. **Hormonal effects**
   a. Adrenal insufficiency—common without replacement hydrocortisone in patients with normal adrenal glands.
   b. Hypothyroidism—uncommon.
5. **Neurologic effects**
   a. Lethargy is common. Although usually mild and transient, occasionally it is quite severe.
   b. Vertigo, nystagmus, and ataxia—uncommon.
6. **Miscellaneous effects**
   a. Facial flushing—uncommon.
   b. Periorbital edema—uncommon.

Androgens

Other names. Fluoxymesterone (Halotestin®), testolactone (Teslac®), others

Mechanism of action. Mechanism of antitumor effects is not clear.

Primary indications. Breast carcinoma.

Usual dosage and schedule
1. **Fluoxymesterone:** 20 to 30 mg PO daily in 4 divided doses.
2. **Testolactone:** 1000 mg PO daily in 4 divided doses.

Special precautions. Hypercalcemia may occur with initial therapy.

Toxicity
1. **Myelosuppression.** None. Erythropoiesis is stimulated.
2. **Nausea and vomiting** are mild and dose related.
3. **Mucocutaneous.** Acne.
4. **Miscellaneous effects**
   a. Masculinization, including an increase in facial and body hair, deepening of voice, acne, baldness, and clitoral hypertrophy, is common, but may be minimized by dose attenuation.
   b. Intrahepatic biliary stasis with hyperbilirubinemia is uncommon but may occur at high androgen doses (17 methyl derivatives only).
   c. Fluid retention may occur, although it is less severe with androgens than with estrogens—occasional.

Asparaginase

Other names. L-Asparaginase, Elspar®

Mechanism of action. Hydrolysis of serum asparagine occurs which deprives leukemia cells of the required amino acid. Normal cells are spared because they generally have the ability to synthesize their own asparagine.

Primary indication. Acute lymphocytic leukemia, for induction therapy only.

Usual dosage and schedule. Both schedules are usually used in combination with other drugs (see Special precautions 2). These schedules are only two of many acceptable dosing schedules.
1. 20,000 to 40,000 IU/m^2 IV daily for 10 to 14 days *or*
2. 6000 IU/m^2 IM every 3 days.

Special precautions
1. Be prepared to treat anaphylaxis at each administration of the drug. Epinephrine, antihistamines, corticosteroids, and life-support equipment should be readily available.
2. Do not give concurrently with or immediately before vincristine because of possible increased vincristine toxicity.

Toxicity
1. **Myelosuppression.** Occasional.
2. **Nausea and vomiting** are occasionally seen and are usually mild.
3. **Mucocutaneous.** No toxicity occurs except as a sign of hypersensitivity.
4. **Anaphylaxis.** Mild to severe hypersensitivity reactions, including anaphylaxis, occur in 20 to 30 percent of patients. They are less likely to occur during the first few days of treatment and are particularly common with intermittent schedules or repeat cycles. If the patient develops hy-

persensitivity to the *Escherichia coli* derived enzyme (Elspar®), *Erwinia* derived asparaginase may be safely substituted since the two enzyme preparations are not cross-reactive. Note that hypersensitivity may also develop to *Erwinia* derived asparaginase, and continued preparedness to treat anaphylaxis must be maintained.

5. **Miscellaneous effects**
   a. Mild fever and malaise is common and may occasionally progress to severe chills and malignant hyperthermia.
   b. Hepatotoxicity is common and occasionally severe. Abnormalities observed include elevation of SGOT, alkaline phosphatase, and bilirubin; depression of hepatic derived clotting factors and albumin; and hepatocellular fatty metamorphosis.
   c. Renal failure is rare.
   d. Pancreatic endocrine and exocrine dysfunction, often with manifestations of pancreatitis—occasional. Nonketotic hyperglycemia is uncommon.
   e. CNS effects consisting of depression, somnolence, fatigue, confusion, agitation, hallucinations, or coma—occasional. These are usually reversible following discontinuation of the drug.

Azacytidine (Investigational)

Other names. 5-Azacytidine, 5 aza-C, ladakamycin

Mechanism of action. A pyrimidine analog antimetabolite that causes interference with nucleic acid synthesis and is incorporated into both DNA and RNA, where it acts as a false pyrimidine.

Primary indication. Acute nonlymphocytic leukemia.

Usual dosage and schedule
1. 100 mg/m^2 IV push q8h for 5 days *or*
2. 150 to 200 mg/m^2 IV daily as continuous infusion for 5 days.

Special precautions. Because of drug instability, dose should be prepared immediately before use and discarded after 8 hours. Infusions should be freshly prepared with Ringer's lactate solution and changed every 8 hours.

Toxicity
1. **Myelosuppression** is severe in all patients, with leukocyte nadir occurring at 12 to 14 days. Occasionally, suppression is prolonged beyond several weeks.
2. **Nausea and vomiting** are common. Continuous infusion lessens nausea and vomiting.
3. **Mucocutaneous.** Stomatitis and rash—occasional.
4. **Miscellaneous effects**
   a. Diarrhea—common.
   b. Neurologic problems with muscle pain, weakness, lethargy, and coma—uncommon.
   c. Hepatotoxicity—rare.
   d. Transient fever—occasional.

Bleomycin

Other name. Blenoxane®

Mechanism of action. Bleomycin binds to DNA, causes single and double strand scission, and inhibits further DNA, RNA, and protein synthesis.

Primary indications
1. Testis, head and neck, penis, cervix, vulva, anus, skin, and lung carcinomas.
2. Hodgkin's and non-Hodgkin's lymphomas.

Usual dosage and schedule
1. 10 to 20 units/m^2 IV or IM twice a week *or*
2. 30 units IV push, then 15 units/m^2/24 hr as continuous infusion for 4 to 6 days is commonly used in combination with other drugs for testicular cancer.

Special precautions
1. In patients with lymphoma, a test dose of 1 or 2 units should be given IM prior to the first dose of bleomycin because of the possibility of anaphylactoid, acute pulmonary, or severe hyperpyrexic responses. If no acute reaction occurs within 4 hours, regular dosing may begin.
2. Reduce dose for renal failure.

Serum Creatinine	Full Dose (%)
2.5–4	25
4–6	20
6–10	10

3. The cumulative lifetime dose should not exceed 400 units because of the dose-related incidence of severe pulmonary fibrosis. Smaller limits may be appropriate for older patients or those with pre-existing pulmonary disease. Frequent evaluation of pulmonary status, including symptoms of cough or dyspnea, rales, infiltrates on chest x-ray film, and pulmonary function studies are recommended to avert serious pulmonary sequelae.

Toxicity
1. **Myelosuppression.** Significant depression of counts is uncommon. This factor permits bleomycin to be used in full doses with myelosuppressive drugs.
2. **Nausea and vomiting** are occasional and self-limiting.
3. **Mucocutaneous.** Alopecia, stomatitis, erythema, edema, thickening of nail bed, and hyperpigmentation and desquamation of skin are common.
4. **Pulmonary**
   a. An acute anaphylactoid or pulmonary edema-like response—occasional in patients with lymphoma (see Special Precautions).
   b. Dose-related pneumonitis with cough, dyspnea, rales, and infiltrates, progressing to pulmonary fibrosis.
5. **Fever.** Common. On occasion severe hyperpyrexia, diaphoresis, dehydration, and hypotension have occurred and resulted in renal failure and death. Antipyretics help control fever.
6. **Miscellaneous effects**
   a. Lethargy, headache, and joint swelling—rare.
   b. IM or SC injection may cause pain at injection site.

Busulfan

Other name. Myleran®

Mechanism of action. Bifunctional alkylating agent. Its effect may be greater on cellular thiol groups than on nucleic acids.

Primary indication. Chronic granulocytic leukemia.

Usual dosage and schedule. 3 to 4 mg/m^2 PO daily for remission induction in adults until the leukocyte count is 50 percent of the original level, then 1 to 2 mg/m^2 daily. Busulfan may be given continuously or intermittently.

Special precautions. Obtain complete blood count weekly while patient is on therapy. If leukocyte count falls rapidly to less than 15,000, discontinue therapy until nadir is reached and rising counts indicate need for further treatment.

Toxicity
1. **Myelosuppression** is dose limiting. A fall in the leukocyte count may not begin for 2 weeks after starting therapy, and it is likely to continue for 2 weeks after therapy has been stopped. Recovery of marrow function may be delayed for 3 to 6 weeks after the drug has been discontinued.
2. **Nausea and vomiting** are rare.
3. **Mucocutaneous.** Hyperpigmentation occurs occasionally, particularly in skin creases.
4. **Pulmonary.** Interstitial pulmonary fibrosis is rare and is an indication to discontinue drug. Corticosteroids may improve symptoms and minimize permanent lung damage.
5. **Metabolic.** Adrenal insufficiency syndrome—rare. Hyperuricemia may occur when the leukemia cell count is rapidly reduced. Ovarian suppression and amenorrhea are common.
6. **Miscellaneous effects.** Secondary neoplasia is possible.

Carmustine

Other names. BCNU, BiCNU®

Mechanism of action. Alkylation and carbamoylation by carmustine metabolites interfere with the synthesis and function of DNA, RNA, and proteins. Carmustine is lipid soluble and easily enters into the brain.

Primary indications
1. Lung, colorectal, and stomach carcinomas.
2. Hodgkin's and non-Hodgkin's lymphomas.
3. Brain tumors.
4. Multiple myeloma.
5. Melanoma.

Usual dosage and schedule. 75 to 100 mg/m^2 IV days 1 and 2 every 6 to 8 weeks.

Special precautions. Because of delayed myelosuppression (3–6 weeks), do not administer drug more often than every 6 weeks. Await a return of normal platelet and granulocyte counts before repeating therapy.

Toxicity
1. **Myelosuppression** is delayed and often biphasic with nadir at 3 to 6 weeks, and may be cumulative with successive doses. Recovery may be protracted for several months.
2. **Nausea and vomiting** begin 2 hours after therapy and last for 4 to 6 hours—common.
3. **Mucocutaneous**
   a. Facial flushing and burning sensation at IV site may be due to alcohol used to reconstitute the drug—common with rapid injection.
   b. Hyperpigmentation of skin following accidental contact—common.

4. **Miscellaneous effects**
   a. Hepatotoxicity and renal toxicity—uncommon, but can be severe.
   b. Pulmonary fibrosis—uncommon.
   c. Secondary neoplasia—possible.

Chlorambucil

Other name. Leukeran®

Mechanism of action. Classic alkylating agent, with primary effect on preformed DNA.

Primary indications
1. Chronic lymphocytic leukemia.
2. Non-Hodgkin's lymphoma of favorable histologic type.

Usual dosage and schedule
1. 3 to 4 mg/m^2 PO daily until a response is seen or cytopenias occur; then, if necessary, maintain with 1 to 2 mg/m^2 PO daily.
2. 30 mg/m^2 PO once every 2 weeks (usually with prednisone, 80 mg/m^2 PO days 1–5).

Special precautions. Increased toxicity may occur with prior barbiturate use.

Toxicity
1. **Myelosuppression** is dose limiting and may be prolonged.
2. **Nausea and vomiting** may be seen with higher doses, but are uncommon.
3. **Mucocutaneous.** None.
4. **Miscellaneous effects**
   a. Liver function abnormalities—rare.
   b. Secondary neoplasia—possible.
   c. Amenorrhea and azoospermia—common.
   d. Drug fever or rash—uncommon.

Chlorozotocin (Investigational)

Other name. DCNU

Mechanism of action. Alkylation by chlorozotocin metabolites interferes with structure and function of DNA and RNA. Glucose moiety attaches to the nitrosourea to diminish myelotoxicity.

Primary indication. Pancreatic islet cell carcinoma.

Usual dosage and schedule. 150 mg/m^2 IV by rapid injection every 6 to 7 weeks.

Special precautions. None.

Toxicity
1. **Myelosuppression.** Thrombocytopenia is dose limiting with nadir at about 4 weeks. Leukopenia is less severe.
2. **Nausea and vomiting** are common, but mild, beginning in 1 to 2 hours and lasting 4 to 6 hours.
3. **Mucocutaneous.** Not observed.

4. Miscellaneous effects
  a. Transient mild hepatotoxicity—common.
  b. Uncontrolled diabetes with ketoacidosis in pancreatic islet cell carcinoma—occasional.
  c. Interstitial pulmonary fibrosis—uncommon.

Cisplatin

Other names. *Cis*-diamminedichloroplatinum (II), DDP, CDDP, Platinol®

Mechanism of action. Similar to alkylating agents with respect to binding and cross-linking strands of DNA.

Primary indications. Testis, ovary, bladder, head and neck, and lung carcinomas.

Usual dosage and schedule
1. 40 to 120 mg/m^2 IV day 1 as push or infusion every 3 weeks.
2. 15 to 20 mg/m^2 IV days 1 to 5 as push or infusion every 3 to 4 weeks.

Special precautions. Do not administer if creatinine is greater than 1.5 mg/100 ml. Irreversible renal tubular damage may occur if vigorous diuresis is not maintained, particularly with higher doses (> 40 mg/m^2) and with additional concurrent nephrotoxic drugs, such as the aminoglycosides. At higher doses, diuresis with furosemide, mannitol, or both together with vigorous hydration is mandatory.
1. An acceptable method for hydration in patients without cardiovascular impairment for cisplatin doses up to 80 mg/m^2 is as follows:
  a. Have the patient void and begin an infusion of 2 liters of 5% dextrose in half-normal saline with 10 mEq of potassium chloride/liter and run at the rate of 1000 ml/hr.
  b. As soon as the infusion is started, give furosemide 40-mg IV push.
  c. After 30 minutes, if the patient has voided at least 250 ml, give mannitol 12.5-g IV push. If the patient is unable to void at a rate of 500 ml/hr, no cisplatin should be given.
  d. Following the mannitol, give the cisplatin IV push or as a 15- to 30-minute infusion through the sidearm of the first IV or by a second IV.
  e. Give additional mannitol or furosemide to maintain a urine flow of greater than 500 ml/hr for the first 2 hours or if the patient shows any evidence of congestive heart failure.
  f. At the end of the 2-liter infusion, the IV may be discontinued if the patient is to go home, or kept open until the vomiting stops if the patient is to remain hospitalized.
2. For doses greater than 80 mg/m^2 the following schedule is recommended:
  a. Have the patient void and begin an infusion of 2 liters of 5% dextrose in half-normal saline with 10 mEq potassium chloride/liter to run at 1000 ml/hr.
  b. As soon as the infusion is started, give furosemide 40-mg IV push.
  c. At 2 hours, if the patient has voided at least 1000 ml, give mannitol 12.5-g IV push and furosemide 40-mg IV push. If the patient has been unable to void at a rate of 500 ml/hr, no cisplatin should be given.
  d. Following the mannitol and additional furosemide, give cisplatin by a 30-minute infusion.

e. At the end of the cisplatin infusion, restart an infusion of 5% dextrose in half-normal saline with 10 mEq potassium chloride/liter at 500 ml/hr for 4 more hours. For the next 24 hours, give at least 4 liters of fluid orally or IV.

Toxicity
1. **Myelosuppression** is mild to moderate, depending on the dose. Relative lack of myelosuppression allows cisplatin to be used in full doses with more myelosuppressive drugs.
2. **Nausea and vomiting.** Severe and often intractable vomiting regularly begins within 1 hour of starting cisplatin and may last 8 to 12 hours. Higher than usual doses of antiemetics may partially ameliorate these symptoms.
3. **Mucocutaneous.** Not seen.
4. **Renal tubular damage.** Irreversible nephrotoxicity may occur, particularly if adequate attention is not given to achieving sufficient hydration and diuresis.
5. **Ototoxicity.** High tone hearing loss is common, but significant hearing loss in vocal frequencies is only occasional. Tinnitus is uncommon.
6. **Anaphylaxis** may occur after several doses. Responds to epinephrine, antihistamines, and corticosteroids.
7. **Miscellaneous effects**
   a. Peripheral neuropathies—rare.
   b. Hyperuricemia—uncommon; parallels renal failure.

Corticosteroids

Other names. Prednisone, dexamethasone (Decadron®), and others

Mechanism of action. Unknown, but apparently related to the presence of glucocorticoid receptors in tumor cells.

Primary indications
1. Carcinoma of the breast.
2. Acute and chronic lymphocytic leukemia.
3. Hodgkin's and non-Hodgkin's lymphomas.
4. Multiple myeloma.
5. Cerebral edema.

Usual dosage and schedule
1. **Prednisone:** dose varies with neoplasm and combination. Typical regimen *except* for acute lymphocytic leukemia is as follows:
   a. 40 mg/m^2 PO days 1 to 14 every 4 weeks *or*
   b. 100 mg/m^2 PO days 1 to 5 every 4 weeks.
2. **Prednisone:** for acute lymphocytic leukemia: 40 to 50 mg/m^2 PO daily for 28 days.
3. **Dexamethasone:** for cerebral edema: 16 to 32 mg PO daily to start, then reduce to lowest dose at which symptoms remain controlled.

Special precautions. None.

Toxicity
1. **Myelosuppression.** None.
2. **Nausea and vomiting.** None.
3. **Mucocutaneous.** Acne; increased risk for oral, rectal, and vaginal thrush. Thinning of skin and striae develop with continuous use.

4. **Suppression of adrenal-pituitary axis** may lead to adrenal insufficiency when corticosteroids are withdrawn, which is not common on intermittent schedules.
5. **Metabolic effects** include potassium depletion, sodium and fluid retention, diabetes, increased appetite, loss of mucle mass, myopathy, weight gain, osteoporosis, and development of cushingoid features. Their frequency depends both on dose and duration of therapy.
6. **Miscellaneous effects**
   a. Epigastric pain, extreme hunger, and occasional peptic ulceration with bleeding may occur. Antacids are recommended as prophylaxis.
   b. CNS effects including euphoria, depression, and sleeplessness, which may progress to dementia or frank psychosis, are common.
   c. Increased susceptibility to infection is common.
   d. Subcapsular cataracts in patients on long-term therapy are uncommon.

Cyclophosphamide

Other names. CTX, Cytoxan®

Mechanism of action. Metabolism of cyclophosphamide by hepatic microsomal enzymes produces active alkylating metabolites. Cyclophosphamide's primary effect is probably on DNA.

Primary indications
1. Breast, lung, ovary, testis, and bladder carcinomas.
2. Bone and soft tissue sarcomas.
3. Hodgkin's and non-Hodgkin's lymphomas.
4. Acute and chronic lymphocytic leukemias.
5. Neuroblastoma and Wilms' tumor of childhood.
6. Multiple myeloma.

Usual dosage and schedule
1. 1000 to 1500 mg/m^2 IV every 3 to 4 weeks *or*
2. 400 mg/m^2 PO days 1 to 5 every 3 to 4 weeks *or*
3. 60 to 120 mg/m^2 PO daily.

Special precautions. Maintain ample fluid intake and have patient empty bladder several times daily to diminish likelihood of cystitis.

Toxicity
1. **Myelosuppression** is dose limiting. Platelets are relatively spared. Nadir is reached about 10 to 14 days after IV dose with recovery by day 21.
2. **Nausea and vomiting** are seen frequently with large IV doses, less commonly after oral doses. Symptoms begin several hours after treatment, and are usually over by the next day.
3. **Mucocutaneous.** Reversible alopecia is common, usually starting after 2 to 3 weeks. Skin and nails may become darker; mucositis is uncommon.
4. **Bladder.** Hemorrhagic or nonhemorrhagic cystitis may occur in 5 to 10 percent of patients treated. It is usually reversible on discontinuation of the drug, but it may persist and lead to fibrosis or death. Frequency is diminished by ample fluid intake.
5. **Miscellaneous effects**
   a. Immunosuppression—common.
   b. Amenorrhea and azoospermia—common.
   c. Inhibition of antidiuretic hormone—only of significance with very large doses.

d. Interstitial pulmonary fibrosis—rare.
e. Secondary neoplasia—possible.

Cytarabine

Other names. Cytosine arabinoside, ara-C, Cytosar-U®

Mechanism of action. A pyrimidine analog antimetabolite that, when phosphorylated to ara-cytosinetriphosphate (ara-CTP), is a competitive inhibitor of DNA polymerase.

Primary indication. Acute nonlymphocytic leukemia.

Usual dosage and schedule
1. **For induction:** 100 to 200 mg/m^2 IV daily as a continuous infusion for 5 to 10 days (in combination with other drugs).
2. **For maintenance:** 100 mg/m^2 SC every 12 hours for 4 or 5 days every 3 to 4 weeks (with other drugs).
3. **Intrathecally:** 40 to 50 mg/m^2 every 4 days in preservative-free buffered isotonic diluent.

Special precautions. None.

Toxicity
1. **Myelosuppression.** Dose-limiting leukopenia and thrombocytopenia occur with nadir 7 to 10 days after treatment has ended and recovery in the following 2 weeks, depending on the degree of suppression. Megaloblastosis is common.
2. **Nausea and vomiting** are common, particularly if the drug is given as a push or rapid infusion.
3. **Mucocutaneous.** Stomatitis is occasional.
4. **Miscellaneous effects**
   a. Flulike syndrome with fever, arthralgia, and sometimes a rash—occasional.
   b. Transient mild hepatic dysfunction—occasional.

Dacarbazine

Other names. Imidazole carboxamide, DIC, DTIC-DOME®

Mechanism of action. Uncertain, but probably interacts with preformed macromolecules by alkylation.

Primary indications
1. Melanoma.
2. All soft tissue sarcomas.
3. Hodgkin's lymphoma.

Usual dosage and schedule
1. 150 to 250 mg/m^2 IV push or rapid infusion days 1 to 5 every 3 to 4 weeks
   or
2. 400 to 500 mg/m^2 IV push or rapid infusion days 1 and 2 every 3 to 4 weeks.

Special precautions
1. Administer cautiously to avoid extravasation as tissue damage may occur.
2. Venous pain along the injection site may be reduced by diluting dacar-

bazine in 100 to 200 ml of 5% dextrose in water and infusing over 30 minutes rather than injecting rapidly. Ice application may also reduce pain.

Toxicity
1. **Myelosuppression** is mild to moderate in degree. This factor allows dacarbazine to be used in full doses with other myelosuppressive drugs.
2. **Nausea and vomiting** are common and severe, but decrease in intensity with each subsequent daily dose. Onset is within 1 to 3 hours with duration up to 12 hours.
3. **Mucocutaneous**
   a. Moderately severe tissue damage if extravasation occurs.
   b. Alopecia—uncommon.
   c. Erythematous or urticarial rash—uncommon.
4. **Miscellaneous effects.** Flulike syndrome with fever, myalgia, and malaise lasting several days is uncommon.

Dactinomycin

Other names. Actinomycin D, act-D, Cosmegen®

Mechanism of action. Binds to DNA and inhibits DNA-dependent RNA synthesis.

Primary indications
1. Gestational trophoblastic and testis carcinomas.
2. Wilms' tumor, rhabdomyosarcoma, and Ewing's sarcoma of childhood.

Usual dosage and schedule
1. **Children.** 0.4 to 0.45 mg/m^2 (up to a maximum of 0.5 mg) IV daily for 5 days every 3 to 5 weeks.
2. **Adults**
   a. 0.4 to 0.45 mg/m^2 IV days 1 to 5 every 2 to 3 weeks.
   b. 0.5 mg IV daily for 5 days every 3 to 5 weeks.
   c. 1 mg/m^2 IV day 1 every 4 weeks (in combination with cyclophosphamide, vinblastine, and bleomycin).

Special precautions. Administer by slow IV push through the sidearm of a running IV being careful to avoid extravasation, which causes severe soft tissue damage.

Toxicity
1. **Myelosuppression** may be dose limiting and severe. It begins within the first week of treatment, but the nadir may not be reached for 21 days.
2. **Nausea and vomiting.** Severe vomiting often occurs during the first few hours after drug administration and lasts for up to 24 hours.
3. **Mucocutaneous**
   a. Erythema, hyperpigmentation, and desquamation of the skin potentiation by previous or concurrent radiotherapy are common.
   b. Oropharyngeal mucositis is potentiated by previous or concurrent radiotherapy.
   c. Alopecia is common.
   d. Moderately severe tissue damage occurs with extravasation.
4. **Miscellaneous effects.** Mental depression is rare.

Daunorubicin

Other names. Daunomycin, rubidomycin, DNR, Cerubidine®

Mechanism of action. Binds to DNA and inhibits DNA replication and DNA-dependent RNA synthesis.

Primary indication. Acute nonlymphocytic leukemia.

Usual dosage and schedule
1. 60 mg/m^2 IV push days 1, 2, and 3 every 2 weeks as induction therapy for 1 or 2 cycles in combination with other drugs.
2. 45 mg/m^2 IV push days 1 and 2 every 4 weeks as consolidation therapy for 1 or 2 cycles in combination with other drugs.

Special precautions
1. Administer over several minutes into the sidearm of a running IV infusion, taking precautions to avoid extravasation.
2. Reduce dose if patient has impaired liver or renal function.

Serum Bilirubin	Serum Creatinine	Full Dose (%)
1.2–3.0 mg/100 ml	—	75
> 3.0 mg/100 ml	> 3.0 mg/100 ml	50

3. Do not exceed cumulative dosage of 550 mg/m^2.

Toxicity
1. **Myelosuppression.** Dose-limiting pancytopenia with nadir at 1 to 2 weeks.
2. **Nausea and vomiting** may occur on the day of administration in one half of patients.
3. **Mucocutaneous.** Alopecia is common, but stomatitis is rare. Severe local tissue damage may progress to skin ulceration and necrosis may occur with subcutaneous extravasation.
4. **Cardiac.** Potentially irreversible congestive heart failure may occur owing to cardiomyopathy. The incidence is highly dependent on the lifetime cumulative dose, which should not exceed 550 mg/m^2. Congestive heart failure may be predicted by serial measurement of left ventricular function or endomyocardial biopsy. Transient ECG changes are common and not usually serious.
5. **Miscellaneous effects**
   a. Red urine caused by the drug and its metabolites—common.
   b. Chemical phlebitis and phlebothrombosis of veins used for injection—common.

Dibromodulcitol (Investigational)

Other names. DBD, mitolactol

Mechanism of action. A halogenated hexitol, dibromodulcitol acts, at least in part, as an alkylating agent with efects on DNA, RNA, and protein synthesis.

Primary indications
1. Breast and lung carcinomas.
2. Melanoma.
3. Hodgkin's and non-Hodgkin's lymphomas.

Usual dosage and schedule
1. **As a single agent:** 100 to 130 mg/m^2 PO daily until mild hematologic suppression develops.
2. **In combination with other drugs:** 130 to 135 mg/m^2 PO daily for 10 days every 28 days.

Special precautions. Use with caution in patients with impaired renal function since renal excretion is the primary mode of elimination of the drug and its metabolites.

Toxicity
1. **Myelosuppression.** Usually dose limiting with thrombocytopenia predominating.
2. **Nausea and vomiting.** Uncommon.
3. **Mucocutaneous.** Skin pigmentation—uncommon.
4. **Miscellaneous effects**
    a. Dyspnea—occasional.
    b. Transient liver enzyme elevation—occasional.
    c. Somnolence or other neurologic problems—uncommon.

Doxorubicin

Other names. ADR, Adriamycin™

Mechanism of action. Binds to DNA and inhibits DNA replication and DNA-dependent RNA synthesis.

Primary indications
1. Breast, bladder, liver, lung, prostate, stomach, and thyroid carcinomas.
2. Bone and soft tissue sarcomas.
3. Hodgkin's and non-Hodgkin's lymphomas.
4. Acute lymphocytic and acute nonlymphocytic leukemias.
5. Wilms' tumor, neuroblastoma, and rhabdomyosarcoma of childhood.

Usual dosage and schedule
1. 60 to 75 mg/m^2 IV every 3 weeks.
2. 30 mg/m^2 IV days 1 and 8 every 4 weeks (in combination with other drugs).

Special precautions
1. Administer over several minutes into the sidearm of a running IV infusion, taking care to avoid extravasation.
2. Reduce or hold dose if patient has impaired liver function.
    a. For bilirubin 1.2 to 3.0: give one half of the normal dose.
    b. For bilirubin greater than 3.0: give one fourth of the normal dose.
3. Do not exceed a lifetime cumulative dose of 550 mg/m^2.

Toxicity
1. **Myelosuppression** is dose limiting for most patients. Nadir WBC and platelet counts occur at 10 to 14 days; recovery by day 21.
2. **Nausea and vomiting** are mild to moderate in about one half of patients.
3. **Mucocutaneous**
    a. Stomatitis—dose dependent.
    b. Alopecia beginning 2 to 5 weeks from start of therapy with recovery following completion of therapy—common.
    c. Recall of skin reaction owing to prior radiotherapy—common.

d. Severe local tissue damage possibly progressing to skin ulceration and necrosis if subcutaneous extravasation occurs—common.

e. Hyperpigmentation of skin overlying veins used for drug injection in which chemical phlebitis has occurred—common.

4. **Cardiac**

a. Potentially irreversible congestive heart failure may occur owing to cardiomyopathy. The incidence is highly dependent on the lifetime cumulative dose, which should not exceed 550 mg/m^2. This limit is lower (450 mg/m^2) if patient has received prior chest radiotherapy or is receiving cyclophosphamide concomitantly. Congestive heart failure may be predicted by serial measurement of left ventricular function or endomyocardial biopsy.

b. Transient ECG changes are common and not usually serious.

5. **Miscellaneous effects**

a. Red urine owing to drug and its metabolites—common.

b. Chemical phlebitis and phlebosclerosis of veins used for injection, particularly if a vein is used repeatedly—common.

c. Fever and chills and urticaria—uncommon.

Estramustine

Other name. Estracyt®, Emcyt®

Mechanism of action. A chemical combination of mechlorethamine and estradiol phosphate, estramustine is believed to selectively enter cells with estrogen receptors where it acts as an alkylating agent.

Primary indication. Metastatic prostate carcinoma.

Usual dosage and schedule. 600 mg/m^2 PO daily in 3 divided doses.

Special precautions. Take with meals and antacids to lessen gastrointestinal disturbances.

Toxicity

1. **Myelosuppression** occurs only occasionally.

2. **Nausea and vomiting** are commonly seen soon after starting treatment, but usually lessen with continued therapy and antiemetices. If persistent and severe, it may be necessary to discontinue the drug.

3. **Mucocutaneous.** Rash with fever is rare.

4. **Miscellaneous effects**

a. Congestive heart failure—must be watched for in patients with pre-existing cardiac disease.

b. Gynecomastia—occasional.

Estrogens

Other names. Diethylstilbestrol (DES), chlorotrianisene (TACE®), diethylstilbestrol diphosphate (Stilphostrol®), and others

Mechanism of action. Unknown, but in breast cancer, responses are related to the presence of cytoplasmic estrogen receptors.

Primary indications. Breast and prostate carcinomas.

Usual dosage and schedule
1. **DES**
   a. Prostate carcinoma. 1 to 3 mg PO daily.
   b. Breast carcinoma. 3 to 15 mg PO daily in 3 divided doses.
2. **Chlorotrianisene.** 12 to 25 mg PO daily (prostate only).
3. **Diethylstilbestrol diphosphate.** 500 to 1000 mg IV daily for 5 to 7 days, then 250 to 500 mg IV 1 to 2 times weekly.

Special precautions
1. Acute fluid retention and pulmonary edema are possible, particularly with high-dose IV therapy.
2. Hypercalcemia may occur with initial therapy.

Toxicity
1. **Myelosuppression.** None.
2. **Nausea and vomiting** are common at beginning of therapy, but diminish or stop with continued treatment. Severity may be lessened by beginning treatment with doses lower than those recommended.
3. **Mucocutaneous.** Darkening of nipples—common.
4. **Miscellaneous effects**
   a. Peripheral edema owing to sodium retention is common but congestive heart failure occurs in less than 5 percent of patients.
   b. Vaginal bleeding and menstrual irregularities occur in 15 to 20 percent of patients.
   c. Diarrhea is uncommon.
   d. Any patient on estrogens may be at higher risk than normal for thromboemboli. An increase in cardiovascular deaths has been seen in male patients given DES 5 mg daily for prostate carcinoma.
   e. Increased bone pain, tumor pain, and local disease flare are associated with both good tumor response and tumor progression.
   f. Feminization occurs in male patients.

Etoposide (Investigational)

Other names. Epipodophyllotoxin, VP-16, VP-16-213

Mechanism of action. Arrests cells in late S or G_2 phases, probably by producing single-strand breaks in DNA.

Primary indications
1. Small-cell anaplastic lung carcinoma.
2. Acute nonlymphocytic leukemia.

Usual dosage and schedule
1. 50 to 100 mg/m^2 IV days 1 to 5 every 2 to 4 weeks.
2. 125 to 140 mg/m^2 IV days 1, 3, and 5 every 5 weeks.
3. 200 mg/m^2 IV weekly.

Special precautions
1. Administer as a 30- to 60-minute infusion to avoid severe hypotension. Monitor blood pressure during infusion.
2. Take care to avoid extravasation.
3. Must be diluted in 20 to 50 volumes (100–250 ml) of isotonic saline before use.

Toxicity

1. **Myelosuppression.** Dose-limiting leukopenia and less severe thrombocytopenia have a nadir at 16 days with recovery by day 20 to 22.
2. **Nausea and vomiting** are usually minor problems in about one third of patients.
3. **Mucocutaneous**
   a. Alopecia—common.
   b. Stomatitis—rare.
4. **Hypotension** occurs if the drug is infused in less than 30 minutes.
5. **Miscellaneous effects**
   a. Severe allergic reactions, including bronchospasm, wheezing, and anaphylaxis—rare.
   b. Chemical phlebitis—uncommon.

Floxuridine

Other name. FUDR®

Mechanism of action. A pyrimidine antimetabolite that, when converted to the active nucleotide, inhibits the enzyme thymidylate synthetase.

Primary indications. Hepatic metastasis of gastrointestinal carcinoma.

Usual dosage and schedule. 8 to 20 mg/m^2 daily as a continuous hepatic artery infusion for 2 to 6 weeks. A dose of 12 mg/m^2 daily for 2 weeks followed by a 2-week rest is usually tolerated well.

Special precautions

1. Reduce dose in patients with compromised liver function.
2. For intraarterial infusion, add 5000 units of heparin to 1 liter of 5% dextrose in water together with the daily dose of floxuridine. The catheter position should be checked with dye injection every few days to ensure that it has not moved and that the hepatic artery has not thrombosed. Ulcerlike pain or other significant gastrointestinal symptoms are indications to discontinue intraarterial therapy as hemorrhage or perforation may occur.

Toxicity

1. **Myelosuppression** is uncommon using the intermittent 12 mg/m^2 dosage.
2. **Nausea and vomiting** are uncommon unless the hepatic artery catheter has become displaced and the stomach and duodenum are being infused.
3. **Mucocutaneous**
   a. Stomatitis is an early sign of severe toxicity. It progresses from soreness and erythema to frank ulceration, which may become hemorrhagic in a small number of patients. Esophagitis, proctitis, and diarrhea may also occur.
   b. Partial alopecia is uncommon.
   c. Hyperpigmentation of skin over face, hands, and veins used for infusion—occasional.
   d. Maculopapular rash is uncommon.
   e. Sun exposure tends to increase skin reactions.
4. **Miscellaneous effects**
   a. Neurotoxicity, including headache, minor visual disturbances, and cerebellar ataxia—rare.

b. Increased lacrimation—uncommon.
c. Abdominal cramps and pain are common if the catheter is displaced and the stomach and duodenum are being infused. This can progress to frank gastritis or duodenal ulcer.

Fluorouracil

Other names. 5-FU, Fluorouracil®, Adrucil®, 5-fluorouracil

Mechanism of action. A pyrimidine antimetabolite that, when converted to the active nucleotide, inhibits the enzyme thymidylate synthetase and thereby blocks DNA synthesis.

Primary indications
1. Breast, colorectal, stomach, pancreas, esophagus, liver, and bladder carcinomas.
2. Basal cell carcinoma of skin (topically).

Usual dosage and schedule
1. **Systemic**
   a. 500 mg/m^2 IV days 1 to 5 every 4 weeks *or*
   b. 500 to 600 mg/m^2 IV weekly.
2. **Intracavitary.** 500 to 1000 mg for pericardial, 2000 to 3000 mg for pleural or peritoneal effusions.
3. **Intraarterial** (liver). 800 to 1200 mg/m^2 as a continuous infusion days 1 to 4, followed by 600 mg/m^2 as a continuous infusion days 5 to 21.

Special precautions
1. Reduce dose in patients with compromised liver function.
2. For intraarterial infusion, add 5000 units of heparin to 1 liter of 5% dextrose in water together with the daily dose of fluorouracil. The catheter position should be checked with dye injection every few days to ensure that it has not moved and that the hepatic artery has not thrombosed. Ulcerlike pain or other significant gastrointestinal symptoms are indications to discontinue intraarterial therapy as hemorrhage or perforation may occur.

Toxicity
1. **Myelosuppression** is dose limiting with nadir at 10 to 14 days after last dose and recovery by 21 days.
2. **Nausea and vomiting** may be seen, but are not usually severe.
3. **Mucocutaneous**
   a. Stomatitis is an early sign of severe toxicity. It progresses from soreness and erythema to frank ulceration, which may become hemorrhagic in a small number of patients. Esophagitis, proctitis, and diarrhea may also occur.
   b. Partial alopecia is uncommon.
   c. Hyperpigmentation of skin over face, hands, and veins used for infusion—occasional.
   d. Maculopapular rash is uncommon.
   e. Sun exposure tends to increase skin reactions.
4. **Miscellaneous effects**
   a. Neurotoxicity, including headache, minor visual disturbances, and cerebellar ataxia—rare.
   b. Increased lacrimation—uncommon.

Hexamethylmelamine (Investigational)

Other name. HXM

Mechanism of action. Unknown. Although it structurally resembles the known alkylating agent triethylenemelamine, it has some antimetabolite characteristics.

Primary indication. Carcinoma of the ovary.

Usual dosage and schedule
1. 200 to 320 mg/m^2 PO daily in 3 to 4 divided doses for 21 days every 6 weeks when used as a single agent.
2. 150 to 200 mg/m^2 PO daily in 3 to 4 divided doses for 2 out of 3 or 4 weeks when used in combination.

Special precautions. None.

Toxicity
1. **Myelosuppression.** Dose-limiting leukopenia and thrombocytopenia are uncommon.
2. **Nausea and vomiting** are usually dose limiting and associated with anorexia, diarrhea, and abdominal cramps. Tolerance may develop.
3. **Mucocutaneous.** Alopecia, skin rash, and pruritus are rare.
4. **Miscellaneous effects**
   a. Peripheral neuropathies—occasional.
   b. CNS effects, including agitation, confusion, hallucinations, depression, and parkinsonianlike symptoms—less common with recommended intermittent schedule than with continuous treatment.

Hydroxyurea

Other name. Hydrea®

Mechanism of action. Interferes with DNA synthesis, at least in part by inhibiting the enzymatic conversion of ribonucleotides to deoxyribonucleotides.

Primary indications
1. Head and neck carcinomas.
2. Chronic granulocytic leukemia; acute lymphocytic and acute nonlymphocytic leukemia with high blast counts.

Usual dosage and schedule
1. 800 to 2000 mg/m^2 PO as a single daily dose *or*
2. 3200 mg/m^2 PO as a single dose every third day (not for leukemias).

Special precautions. The daily dose must be adjusted for blood counts.

Toxicity
1. **Myelosuppression** occurs at doses greater than 1600 mg/m^2 daily by day 10. Recovery is usually prompt.
2. **Nausea and vomiting** are common at higher doses.
3. **Mucocutaneous.** Stomatitis is rare. Maculopapular rash may be seen. Inflammation of mucous membranes caused by radiation may be exaggerated.

4. **Miscellaneous effects**
    a. Temporary renal function impairment or dysuria—uncommon.
    b. CNS disturbances—rare.

Lomustine

Other names. CCNU, CeeNU®

Mechanism of action. Alkylation and carbamoylation by lomustine metabolites interfere with the synthesis and function of DNA, RNA, and proteins. Lomustine is lipid soluble and easily enters into the brain.

Primary indications
1. Lung and kidney carcinomas.
2. Hodgkin's and non-Hodgkin's lymphomas.
3. Brain tumors.

Usual dosage and schedule. 100 to 130 mg/m^2 PO once every 6 to 8 weeks (lower dose used for patients with compromised bone marrow function).

Special precautions. Because of delayed myelosuppression (3–6 weeks), do not treat more often than every 6 weeks. Await a return of normal platelet and granulocyte counts before repeating therapy.

Toxicity
1. **Myelosuppression** is universal and dose limiting. Leukopenia and thrombocytopenia are delayed 3 to 6 weeks after therapy begins and may be cumulative with successive doses.
2. **Nausea and vomiting** begin 3 to 6 hours after therapy and last up to 24 hours.
3. **Mucocutaneous.** Stomatitis and alopecia are rare.
4. **Miscellaneous effects**
    a. Confusion, lethargy, and ataxia—rare.
    b. Mild hepatotoxicity—infrequent.
    c. Secondary neoplasia—possible.

Mechlorethamine

Other names. Nitrogen mustard, HN2, Mustargen®

Mechanism of action. Mechlorethamine is a prototype alkylating agent. Its action involves transfer of the alkyl group to amino, carboxyl, hydroxyl, imidazole, phosphate, and sulfhydryl groups within the cell, altering structure and function of DNA (primarily), RNA, and proteins.

Primary indications
1. Hodgkin's and non-Hodgkin's lymphomas.
2. Lung carcinoma.
3. Malignant pleural and, less commonly, peritoneal or pericardial effusions.

Usual dosage and schedule
1. 6 mg/m^2 IV days 1 and 8 every 4 weeks (in MOPP regimen for Hodgkin's disease).
2. 16 mg/m^2 IV day 1 every 4 to 6 weeks.
3. 8 to 16 mg/m^2 by intracavitary injection.

Special precautions

1. Administer over several minutes into the sidearm of a running IV taking care to avoid extravasation.
2. Because mechlorethamine is a potent vesicant, extreme care must be exercised while preparing and administering the drug. Gloves and eye glasses are recommended to protect the preparer. If accidental eye contact should occur, institute copious irrigation with normal saline and follow by prompt ophthalmologic consultation. If accidental skin contact occurs, irrigate the affected part immediately with water for at least 15 minutes and follow by 2.6% sodium thiosulfate solution (⅙ M).
3. Mechlorethamine should be used soon after preparation (within 15–30 minutes) as it will decompose on standing. It *must not* be mixed in the same syringe with any other drug.

Toxicity

1. **Myelosuppression** is dose limiting with nadir at about 1 week and recovery by 3 weeks.
2. **Nausea and vomiting** are universal. They usually begin within the first 3 hours and last for 4 to 8 hours.
3. **Mucocutaneous.** Severe painful inflammation and necrosis are likely if extravasation occurs. May be ameliorated if 2.6% thiosulfate solution (⅙ M) is instilled into the area to neutralize active drug and ice packs are applied locally for 6 to 12 hours. Maculopapular rash is uncommon.
4. **Miscellaneous effects**
   a. Phlebitis and/or thrombosis of the vein used for injection—common.
   b. Amenorrhea and azoospermia—common.
   c. Hyperuricemia with rapid tumor destruction.
   d. Weakness, sleepiness, and headache—uncommon.
   e. Severe allergic reactions, including anaphylaxis—rare.
   f. Secondary neoplasms—possible.

Melphalan

Other names. Phenylalanine mustard, L-sarcolysin, L-PAM, Alkeran®

Mechanism of action. Alkylating agent with primary effect on DNA. Amino acid type structure may result in cellular transport that is different from other alkylating agents.

Primary indications

1. Multiple myeloma.
2. Breast, ovary, and testis (seminoma) carcinomas.

Usual dosage and schedule

1. 8 mg/m^2 PO days 1 to 4 every 4 weeks *or*
2. 10 mg/m^2 PO days 1 to 4 every 6 weeks *or*
3. 3 to 4 mg/m^2 PO daily for 2 to 3 weeks, then 1 to 2 mg/m^2 PO daily for maintenance.

Special precaution. Myelosuppression may be delayed and prolonged to 4 to 6 weeks.

Toxicity

1. **Myelosuppression.** Dose limiting; nadir at day 14 to 21.
2. **Nausea and vomiting.** Uncommon.

3. **Mucocutaneous.** Alopecia, dermatitis, and stomatitis—uncommon.
4. **Miscellaneous effects**
   a. Acute nonlymphocytic leukemia—rare, but well documented.
   b. Pulmonary fibrosis—rare.

Mercaptopurine

Other names. 6-Mercaptopurine, 6-MP, Purinethol®

Mechanism of action. A purine antimetabolite that, when converted to the nucleotide, inhibits the formation of nucleotides necessary for DNA and RNA synthesis.

Primary indications. Acute lymphocytic and juvenile chronic granulocytic leukemias.

Usual dosage and schedule
1. 100 mg/m^2 PO daily if used alone.
2. 50 to 90 mg/m^2 PO daily if used with methotrexate.

Special precautions
1. Decrease dose by 75 percent when used concurrently with allopurinol.
2. Increase interval between doses or reduce dose in patients with renal failure.

Toxicity
1. **Myelosuppression** is common, but mild at recommended doses.
2. **Nausea and vomiting** are uncommon.
3. **Mucocutaneous.** Stomatitis may be seen with very large doses. Dry scaling rash is uncommon.
4. **Miscellaneous effects**
   a. Intrahepatic cholestasis and mild focal centrolobular necrosis with jaundice—uncommon.
   b. Diarrhea—rare.
   c. Hyperuricemia with rapid leukemia cell lysis is common.
   d. Fever—uncommon.

Methotrexate

Other names. Amethopterin, MTX, Mexate®

Mechanism of action. Inhibition of dihydrofolate reductase, which results in a block of the reduction of dihydrofolate to tetrahydrofolate. This blockage in turn inhibits the formation of thymidylate and purines and arrests DNA (predominately), RNA, and protein synthesis.

Primary indications
1. Breast, head and neck, gastrointestinal, lung, and gestational trophoblastic carcinomas.
2. Osteosarcomas (high-dose methotrexate).
3. Acute lymphocytic leukemia.
4. Meningeal leukemia or carcinomatosis.

Usual dosage and schedule
1. **Gestational trophoblastic carcinoma.** 15 to 30 mg PO or IM days 1 to 5 every 2 weeks.

2. **Other carcinomas.** 40 to 80 mg/m^2 IV or PO 2 to 4 times monthly with a 7- to 14-day interval between doses.
3. **Acute lymphocytic leukemia.** 15 to 20 mg/m^2 PO or IV weekly (together with mercaptopurine).
4. **Osteogenic sarcoma.** Up to 10 g/m^2 with leucovorin rescue (high-dose methotrexate). This usage is investigational and should not be used outside of a research setting.
5. **Intrathecally.** 12 mg/m^2 (not >20 mg) twice weekly.

Special precautions
1. High-dose methotrexate (>80 mg/m^2) is experimental and should be administered only by individuals experienced in its use and at institutions where serum methotrexate levels are readily available.
2. Intrathecal methotrexate must be mixed in buffered physiologic solution containing no preservative.
3. Avoid aspirin, sulfonamides, tetracycline, phenytoin, and other protein-bound drugs that may displace methotrexate and cause an increase in free drug.
4. Oral anticoagulants, such as warfarin, may be potentiated by methotrexate, and prothrombin times should be followed carefully.
5. In patients with renal insufficiency it may be necessary to markedly reduce the dose or discontinue methotrexate therapy.

Toxicity
1. **Myelosuppression** occurs regularly with nadir at 6 to 10 days after a single IV dose. Recovery is rapid.
2. **Nausea and vomiting** occur occasionally at standard doses.
3. **Mucocutaneous**
   a. Mild stomatitis is common and is a sign that a maximum tolerated dose has been reached. Higher doses may result in confluent or hemorrhagic stomal ulcers and bloody diarrhea.
   b. Erythematous rashes, urticaria, and skin pigment changes are uncommon.
   c. Mild alopecia is frequent.
4. **Miscellaneous effects**
   a. Acute hepatocellular injury—uncommon at standard doses.
   b. Hepatic fibrosis—uncommon, but seen at low chronic doses.
   c. Pneumonitis—rare.
   d. Polyserositis—rare.
   e. Renal tubular necrosis—rare at standard doses.
   f. Convulsions and a Guillain-Barré-like syndrome following intrathecal therapy—uncommon.

Mithramycin

Other name. Mithracin®

Mechanism of action. Binds to DNA and inhibits DNA-dependent RNA synthesis.

Primary indications
1. Testis carcinoma.
2. Severe refractory hypercalcemia.

Usual dosage and schedule
1. **Testis carcinoma.** 1 to 2 mg/m^2 IV on alternating days for 3 to 8 doses or until toxicity develops. Repeat in 4 weeks.
2. **Hypercalcemia.** 0.6 to 1 mg/m^2 IV for 1 to 3 days with doses repeated if necessary and tolerated.

Special precautions
1. Administer as IV infusion over ½ to 6 hours to reduce severity of gastrointestinal toxicity.
2. Avoid subcutaneous extravasation.
3. Monitor platelet count, prothrombin time, partial prothrombin time, lactic dehydrogenase, SGOT, and BUN before each dose, particularly with higher dose schedule. Discontinue drug if significant abnormality occurs.

Toxicity
1. **Myelosuppression.** Thrombocytopenia is commonly severe; leukopenia is not usually significant.
2. **Nausea and vomiting** are common.
3. **Mucocutaneous**
   a. Blushing of the face followed by a coarsening of skin folds, hyperpigmentation, and possible desquamation are occasional with alternate day therapy.
   b. Stomatitis—common.
   c. Papular skin rash—uncommon.
   d. Alopecia—uncommon.
4. **Hepatic.** Coagulopathy owing to clotting factor abnormalities and thrombocytopenia is often observed and may be fatal. Prothrombin time, partial thrombin time, SGOT, and lactic dehydrogenase must be monitored during therapy.
5. **Miscellaneous effects**
   a. Diarrhea—common.
   b. CNS toxicity manifested by headache, irritability, and lethargy—dose dependent.
   c. Phlebitis—uncommon.
   d. Renal—more than one half of patients have some abnormality with proteinuria and mild azotemia.
   e. Electrolyte abnormalities—depression of serum calcium, phosphorus, and potassium—common.

Mitomycin

Other names. Mitomycin-C, Mutamycin®

Mechanism of action. Alkylation and cross-linking by mitomycin metabolites interfere with structure and function of DNA.

Primary indications. Stomach and pancreas carcinomas.

Usual dosage and schedule
1. 20 mg/m^2 IV day 1 every 4 to 6 weeks *or*
2. 2 mg/m^2 IV days 1 to 5 and 8 to 12 every 4 to 6 weeks.
3. 10 mg/m^2 IV day 1 every 8 weeks in combination with fluorouracil and doxorubicin for stomach and pancreatic carcinomas.

Special precaution. Administer as slow push or rapid infusion through the sidearm of a rapidly running IV taking care to avoid extravasation.

Toxicity

1. **Myelosuppression** is serious, cumulative, and dose limiting. Nadir is reached usually by 4 weeks, but may be delayed. Recovery is often prolonged over many weeks and occasionally cytopenia never disappears.
2. **Nausea and vomiting** are common at higher doses, but severity is usually mild to moderate.
3. **Mucocutaneous**
   a. Stomatitis and alopecia—common.
   b. Cellulitis at injection site if extravasation occurs—common.
4. **Miscellaneous effects**
   a. Renal toxicity—uncommon.
   b. Pulmonary toxicity—uncommon, but may be severe.
   c. Fever—uncommon.
   d. Secondary neoplasia—possible.

Mitotane

Other names. o,p'-DDD, Lysodren®

Mechanism of action. Suppresses adrenal steroid production, modifies peripheral steroid metabolism, and is cytotoxic to adrenal cortical cells.

Primary indication. Adrenocortical carcinoma.

Usual dosage and schedule. Begin with 2 to 6 g PO daily in 3 to 4 divided doses and build to a maximum tolerated daily dose that is usually 8 to 10 g, but it may range from 2 to 16 g. Glucocorticoid and mineralocorticoid replacement during mitotane therapy are necessary to prevent hypoadrenalism. Cortisone acetate, 25 mg PO in the AM and 12.5 mg PO in the PM, and fludrocortisone acetate, 0.1 mg PO in the AM, are recommended.

Special precautions. Patients who experience severe trauma, infection, or shock should be treated with supplemental corticosteroids. Because of the effect of mitotane on peripheral steroid metabolism, larger than usual replacement doses may be necessary.

Toxicity

1. **Myelosuppression.** None.
2. **Nausea and vomiting** are common and may be dose limiting.
3. **Mucocutaneous.** Skin rash occurs occasionally.
4. **CNS effects.** Lethargy, sedation, vertigo, or dizziness are seen in up to 40 percent of patients and may be dose limiting.
5. **Miscellaneous effects.** Albuminuria, hemorrhagic cystitis, hypertension, orthostatic hypotension, and visual disturbances are uncommon.

Procarbazine

Other name. Matulane®

Mechanism of action. Uncertain, but appears to affect preformed DNA, RNA, and protein.

Primary indications
1. Lung carcinoma.
2. Hodgkin's and non-Hodgkin's lymphomas.

Usual dosage and schedule. 100 mg/m^2 PO daily for 7 to 14 days every 4 weeks (in combination with other drugs).

Special precautions. Many food and drug interactions are possible, although their clinical significance may be low.

Drug or Food	Possible Result
Ethanol	Disulfiramlike reactions: nausea, vomiting, visual disturbances, and headache
Sympathomimetics, antidepressants, and tyramine rich foods (cheese, wine, and bananas)	Hypertensive crisis, tremors, excitation, angina, and cardiac palpitations
CNS depressants	Additive depression

Toxicity
1. **Myelosuppression.** Pancytopenia is dose limiting.
2. **Nausea and vomiting** are frequent during first few days until tolerance develops.
3. **Mucocutáneous**
   a. Stomatitis and diarrhea—uncommon.
   b. Alopecia, pruritus, and drug rash—uncommon.
4. **CNS effects.** Paresthesias, neuropathies, headache, dizziness, depression, apprehension, nervousness, insomnia, nightmares, hallucinations, ataxia, confusion, convulsions, and coma have been reported with varying frequency.
5. **Miscellaneous effects**
   a. Secondary neoplasia—possible.
   b. Visual disturbances—rare.
   c. Postural hypotension—rare.

Progestins

Other names. Medroxyprogesterone acetate (Provera®, Depo-Provera®), hydroxyprogesterone caproate (Delalutin®), megestrol acetate (Megace®)

Mechanism of action. Mechanism of antitumor effects is not clear.

Primary indications. Endometrial and breast carcinomas.

Usual dosage and schedule
1. **Medroxyprogesterone acetate.** 1000 to 1500 mg IM weekly or 400 to 800 mg PO twice weekly.
2. **Hydroxyprogesterone caproate.** 1000 to 1500 mg IM weekly.
3. **Megestrol acetate.** 80 to 320 mg PO daily.

Special precautions
1. Acute local hypersensitivity or dyspnea owing to oil in IM preparations—uncommon.
2. Hypercalcemia with initial therapy—occasional.

Toxicity
1. **Myelosuppression.** None.
2. **Nausea and vomiting.** Rare.

3. **Mucocutaneous.** Mild alopecia or skin rash—uncommon.
4. **Miscellaneous effects**
   a. Mild fluid retention—occasional.
   b. Mild liver function abnormalities—occasional.
   c. Menstrual irregularities—common.

Semustine (Investigational)

Other name. Methyl-CCNU

Mechanism of action. Alkylation and carbamoylation by semustine metabolites interfere with the synthesis and function of DNA, RNA, and proteins. Semustine is lipid soluble and easily enters into the brain.

Primary indications
1. Colorectal and stomach carcinomas.
2. Brain tumors.
3. Hodgkin's and non-Hodgkin's lymphomas.
4. Melanoma.

Usual dosage and schedule. 150 to 200 mg/m^2 PO once every 6 to 10 weeks.

Special precautions. Because of delayed myelosuppression (3–6 weeks) do not treat more often than every 6 weeks. Await a return of normal platelet and granulocyte counts before repeating therapy.

Toxicity
1. **Myelosuppression** is dose limiting. Leukopenia and thrombocytopenia are delayed 3 to 6 weeks after therapy begins and may be cumulative with successive doses.
2. **Nausea and vomiting** begin 3 to 6 hours after administration and last up to 24 hours—common.
3. **Mucocutaneous.** Uncommon.
4. **Miscellaneous effects.**
   a. Renal toxicity and hepatotoxicity are uncommon.
   b. Secondary neoplasia is possible.

Streptozocin (Investigational)

Other names. Streptozotocin, Zanosar®

Mechanism of action. Inhibition of DNA synthesis, possibly by interference with pyridine nucleotide synthesis. Streptozocin appears to have some specificity for neoplastic pancreatic endocrine cells. Glucose moiety attached to nitrosourea appears to diminish myelotoxicity.

Primary indications
1. Pancreatic islet cell and pancreatic exocrine carcinomas.
2. Carcinoid tumors.

Usual dosage and schedule
1. 1.0 to 1.5 g/m^2 IV weekly for 6 weeks followed by 4 weeks of observation.
2. 500 mg/m^2 IV days 1 to 5 every 6 weeks.

Special precautions
1. A 30- to 60-minute infusion is recommended to reduce local pain and burning around the vein during treatment.

2. Avoid extravasation.
3. Have 50% glucose available to treat sudden hypoglycemia.

Toxicity
1. **Myelosuppression** is uncommon and mild.
2. **Nausea and vomiting** are common and severe. May become progressively worse over 5-day course of therapy. Standard antiemetics have been of little value.
3. **Mucocutaneous.** Uncommon.
4. **Nephrotoxicity.** Renal toxicity is common. Although it is not clearly dose related, it may limit continued drug use in individual patients. Proteinuria, glucosuria, azotemia, and hypophosphatemia, if persistent or severe, are indications to discontinue therapy. Hydration may ameliorate.
5. **Miscellaneous effects**
   a. Hypoglycemia. In patients with insulinoma, hypoglycemia may be severe (although transient) owing to a burst of insulin release.
   b. Hyperglycemia is uncommon in normal or diabetic patients as normal beta cells are usually insensitive to streptozocin's effect.
   c. Transient mild hepatotoxicity—occasional.

Tamoxifen

Other name. Nolvadex®

Mechanism of action. Tamoxifen is an estrogen antagonist that binds to cytoplasmic estrogen receptors. This complex is probably transported into the nucleus where it affects nucleic acid function.

Primary indication. Breast carcinoma.

Usual dosage and schedule. 10 mg PO twice daily.

Special precautions. Hypercalcemia may be seen during initial therapy.

Toxicity
1. **Myelosuppression** is uncommon and mild.
2. **Nausea and vomiting** occur early in the course of therapy in up to 20 percent of patients, but they abate rapidly as therapy is continued.
3. **Mucocutaneous.** Skin rash and pruritus vulvae are uncommon.
4. **Miscellaneous effects**
   a. Hot flashes—common.
   b. Vaginal bleeding and menstrual irregularity—uncommon.
   c. Lassitude, headache, leg cramps, and dizziness—uncommon.
   d. Peripheral edema—occasional.
   e. Increased bone pain, tumor pain, and local disease flare (associated both with good tumor response and with tumor progression)—occasional.
   f. Diarrhea—occasional.

Thioguanine

Other names. 6-Thioguanine, 6-TG, Tabloid® Brand Thioguanine

Mechanism of action. A purine antimetabolite that, when converted to the active nucleotide, substitutes for the normal guanine nucleotide in DNA synthesis. Thioguanine may also inhibit purine synthesis reactions.

Primary indication. Acute nonlymphocytic leukemia.

Usual dosage and schedule
1. **Induction.** 100 mg/m^2 PO twice daily for 8 to 21 days (with other drugs).
2. **Maintenance**
   a. 40 mg/m^2 PO twice daily days 1 to 4 weekly (with other drugs) *or*
   b. 100 mg/m^2 PO twice daily days 1 to 4 every 3 to 4 weeks (with other drugs).

Special precautions. None (no dose reduction required for concurrent use of allopurinol).

Toxicity
1. **Myelosuppression.** Major dose-limiting toxicity.
2. **Nausea and vomiting.** Occasional, but not severe.
3. **Mucocutaneous**
   a. Stomatitis and diarrhea, which may necessitate reduction of the dose—uncommon.
   b. Drug rash—rare.

Miscellaneous effects. Hepatotoxicity—rare.

Thiotepa

Other names. Triethylenethiophosphoramide, Thiotepa®

Mechanism of action. Alkylating agent similar to mechlorethamine.

Primary indications
1. Superficial papillary carcinoma of urinary bladder.
2. Malignant peritoneal or pleural effusions.

Usual dosage and schedule
1. 60 to 90 mg in 60 to 100 ml of water instilled into the bladder and retained for 2 hours. Dose may be repeated in 2 to 4 weeks as tolerated by blood counts *or*
2. 20 mg intravesically weekly for 3 weeks, then every 3 weeks for 5 weeks.
3. 25 to 30 mg/m^2 in 50 to 100 ml of saline solution as a single intracavitary injection. Dose may be repeated as tolerated by blood counts.

Special precaution. Dose should be reduced in patients with impaired renal function since the drug is primarily excreted in the urine.

Toxicity
1. **Myelosuppression** is dose limiting. Pancytopenia and sepsis may follow intravesical or intracavitary administration. Nadir counts are reached in 1 to 2 weeks, recovery by 4 weeks is usual.
2. **Nausea and vomiting** are uncommon.
3. **Mucocutaneous.** Uncommon. Thiotepa is *not* a vesicant.
4. **Miscellaneous effects**
   a. Local pain, dizziness, headache, and fever—uncommon.
   b. Secondary neoplasms—possible.
   c. Amenorrhea and azoospermia—common.

Vinblastine

Other names. VLB, Velban®

Mechanism of action. Mitotic inhibition with reversible metaphase arrest owing to action on microtubular and spindle contractile proteins.

Primary indications
1. Testicular, gestational trophoblastic, kidney, and breast carcinomas.
2. Hodgkin's and non-Hodgkin's lymphomas.

Usual dosage and schedule
1. 4 to 18 mg/m^2 IV weekly, starting at the lower dose and increasing the dose weekly by 30 to 50 percent until leukopenia of approximately 3000/μl occurs. Then hold therapy until the WBC is greater than or equal to 4000 and treat with one dose level below the dose that caused leukopenia.
2. 6 mg/m^2 IV days 1 and 15 in combination with doxorubicin, bleomycin, and dacarbazine for lymphomas.

Special precautions. Administer as a slow push taking care to avoid extravasation.

Toxicity
1. **Myelosuppression.** Dose-related leukopenia occurs with a nadir of 4 to 10 days and recovery in 7 to 10 days. Severe thrombocytopenia is uncommon.
2. **Nausea and vomiting** are common but not usually severe.
3. **Mucocutaneous**
   a. Extravasation may lead to severe inflammation, pain, and tissue damage. Local infiltration with 50 to 100 mg of hydrocortisone may help.
   b. Mild alopecia is common.
   c. Stomatitis is occasionally severe.
4. **Miscellaneous effects**
   a. Neurotoxicity manifested by (1) constipation, adynamic ileus, and abdominal pain if very high doses are used, or (2) paresthesias, peripheral neuropathy, and jaw pain with lower doses. Neurotoxicity is less frequent with vinblastine than with vincristine.
   b. Transient hepatitis is uncommon.
   c. Depression, headache, convulsions, or orthostatic hypotension is rare.

Vincristine

Other names. VCR, Oncovin®

Mechanism of action. Mitotic inhibition with reversible metaphase arrest owing to drug action on microtubular and spindle contractile proteins.

Primary indications
1. Breast carcinoma.
2. Hodgkin's and non-Hodgkin's lymphomas.
3. Acute lymphocytic leukemia.
4. Wilms' tumor, neuroblastoma, rhabdomyosarcoma, and Ewing's sarcoma of childhood.
5. Multiple myeloma.

Usual dosage and schedule. 1 to 2 mg/m^2 (maximum 2.0–2.2 mg) IV weekly.

Special precautions
1. Administer as a slow IV push, taking care to avoid extravasation.
2. Because neurotoxicity is cumulative, neurologic evaluation should be done before each dose and therapy withheld if severe paresthesias, motor

weakness, or other severe abnormalities occur. Underlying neurologic problems accentuate vincristine's effect.
3. Reduce dose if liver disease is significant.
4. Stool softeners or high-fiber or bulk diets may avert severe constipation.

Toxicity
1. **Myelosuppression** is mild and rarely of clinical significance.
2. **Nausea and vomiting** are not seen unless paralytic ileus occurs.
3. **Mucocutaneous.** Severe local inflammation if extravasation occurs. Alopecia is common.
4. **Neurotoxicity** is dose dependent and dose limiting. Mild paresthesias and decreased deep tendon reflexes are to be expected. More extensive peripheral neuropathies, severe constipation, or ileus are indications to reduce or hold therapy.
5. **Miscellaneous effects**
   a. Uric acid nephropathy owing to rapid tumor cell lysis and release of uric acid is always a potential problem when therapy is first given.
   b. Syndrome of inappropriate antidiuretic hormone is rare.
   c. Jaw pain is uncommon.

Vindesine (Investigational)

Other name. VDS

Mechanism of action. Mitotic inhibition with reversible metaphase arrest owing to action on microtubule and spindle contactile protein.

Primary indications
1. Colorectal, lung, breast, and esophageal carcinomas.
2. Hodgkin's and non-Hodgkin's lymphomas.
3. Acute lymphocytic leukemia and the blast crisis of chronic granulocytic leukemia.
4. Malignant glioma.
5. Melanoma.

Usual dosage and schedule
1. 3 to 4 mg/m^2 IV push or as a 24-hour infusion weekly for induction, then every 2 weeks *or*
2. 1.2 to 2 mg/m^2 IV push or as a continuous infusion days 1 to 5 every 3 weeks.

Special precautions
1. 5-day infusion requires lowest dose.
2. Take care to avoid extravasation.

Toxicity
1. **Myelosuppression.** Leukopenia is common, but not usually severe.
2. **Nausea and vomiting.** Occasional.
3. **Mucocutaneous.** Alopecia is common.
4. **Neurotoxicity** is dose dependent and cumulative, consisting of constipation, paralytic ileus, paresthesia, myalgias, and weakness. Severity is intermediate between vincristine and vinblastine.
5. **Miscellaneous effects**
   a. Chills and fever—occasional.
   b. Phlebitis—occasional.
   c. Confusion and lethargy—rare.

Chemotherapy of
Human Cancer

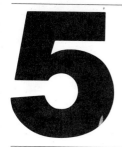

Carcinomas of the Head and Neck

Ronald C. DeConti

The achievement of a management plan resulting in long-term control or cure for many patients with carcinomas of the head and neck remains an elusive, only partially realized goal for surgeons, radiation therapists, and medical oncologists. In the last few decades, important gains in understanding the natural history of these neoplasms have been made, and the individual achievements of radiation, surgical techniques, and chemotherapy have been stressed. However, only recently have these modalities been combined to form new treatment plans, and increased patient benefit that might result from this multidisciplinary effort is now being explored.

This discussion focuses on the squamous cell carcinomas of the lining of the aerodigestive tract, which extends from the lip to the esophagus. These tumors account for approximately 5 percent of the new cancer cases seen in the United States each year. Excluded from this discussion are the melanomas, lymphomas, and sarcomas (which also occur in this area), as well as carcinoma of the thyroid, esophagus, and salivary glands. A cross-sectional view of the anatomic regions with the relative frequency of cancer is shown in Figure 5-1. The large number of potential tumor sites and some difficulties in determining the exact site of origin have led to broad use of these larger subdivision terms in an attempt to avoid confusion and to group the related sites. Table 5-1 lists the major sites within each of these anatomic subdivisions.

I. **Common and divergent characteristics.** Carcinomas of the head and neck are frequently considered together by students, generalists, and medical oncologists as though they represented a single therapeutic problem. A number of factors promote this concept.

A. **Similarities.** In the United States, more than 90 percent of all lesions are squamous cell carcinomas occurring predominantly in men (3 : 1). The majority of patients share common demographic and epidemiologic risk factors; the incidence of head and neck cancer increases with the use of alcohol and tobacco and with advancing age. Head and neck cancers occur in continuity, one with another, and it is occasionally difficult to determine the precise site of origin in the closed confines of the complicated interrelated structures comprising the oral cavity, pharynx, larynx, and sinuses. Further, patterns of spread are similar with local failure, local recurrence, and regional node failures predominating. For most sites, spread below the clavicle is unusual, occurring in only a minority of cases usually as pulmonary involvement. Bone lesions, usually as a result of local extension involving the mandible or floor of the skull, are not uncommon, although widespread bone metastases are unusual. A few patients develop hepatic metastases. Inanition, oral ulcera-

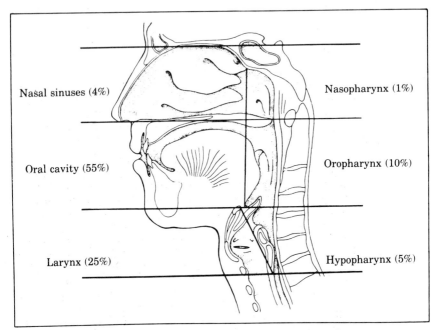

Fig. 5-1. The anatomic divisions of the head and neck are shown. The percentages indicate the relative frequency of carcinoma in these regions.

tion, fistula formation, respiratory difficulty, and aspiration characterize the late course of disease. Recurrence after primary treatment usually occurs within 18 months, and patients who are not cured are usually dead within 3 years of diagnosis.

B. Differences. For the surgeon or radiation therapist, the differences among sites may be more significant than the similarities. Certainly, presenting signs and symptoms differ markedly. For example, patients with an anterior tongue lesion may describe pain, sensation of mass, and limited motion of tongue. For patients with carcinoma of the larynx, hoarseness, dysphagia, or sore throat may predominate. Most importantly, differences in location influence the frequency of nodal spread and the chances for contralateral node involvement. These factors frequently determine optimum treatment planning.

II. Primary treatment. A discussion of the complexity of treatment choices for the multitude of sites where lesions occur is beyond the scope of this chapter. In general, early lesions in most locations are suitable for treatment either by surgery or radiation, and the therapeutic choice is usually made by considering the complications of each treatment, that is, the deformity of definitive surgery or the complications of radiation. With increasing failure rates as tumor bulk increases and the likelihood of pathologic, if not clinical, lymph node involvement by tumor increases, clinicians have begun to investigate combined modality approaches. Radiation may be used electively, preoperatively, or postoperatively after a pathologic assessment of regional nodes provides the opportunity for postsurgical staging assessment. Many

Table 5-1. Upper Aerodigestive Tract Sites

Region	Area	Site
Oral cavity		Lip
		Buccal mucosa
		Lower alveolar ridge
		Upper alveolar ridge
		Retromolar trigone
		Floor of mouth
		Hard palate
		Oral tongue
Pharynx	Nasopharynx	Posterior wall
		Lateral wall
	Oropharynx	Faucial arch
		Tonsillar fossa and tonsil
		Base of tongue
		Pharyngeal wall
	Hypopharynx	Pyriform fossa
		Postcricoid area
		Posterial wall
Larynx	Supraglottis	Ventricular band
		Arytenoid
		Epiglottis
	Glottis	True vocal cords
	Subglottis	Subglottis
Paranasal sinuses		Antrum
		Nasal cavity
		Ethmoid
		Sphenoid
		Frontal

studies have now reported both improved local and regional node control after such multimodality approaches. While substantial progress has been made in improving end results with decreased morbidity and deformity for early stage lesions in many sites, the outcome in advanced stages remains poor: in Stage III disease, the 3- or 5-year survival rate is 20 to 30 percent; in Stage IV disease, there are few long-term survivors.

III. **Staging.** Any consideration of outcome in relation to treatment relies heavily on detailed pretreatment assessment of the extent of the tumor.

A. **The TNM classification.** A complex, site-specific staging system has been devised by the American Joint Committee for Cancer Staging. This system incorporates a TNM classification to identify, both clinically and pathologically, the size of primary tumor (T), the presence and extent of regional node metastases (N), and the presence of distant metastases (M). Table 5-2 illustrates the TNM system for carcinoma of the oral cavity. For lesions of the nasopharynx, hypopharynx, or larynx, fixation or anatomic extensions are substituted for tumor size in determining the extent of the primary lesion.

B. **Stages.** The stage grouping for head and neck cancers is shown in Table 5-3. Stages I and II are determined by the size of the tumor in the absence of nodal involvement or distant metastases. Stage III comprises both large tumors and tumors of any size with early regional node involve-

Table 5-2. TNM Staging System for Carcinomas of the Oral Cavity

T Stage	Primary Tumor
TX	No available information on primary tumor
T_0	No evidence of primary tumor
T_{1S}	Carcinoma in situ
T_1	Greatest diameter of tumor ≤ 2 cm
T_2	Greatest diameter of tumor $> 2 \leq 4$ cm
T_3	Greatest diameter of tumor > 4 cm
T_4	Massive tumor > 4 cm in diameter with deep invasion to involve antrum, pterygoid muscles, base of tongue, or skin of neck
N Stage	Regional Nodal Status
NX	Nodes cannot be assessed
N_0	No clinically positive node
N_1	Single clinically positive homolateral node ≤ 3 cm in diameter
N_2	Single clinically positive homolateral node $> 3 \leq 6$ cm, or multiple clinically positive nodes, none > 6 cm
N_3	Massive homolateral node(s), bilateral nodes, or contralateral nodes
M Stage	Distant Metastasis
MX	Not assessed
M_0	No (known) distant metastasis
M_1	Distant metastasis present

Table 5-3. Stage Grouping for Carcinoma of the Oral Cavity, Pharynx, Larynx, and Paranasal Sinuses

Stage	Groups
I	T_1, N_0, M_0
II	T_2, N_0, M_0
III	T_3, N_0, M_0
	T_1, *or* T_2, *or* T_3, N_1, M_0
IV	T_4, N_0, *or* N_1, M_0
	Any T, N_2, *or* N_3, M_0
	Any T, *any* N, M_1

ment. Stage IV lesions may be huge with local extension or may be of any size with distant metastatic disease. This stage grouping has been uniformly applied to each tumor site to demonstrate gradations in prognosis.

IV. Chemotherapy

A. Prognostic factors. Whether chemotherapy is considered for the treatment of advanced recurrent head and neck cancers or for preoperative induction treatment, a number of similar, single prognostic variables have now been clearly identified (Table 5-4).

1. **Stage of carcinoma.** Small lesions, with minimal regional node involvement, respond better than the massive tumors of stage IV. Within stage IV, bulky nodal lesions are benefited with difficulty, and response rates are lowest for stage IV disease with pulmonary and/or visceral metastases. Since patients with head and neck cancers have

Table 5-4. Factors Prognostic for Response to Chemotherapy

Favorable	Unfavorable
Stage III	Stage IV
No metastatis	Pulmonary metastasis
ECOG performance status 0–1*	ECOG performance status 2–3
No weight loss	Weight loss
Normal immune mechanism	Impaired delayed hypersensitivity
Prior surgery	Prior irradiation
Long disease-free interval	Short disease-free interval
No prior chemotherapy	Prior chemotherapy

*See Table 2-2.

an increased risk of developing second primary neoplasms, the finding of distant metastases in the absence of primary or regional node recurrence should suggest this possibility.

2. **State of health.** Both poor ECOG performance status (see Table 2-2) and weight loss greater than 5 percent have been found to adversely affect prognosis. It is still unclear whether aggressive attempts to improve nutrition or restore cellular immunity after hyperalimentation results in gains in response rate.

3. **Prior treatment.** Many studies have shown the adverse effect of prior x-ray therapy on drug response. This effect has usually been attributed to an impaired tumor blood supply, a large tumor burden, and poor patient performance status. The failure to respond to irradiation or rapid relapse after radiation therapy has also been shown to adversely affect response rates.

B. **Single agent responses.** Only methotrexate, bleomycin, fluorouracil, and cisplatin have been extensively studied as individual agents in head and neck carcinomas, and it is largely from this group that most of the combinations are derived.

1. **Methotrexate.** In efforts to improve its therapeutic index, methotrexate has been investigated in no other solid tumor as extensively as it has been investigated in the management of head and neck cancer.

   a. **IV methotrexate** in doses from 40 to 60 mg/m^2 weekly achieves objective partial response in 25 to 50 percent of patients studied and is probably the most widely accepted conventional single-agent treatment for this group of tumors. Responses may occur after 1 to 2 weeks but usually require 4 to 6 weeks to become evident. Complete responses occur in approximately 7 to 10 percent of patients studied. Median response durations range from 2 to 6 months. Responders survive significantly longer than nonresponders. Treatment is usually given on an outpatient basis and drug-related mortality is less than 4 percent.

   b. **Intraarterial infusions of methotrexate** have been attempted in an effort to improve drug concentrations in tumor tissue and to improve the therapeutic index of treatment, either alone or with the use of systemic leucovorin. Although these techniques have resulted in marginally superior response rates, the lack of a single predominant blood supply, the technical difficulties of the procedure, and the morbidity of problems with clot, embolus, and infection appear to have precluded widespread adoption of this approach, and it is not recommended for general use.

c. **Leucovorin rescue** has made possible the use of moderate doses (240–500 mg/m^2) to high doses (1–3 g/m^2) of methotrexate in attempts to improve response rates. Individual investigators have reported favorable rates with decreased morbidity. The duration of response is not increased, and two comparative trials have demonstrated no advantage to these treatment approaches compared to weekly IV methotrexate. The need for hydration, urinary alkalinization, careful monitoring of renal clearance, and the high cost of treatment have been important factors in limiting general use of this approach, and it is not recommended outside of a research setting.

2. **Bleomycin** has attracted continued interest in head and neck cancers because of its generally mild myelosuppressant effects and the potential for its application in combination with myelosuppressive chemotherapy. Bleomycin, 10 to 30 mg/m^2, is usually given weekly, biweekly, or on a 5-day per month schedule by IM and IV injections. These approaches have the advantage of being convenient for outpatient use. Tumor response rarely occurs at cumulative doses of less than 200 mg/m^2, and response most often requires a total dose of 300 mg/m^2, doses that will usually have produced significant mucosal toxicity. Response rates range between 15 to 25 percent and are generally inferior in duration to those achieved with methotrexate. In general, the mucosal toxicity that accompanies the use of bleomycin is more frequent and severe than that produced with the use of a weekly methotrexate schedule.

3. **Cisplatin.** Cisplatin, 40 to 50 mg/m^2, is given IV on an every 3-week schedule. Higher doses result in the increased risks of renal toxicity unless special precautions are taken. Doses of 80 to 120 mg/m^2 may be tolerated if preceded by hydration and accompanied by furosemide and mannitol for diuresis to protect renal function (see Chap. 4). Cisplatin produces objective antitumor responses in approximately 25 percent of patients, many of whom have previously been treated with other antineoplastic drugs. Occasionally, dramatic tumor responses occur, although the frequency of complete remission is still low. Its major side effects are severe nausea, vomiting, tinnitus, occasional high-tone deafness, and most significantly, renal toxicity with, in some cases, progressive loss in creatinine clearance.

4. **Other drugs.** Of the remaining agents for which some information is available, fluorouracil may be of somewhat greater value for oral cavity lesions than other agents. The 23 percent response rate for doxorubicin (Adriamycin™) alone, although based on a small number of patients, has prompted the trial of this drug in several combinations without convincing results to date.

C. **Combination chemotherapy responses.** Multiple attempts have been made to improve single agent response rates with combination chemotherapy. A number of studies using methotrexate, bleomycin, and cisplatin in a variety of schedules have now been reported. The Eastern Cooperative Oncology Group, in a comparison of methotrexate, bleomycin, and cisplatin with weekly methotrexate, demonstrated a clear-cut advantage for combination chemotherapy. Forty-three percent of patients with advanced disease responded to an outpatient program using methotrexate, bleomycin, and cisplatin, compared to 26 percent using methotrexate alone. Complete remissions were achieved in 18 percent for combination chemotherapy and for 7 percent with methotrexate alone. The median duration of response was the same in both treatment groups, and no survival advantage was demonstrated for the combination treatment. Although neither response rate is exceptional, the careful randomization and stratification procedures used lend weight to the result. This program stands as the most controlled prospective trial to show an advantage to combination chemotherapy in the treatment of recurrent disease.

D. Combined modality treatment. Attempts to increase tumor destruction with drugs prior to definitive therapy are not new, although new developments in chemotherapy have reawakened enthusiasm for this approach.

1. **Drugs before radiation or surgery**

   a. **Methotrexate.** In several small single institution studies, both moderate and high-dose methotrexate with leucovorin rescue were given for several doses or cycles in advance of radiation or surgery. These schedules have shown response rates approximating 75 percent and have avoided the problems of oral mucositis and ulceration reported by the older studies of concomitant chemotherapy. No data are available to allow comparisons of these rescue programs with weekly methotrexate schedules.

   b. **Combination chemotherapy.** A number of combination drug therapy programs have been developed as initial therapy for advanced local–regional disease. These programs are intended either to reduce tumor bulk and allow more effective radiotherapy or to improve resectability of advanced lesions. In general, these programs use high-dose cisplatin in conjunction with hydration and diuretics (see Chap. 4) combined with 3 to 5 days of bleomycin, usually by infusion. Vincristine is frequently included; methotrexate is usually omitted. These programs produce high response rates (67%–94%). In six studies composed of 215 patients, complete clinical disappearance of tumor was achieved in 19 to 28 percent of patients and partial response was achieved in 48 to 74 percent. After 1 to 2 cycles of drug treatment, surgery and/or irradiation follows. The number of patients with advanced local–regional disease who were made disease-free is greater than expected based on pretreatment staging expectations, but the long-range impact of these programs on survival remains to be clarified.

2. **Drugs as posttreatment adjuvant.** Whereas the most recent emphasis in head and neck cancer has been on achieving gains in early tumor control, little attention has been paid to the potential of postoperative or postradiation therapy adjuvant drug studies. The available clinical evidence now demonstrates efficacy for two different

types of induction chemotherapy, that is, programs using cisplatin, vincristine, and bleomycin combinations, and drug treatment programs with methotrexate. If the lessons of tumor biology and experience in human acute leukemia and breast carcinoma apply, pursuit of a comprehensive treatment program using these agents to best kinetic and clinical advantage will offer increased opportunity to benefit larger numbers of patients with head and neck cancer than are generally benefited today, even without new gains in theoretic knowledge or development of more potent drugs.

E. **Pretreatment patient assessment.** The extent of evaluation required to determine the suitability of a patient for chemotherapy depends, to a considerable degree, on the intent and type of program to be employed. The major organ systems affected by the antineoplastic drugs under consideration are bone marrow, lungs, and kidneys. Any pretreatment assessment should consider not only careful evaluation of the size and extent of tumor, but also the presence of comorbid disease processes involving these organ systems. A careful history, review of systems, physical assessment, and routine laboratory data may provide clues in these areas.

1. **Bone marrow function.** Chronic alcoholism and malnutrition or the effect of the tumor on diet may contribute to the high incidence of folate deficiency seen in this population. Because of the additive effect of this deficiency and the inhibition of folate metabolism by methotrexate, there is often an increased sensitivity to even small doses of methotrexate with marked clinical toxicity.

2. **Pulmonary function.** Chronic obstructive pulmonary disease is common in this group of patients. Moderate to severe pretreatment reductions in timed forced expiratory volumes may be reduced further with treatment with bleomycin. It is recommended that if clinical assessment suggests impaired pulmonary reserve and bleomycin is to be part of the treatment program, pretreatment pulmonary function studies should be performed.

3. **Renal function.** Both cisplatin and methotrexate affect renal function. The major cumulative toxicity of cisplatin is renal. Unfortunately, there may be considerable impairment of renal function before a rise in serum creatinine concentration occurs; doses of cisplatin, 80 to 120 mg/m^2, require serial determination of creatinine clearance to assess the cumulative effects of the drug on renal function.

Limited excretion of methotrexate prolongs the duration of high serum concentration of drugs and extends the duration of impaired DNA synthesis for normal as well as neoplastic tissues. Weekly IV methotrexate is usually given in the advanced disease situation after a normal serum creatinine determination. A careful clinical assessment at the time of each dose is probably more reliable than serial determinations in this situation. Most episodes of serious methotrexate toxicity relate to failure to appreciate intercurrent events that limit excretion of these relatively low doses of the drug. The most common of these toxicities is probably dehydration, which is related to progressive disease, increasingly poor oral intake, nausea, and vomiting, or mucositis that may have been caused by prior drug treatment.

Table 5-5. Selected Drug Treatment Programs in Head and Neck Cancer

Intent	Suitabiity	Scheme
Cytoreductive induction treatment	Advanced stage, no prior treatment	Cisplatin, 100 mg/m^2 IV day 1 with induced diuresis Bleomycin, 30 units/day as 24-hr infusion days 2–5 Vincristine, 1 mg IV days 2 and 5 Cycle repeats in 3 weeks
Palliation	Prior treatment	Methotrexate, 40 mg/m^2 IM days 1 and 15 Bleomycin, 10 units IM days 1, 8, and 15 Cisplatin, 50 mg/m^2 IV day 4 with induced diuresis Cycle repeats in 3 weeks
Palliation	Prior treatment and contraindications to combination drugs	Methotrexate, 40–60 mg/m^2 IV weekly

The addition of any drug that further alters renal clearance of methotrexate may tip the balance. Aspirin, sulfonamides, phenytoin, cefoxitin, and gentamicin may all decrease methotrexate clearance and increase toxicity. Careful interval patient assessment with these considerations in mind will help avoid these pitfalls.

F. Selected treatment plans. The plans of drug administration for three types of drug treatment programs are displayed in Table 5-5.

  1. Cytoreductive induction treatment

    a. Selection of patients. This treatment is designed to reduce tumor bulk prior to surgery or radiotherapy in patients with advanced stage disease and with no prior therapy. The induction treatment regimen is intended for hospitalized patients following an assessment of the extent of their tumor and an evaluation to exclude comorbid disease processes that might unacceptably increase the risks of treatment.

    b. Administration. Oral hydration is begun the evening before treatment. On the morning of treatment an IV infusion of 5% dextrose in half-normal saline with 20 mEq of potassium chloride/liter is begun at a rate of 200 ml/hr. Furosemide, 40 mg, and mannitol, 12.5 g, are given IV after the first liter. The patient should be voiding freely. Immediately thereafter, cisplatin, 100 mg/m^2, is added to a calibrated solution set and given over a 30-minute period and the second liter of fluid is continued. Chlorpromazine or prochlorperazine is given on a 4 to 6-hour schedule to alleviate nausea or vomiting. The volume of subsequent IV fluids for the day is judged by the extent of nausea and vomiting and urinary excretion. On day 2, vincristine, 1 mg, is given IV push and bleomycin infusion is begun. Bleomycin, 15 units, is added to each of 2 liters of 5% dextrose in half-normal saline with 20 mEq of potassium chloride to be administered q24-h. The continuous infusion is maintained for 4 days. On day 5, vincristine, 1 mg, is given IV push. If adequate oral intake has not been resumed, additional IV fluids may be given. An infusion pump may be used to help assure an even rate of flow.

The patient may be discharged after completion of the treatment course, depending on both tolerance to the drug and ability to eat and drink. An interim clinic visit before a second induction course is recommended as a safeguard. A second course of treatment is planned on day 21, but should be administered only after hematologic values and serum creatinine are normal, and no pulmonary symptoms are reported. If tumor regression is continuing on day 42 after two cycles of treatment, a third cycle may be considered, although the cumulative risks of renal and pulmonary toxicity increase with continued treatment. At this point radiation, surgery, or both should be considered once again.

2. **Combination chemotherapy for advanced recurrent disease.** In advanced, recurrent disease, either elect one or two courses of induction treatment (see **IV.F.1**) followed by an intermittent program with lesser doses of drug, or initiate treatment on an outpatient basis using a combination drug program as described in Table 5-5. Methotrexate, 40 mg/m^2, and bleomycin, 10 units, are given IM or IV on day 1. On day 4, cisplatin is given as an IV bolus at 50 mg/m^2. Cisplatin is given approximately 30 minutes after starting a 2-hour infusion of 2 liters of 5% dextrose in half-normal saline with 20 mEq of potassium chloride/liter. Furosemide, 40 mg, is given IV at the start of the infusion and mannitol, 12.5 mg, is given just before the administration of cisplatin. Antiemetics are given as necessary. On day 8, bleomycin is given at a dose of 10 units and on day 15 both methotrexate and bleomycin are repeated.

Dosages of methotrexate and cisplatin are reduced 50 percent for mild myelosuppression. Drugs are withheld if more severe myelosuppression occurs; treatment is resumed as soon as peripheral blood counts recover. Methotrexate and bleomycin are withheld if stomatitis is present. Complete blood counts, including platelets, should be done on a weekly basis. Serum creatinine levels are measured on day 8 of each cycle to ensure adequate renal function before the next dose of methotrexate, and creatinine clearance should be measured if creatinine levels rise 50 percent or more.

3. **Methotrexate alone for advanced disease**

   a. **Selection of patients.** With one study showing an increased response rate for a combination of methotrexate, bleomycin, and cisplatin compared to methotrexate alone, the latter program should probably be reserved for selected patients: patients in relapse after induction treatment programs without methotrexate, patients who refuse treatment with cisplatin or bleomycin, patients whose pulmonary function excludes a bleomycin treatment program, and finally, that portion of the head and neck patient population whose reliability and follow-up opportunities are poor.

   b. **Treatment regimens.** The usual starting dose is 40 mg/m^2, but if advanced age, anemia, borderline renal function, or other factors suggest sensitivity to methotrexate, the initial dose may be reduced as low as 20 mg/m^2. Blood counts are done weekly, and if there is no evidence of mucositis or myelosuppression, the dose is escalated to a maximum of 60 mg/m^2. Most patients will tolerate this treatment with minimal nausea and vomiting; a few will require antiemetics. Careful attention to oral hygiene may be helpful in preventing or reducing the severity of mucositis. Candidiasis should be suspected and, if present, treated with mycostatin. If mucositis or myelosuppression occurs, treatments are delayed until they clear and blood counts are normal.

G. Problems in supportive care

1. **Support systems.** Patients with head and neck cancer tend to be elderly men, often social reprobates, recluses, heavy smokers and drinkers, and occasionally, frank derelicts. They are frequently divorced or separated from their families, and many live alone, often in reduced circumstances. Lack of family, friends, resources, and initiative are often an impediment to adequate care—especially in advanced disease situations where close follow-up, regular clinic visits, and adherence to treatment schedules are important. They desperately need a primary care giver in the home or closely allied with the home to promote their well-being and optimal utilization of medical care and to derive advantage from the health care delivery system. Social service, ministerial help, patient-care support groups, Alcoholics Anonymous, and any other social care groups should be enlisted as appropriate to help the patient cope with illness.

2. **Nutrition.** Gradual, progressive weight loss and inanition are common factors in the relentless illness of many patients. Their nutrition is generally inadequate, and repetitive efforts at reinforcing the need for a high-calorie diet, as free of alcohol as possible, must be given. Depending on the location of the tumor and the particular problems with swallowing, efforts need to be extended on a regular basis to ensure adequate patient nutrition. Many patients, or their families, need to be instructed in the use of blended foods, the use of high-protein supplements, or both. Some patients will benefit from the use of a pediatric feeding tube when deformities in the anatomy prevent adequate swallowing. In selected patients a gastrostomy tube feeding may be appropriate, especially early in the patient's clinical course when it is to be hoped that this may only be a temporary expedient. Most patients will benefit from any attempts at oral hyperalimentation. The role of IV hyperalimentation is not clear and needs to be considered early in the management course during the perioperative or radiation therapy period when induction treatment is taking place. Its role in maintaining patients in the advanced disease state is still unclear. Efforts to maintain nutrition need to be reinforced at every opportunity with the family, the care giver, and the patient. Dietary advice or consultation with a dietetic department should be offered freely.

3. **Mouth care** may be an important problem for some patients with head and neck cancer. Many patients have difficulty with secretions. Xerostomia may be produced by radiation therapy and need treatment with artificial saliva. At the opposite extreme, patients with posterior tongue lesions may have edema and swelling that precludes

adequate swallowing, and the pooling of secretions and subsequent aspiration becomes a problem. These patients may benefit from the use of suction to drain their secretions. Cleansing mouthwash may be appropriate, and efforts at dental hygiene need to be maintained. Radiation-induced bone necrosis or fistulas need to be cleaned or debrided and occasionally packed with toothpaste or other material to promote comfort.

4. **Hypercalcemia** in patients with epidermoid carcinoma of the head and neck is a common situation. As many as 23 percent of patients with advanced recurrent head and neck cancers may experience hypercalcemia before their death. In general, this phenomenon accompanies late-stage recurrent tumor, often with little evidence of bone involvement. Dehydration, all too common in these patients, may be a precipitating factor, and in many patients hypercalcemia is mild and easily controlled with hydration, saline diuresis, or both. Although hydration, saline diuresis, or reduction in tumor achieved with radiation, drug, or surgery frequently reverses this phenomenon, a few patients will require mithramycin for adequate treatment.

5. **Pneumonia.** The anatomic deformities induced by operation, recurrent tumor, or both make patients with head and neck cancer highly susceptible to aspiration of pooled secretions. Fever, tachycardia, tachypnea, rales, and infiltrates in the lung are the usual findings and are often confused with bacterial pneumonia. Knowledge of the aspiration or observation of the event may be the only decisive method of proving the diagnosis. Immediate recognition of an aspiration should suggest treatment with steroids, antibiotics, or both.

6. **Granulocytopenia.** The greatest concern is for the need to quickly identify pulmonary infection in the presence of drug-induced granulocytopenia. The mortality from pneumonia and sepsis is high in this situation. Appropriate cultures need to be obtained in an effort to document infection and help distinguish the problem from aspiration. Fever, in a granulocytopenic patient, should be promptly treated with broad spectrum antibiotics without awaiting results of the cultures (see Chap. 25).

Selected Reading

American Joint Committee in Cancer. Staging Cancer at Head and Neck Sites. *Manual for Staging of Cancer,* 1978, p. 27.

Kramer, S. (Ed.). Head and neck cancers. *Semin. Oncol.* 4:353, 1977.

Carcinoma of the Lung

Robert B. Livingston

I. Introduction

A. Incidence. Carcinoma of the lung is the most common malignancy seen in the United States (excluding nonmelanoma skin cancers) and accounts for one of eight cancers diagnosed. With more than 100,000 deaths occurring yearly in the United States from lung cancer, it takes nearly twice the toll of any other malignancy and is responsible for one of every four cancer deaths.

B. Treatment modalities. The majority of patients are inoperable at the time of diagnosis because of either the extent of local invasion or the presence of distant metastasis. Of those patients who are operable and resectable, the majority will have local or distant recurrence. Therefore, less than 10 percent of all patients with lung cancer are curable by surgery. Although radiotherapy plays an important palliative role in lung cancer, it is uncommonly curative and is effective primarily for limited regional disease or isolated metastases. For these reasons, there is a great need for effective chemotherapy to help the great majority of patients who cannot be cured with other modalities.

C. Cell types. The role of chemotherapy in lung cancer differs according to the cell type. The four primary types of lung cancer are *squamous cell carcinoma, adenocarcinoma, large-cell anaplastic carcinoma,* and *small-cell anaplastic carcinoma* (sometimes referred to as *oat-cell carcinoma,* which is actually a subtype of small-cell anaplastic carcinoma). Because the biologic behavior and response to treatment of the small-cell carcinomas are so different from the other three types, a separation into two broad categories—small-cell carcinoma and non-small-cell carcinoma (squamous cell, adenocarcinoma, and large cell anaplastic)—is necessary for any discussion of treatment.

Chemotherapy is now the main modality of treatment for small-cell (oat-cell) carcinoma of the lung. In patients with other histologies, it is used in clinical practice only for palliation. For purposes of selecting treatment and comparing responses, patients who have cancers in either histologic grouping (small- or non-small-cell) are further separated on the basis of the extent of their disease into the categories of extensive disease or limited (regional) disease. The term *extensive* is used to imply clinical evidence of dissemination beyond the hemithorax and its regional node drainage (mediastinal, scalene, and supraclavicular). The term *limited* or *regional* is used to describe disease that is within these boundaries clinically, but inoperable.

II. Small-cell carcinoma

A. General considerations and aims of therapy.
Small-cell anaplastic carcinoma of the lung accounts for about 25 percent of lung cancer in the United States. Most cases are related to cigarette smoking. The tumor mass is typically central on location (mediastinal or perihilar) on chest x-ray film. Pretreatment evaluation of the patient should include a complete blood count, liver function tests, a bone marrow aspiration and biopsy, computed tomography of the brain (or a radionuclide brain scan), a bone scan, and a liver scan. If none of these tests reveal spread of the disease beyond the lung and regional nodes, the disease is deemed to be clinically limited. Clinically limited disease occurs in about one third of patients with small-cell carcinoma, despite the fact that microscopic or submicroscopic hematogenous spread is almost universal at the time of diagnosis. In this group, complete response (CR) with combined chemotherapy and radiation can be expected in 40 to 60 percent of patients, with long-term disease-free survival rates of 10 to 15 percent. For patients with extensive disease, CR is achieved in only 10 to 15 percent, although the majority will have a partial response (PR), symptomatic improvement, and some prolongation of survival. Median survivals are in the range of 6 to 12 months, respectively, for extensive and limited disease using best standard treatment; with supportive care only, the respective figures are about 6 to 12 weeks.

B. Remission induction.
As in acute leukemia and the lymphomas, patients should be placed on allopurinol, 300 mg/day, during the first treatment cycle to avert problems related to hyperuricemia associated with massive tumor lysis.

A number of combination drug programs are effective and superior to treatment with the most active single agent, cyclophosphamide, used alone. Two of the most common induction programs are listed here:

1. VAC
  a. Vincristine, 2 mg IV day 1

  b. Doxorubicin (Adriamycin™), 50 mg/m^2 IV day 1

  c. Cyclophosphamide, 750 mg/m^2 IV day 1

Repeat every 3 weeks for four cycles.

2. "High" CMC-VAP
  a. Cyclophosphamide, 1500 mg/m^2 IV day 1 and 1000 mg/m^2 IV day 21

  b. Methotrexate, 15 mg/m^2 PO twice weekly for 5 weeks

  c. Lomustine (CCNU), 100 mg/m^2 PO day 1

  d. Vincristine, 2 mg IV days 42 and 63

  e. Doxorubicin (Adriamycin™), 60 mg/m^2 IV days 42 and 63

  f. Procarbazine, 100 mg/m^2 PO days 42 to 51 and 63 to 72

C. Radiation therapy and CNS prophylaxis.
After the maximal response to induction chemotherapy has been achieved (usually 8–12 weeks from the start of treatment), responding patients should have prophylactic

whole brain irradiation to prevent isolated relapse at that site, which will otherwise occur in 20 to 40 percent of patients, regardless of whether chemotherapy that crosses the blood-brain barrier was employed. The usual dose is 3000 rad in 2 weeks.

Although more controversial, many oncologists also stop chemotherapy at this point to administer chest irradiation; in both limited and extensive disease, the incidence of relapse at the primary site is otherwise likely to be very high. Exact doses and duration of such radiation are the subject of current research protocols.

D. Treatment during remission. Although widely used, the role of *maintenance* chemotherapy has not been determined. If administered, common regimens employ cyclophosphamide in doses of 750 to 1000 mg/m^2 every 4 weeks, with or without doxorubicin (Adriamycin™), vincristine, or methotrexate. As in other diseases, total doses of doxorubicin (Adriamycin™) above 450 to 550 mg/m^2 cannot be exceeded owing to the risk of cardiomyopathy. (The lower dose must be used if mediastinal radiation is given.)

It now appears that *reinduction* at 6 and 12 months into therapy with a single cycle of the induction regimen produces prolongation of response and survival, especially for those patients who achieve a complete response.

E. Complications

1. Paraneoplastic syndromes. The most common paraneoplastic syndrome is the *syndrome of inappropriate antidiuretic hormone (SIADH)*, which can be managed supportively with demeclocycline (300 mg tid) while induction therapy is administered. Less common paraneoplastic problems associated with small-cell carcinoma include pseudomyasthenia (Eaton-Lambert syndrome), hyperadrenocorticism owing to ectopic ACTH, and galactorrhea or gynecomastia.

2. Complications of treatment

   a. Myelotoxicity. The major risks of chemotherapy are infection related to leukopenia and bleeding from thrombocytopenia. Nadir granulocyte and platelet counts are usually seen 10 to 14 days after chemotherapy has been given (except for lomustine, which produces effects delayed 3–5 weeks), and both patient and doctor should be alert to the significance of an elevated temperature or, less commonly, hemorrhage during this nadir period. Any patient with a temperature of 38.2 C (101 F) or greater who is more than a few days postchemotherapy should be seen in the emergency room for a physical examination, chest x-ray, complete blood count (including platelets and differential), and appropriate cultures. If the granulocytes are less than 1000/mm^3, the patient should be hospitalized and treated empirically with broad-spectrum antibiotics, even if no clinical site of infection is identified.

   b. Other chemotherapy-related complications

   (1) Alopecia from cyclophosphamide and doxorubicin (Adriamycin™).

   (2) Stomatitis from methotrexate and occasionally doxorubicin (Adriamycin™).

(3) Peripheral neuropathy and constipation from vincristine (may be avoided by routine administration of psyllium hydrophilic mucilloid [Metamucil®], or milk of magnesia at bedtime).

(4) Necrosis of skin with underlying slough of the soft tissues secondary to inadvertent extravasation of doxorubcin (Adriamycin™) or vincristine. This disastrous complication can be avoided by meticulous care to ensure an adequate IV, which should include use of a fresh site, avoidance of the dorsum of the hand or wrist veins if possible, and checking for a blood return, as well as flushing the IV line immediately after drug administration.

c. **Complications of radiation therapy** to the brain include alopecia, redness and itching of the scalp, and external otitis, especially at doses of more than 3000 rad. Occasionally, patients will complain of weakness or somnolence after whole brain irradiation, but these symptoms are usually transient and minor. Complications of chest irradiation include symptomatic esophagitis (most patients) and clinically significant pneumonitis (about 5%–10%) or transverse myelitis. The latter complication should not occur if posterior portals are blocked to prevent cord irradiation of a total dose greater than 4500 rad. If doxorubicin (Adriamycin™) is given concomitantly with chest irradiation, esophagitis may be quite severe, even resulting in permanent esophageal strictures, unless the dose of both is reduced.

F. **Recurrence and treatment of refractory disease.** No consistently useful chemotherapy regimen is available to treat recurrences. Occasional patients, especially if they are still fully ambulatory at the time of relapse, will respond to doxorubicin (Adriamycin™), vincristine, cisplatin, mitomycin, or etoposide (VP-16), if these agents were not employed in their previous regimen. Radiation therapy is useful to palliate hemoptysis, painful bony lesions, and brain metastases but will not prolong survival. Median survival after relapse is only 6 to 12 weeks; patients who have "chest only" recurrence may live somewhat longer.

III. Non-small-cell carcinoma

A. **General considerations and aims of therapy.** At the present time, surgery, alone or combined with subsequent radiation therapy, is the treatment of choice for resectable disease. For patients with limited inoperable disease, radiation therapy alone is the treatment of choice; the addition of chemotherapy to radiation therapy is of experimental interest, but not part of routine clinical practice. Chemotherapy is used in the treatment of patients with extensive disease. Its goals are to palliate symptoms and prolong survival; extended disease-free survival (more than 2 years) with chemotherapy in this setting has been reported, but remains anecdotal. At the present time, only fully ambulatory patients are appropriate candidates for chemotherapy.

B. **Chemotherapy programs.** No regimen of reproducible, established benefit exists for treatment of extensive non-small-cell lung cancer. Two widely used programs, each of which produces objective response in 25 to 40 percent of patients and modest prolongation of survival in responders, are listed here.

1. CAP

   a. Cyclophosphamide, 400 mg/m^2 IV day 1

   b. Doxorubicin (Adriamycin™), 40 mg/m^2 IV day 1

   c. Cisplatin, 40 mg/m^2 IV day 1 (with prehydration and diuresis)

   Repeat cycle monthly.

2. FOMi

   a. Fluorouracil, 300 mg/m^2 IV days 1 to 4

   b. Vincristine (Oncovin®), 2 mg IV day 1

   c. Mitomycin, 10 mg/m^2 day 1

   Repeat cycle monthly.

The CAP program has the advantage of being a 1-day regimen, but has the disadvantage of severe, often prolonged nausea and vomiting from the doxorubicin (Adriamycin™) and especially the cisplatin. IV prehydration with 500 to 1000 ml of normal saline, with or without concomitant mannitol, 12.5 g, should be given with cisplatin to help minimize renal damage from this drug. The FOMi program has the advantage of being quite well tolerated by most patients, but has the disadvantage of requiring 4 consecutive days for administration. Other programs currently under investigation, often using mitomycin, cisplatin, the investigational vinca alkaloid vindesine, or vinblastine in some combination with or without doxorubicin (Adriamycin™) or etoposide (VP-16), may prove to be more effective than either CAP or FOMi.

C. Role of radiation therapy. As the chance of a *local* response to radiation therapy is much higher than the chance of a *local* response to systemically administered drugs in patients with non-small-cell carcinoma, radiation should be locally employed as a palliative modality. It usually is beneficial in the treatment of painful bony lesions and hemoptysis, but it is less often helpful to treat malignant effusions, atelectasis, or lobar collapse secondary to bronchial obstruction or brain metastasis. It should be employed in preference to decompressive surgery for most patients with extradural cord compression.

D. Complications

   1. Paraneoplastic syndromes. The most common of these syndromes is hypercalcemia (almost never seen with small-cell carcinoma), especially if the tumor is of squamous histology. This occurrence may be caused by ectopic parathyroid hormone, in which event it will only respond definitively to measures directed at the tumor, or it may be caused by excessive prostaglandin production from the tumor. In the latter case, hypercalcemia *may* respond to indomethacin, 50 mg tid, or aspirin, 600 mg qid. IV hydration and oral phosphates should be administered in either case. Other paraneoplastic syndromes include hypertrophic osteoarthropathy and a variety of neurologic syndromes (but not Eaton-Lambert), which are likely to improve only if the tumor is controlled.

   2. Treatment-related complications. Leukopenia and thrombocytopenia complications may be seen, as outlined under small-cell carcinoma. With cisplatin use, hemolytic anemia may be seen, occasionally requiring blood transfusions. With repeated administration of mitomycin, thrombocytopenia of a cumulative nature is seen, such that the dose of the agent must be reduced and/or the interval between its administration widened, often to 6 or 8 weeks. Occasionally, mitomycin may also cause symptomatic pulmonary reactions and (rarely) a syndrome of hypertension and renal damage. The vinca alkaloids all produce constipation and peripheral neuropathy in varying degrees, with vincristine and vindesine being the worst offenders.

E. Recurrence and treatment of refractory disease. Chemotherapy of established efficacy is not available in this setting. Appropriate patients, preferably those who are fully ambulatory, may be candidates for trials of new agents in phase II trials.

Selected Reading

Hansen, H. H. et al. Combination chemotherapy of advanced lung cancer. A randomized trial. *Cancer* 38:2201, 1976.

Lanzotti, V. J. et al. Bleomycin (NSC-125066) followed by cyclophosphamide (NSC-26271), vincristine (NSC-67574), methotrexate (NSC-740), and 5-fluorouracil (NSC-19893) for non-oat-cell bronchogenic carcinoma. *Cancer Treat. Rep.* 60:61, 1976.

Livingston, R. B. The management of disseminated non-small-cell lung cancer. In S. K. Carter, E. Glatstein, and R. B. Livingston (Eds.), *Principles of Cancer Treatment.* New York: McGraw-Hill, 1981. Pp. 382–387.

Livingston, R. B. Small cell carcinoma of the lung. *Blood* 56:575, 1980.

Livingston, R. B. et al. Comparative trial of combination chemotherapy in extensive squamous carcinoma of the lung. A Southwest Oncology Group study. *Cancer Treat. Rep.* 61:1623, 1977.

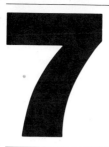

Carcinomas of the Gastrointestinal Tract

John C. Marsh

Cancers of the gastrointestinal (GI) tract (esophagus, stomach, small and large intestine) account for nearly 20 percent of all cancer in the United States and about 21 percent of cancer deaths. Colon cancer is by far the most common of these malignancies, with cancer of the rectum, stomach, esophagus, and small intestine occurring in decreasing frequency. Surgery continues to be the only curative modality, but radiation therapy and chemotherapy have important palliative roles and, in certain adjuvant situations, may improve the cure rate produced by surgery. Chemotherapy alone is not curative; drugs produce objective remissions in only a minority of patients. However, there is little question that meaningful palliation and an increase in survival can be achieved in patients who respond to chemotherapy. Controlled clinical trials, often by interinstitutional cooperative groups, have been useful in defining the natural history and therapeutic benefit of various treatment modalities.

I. Carcinoma of the esophagus

A. General considerations and aims of therapy

1. **Epidemiology.** Cancer of the esophagus is nearly always of the epidermoid variety and accounts for slightly more than 1 percent of cancers. It is three times more common in men than in women (it seems to be increasingly frequent in black men) and is often associated with excessive alcohol and tobacco use. The average patient's age is in the 60s. In certain parts of China, it occurs with extraordinary frequency and is the most common cancer. The high incidence of cancer of the esophagus is thought to be related to dietary habits of the region, perhaps to fungal contamination of pickled vegetables. In this country, the etiology is unknown, although the epidemiology resembles that of squamous cell carcinomas of the oral cavity and upper airway.

2. **Clinical picture and evaluation.** The tumor is usually associated with progressive and persistent dysphagia. Pain, hoarseness, and chronic cough are unfavorable manifestations that indicate spread to regional structures, such as mediastinal nerves, recurrent laryngeal nerve, and fistula formation between the esophagus and the airway. The most common sites of distant metastases are the lungs and liver. Diagnosis is usually made by barium swallow, endoscopy, or lavage cytology. Careful evaluation of the lungs and liver by x-rays and scans is needed for staging following a tissue diagnosis.

3. **Treatment and prognosis.** About one half of patients are operable and one half of these are actually resectable. The overall 5-year sur-

vival is in the range of 5 percent, which means that the majority of patients, if they are to benefit at all, will require radiation therapy of local disease. Many surgeons feel that only lesions of the lower one third of the esophagus are amenable to surgical resection and cure. Radiotherapy and surgery are often combined. The prognosis is also related to the size of the lesion and the depth of penetration of the esophageal wall. Patients are more likely to die of local disease or local recurrence than of distant metastases. The carcinoembryonic antigen (CEA) may be elevated in up to 70 percent of patients. The overall median survival is less than 1 year.

B. Treatment of advanced disease

1. **Standard drugs.** The treatment of cancer of the esophagus with drugs has not been particularly successful. Several agents have been defined as having some activity when used as single agents, including fluorouracil, lomustine, and bleomycin—each of which yields about a 15 percent response rate.

   a. As a first choice for patients with normal marrow function, give fluorouracil, 500 mg/m² IV push days 1 to 5 every 4 to 5 weeks.

   b. For patients with marrow compromise give bleomycin, 15 units/m² IM or IV twice weekly.

   Responses are generally short and range from 5 to 26 weeks (median is 14 weeks); the survival of all treated patients is likely to be less than 4 months.

2. **Investigational drugs and programs.** Mitoguazone dihydrochloride (methyl GAG), an inhibitor of spermidine biosynthesis, has been associated with a good response rate (10/21), but the duration was quite brief and the toxicity was excessive.

   One of the most encouraging reports has come from the Southwestern Oncology Group. Nineteen patients were given cisplatin, 50 mg/m² IV days 1 and 8, with the cycle repeated at monthly intervals. Two patients had complete responses lasting 8 and 56 weeks, four patients had partial responses lasting 9 to 18 weeks, and two patients had disease stabilization lasting 13 and 19 weeks. If confirmed, these results will certainly make cisplatin the treatment of choice in this disease.

C. Adjuvant therapy.
With so many patients given radiotherapy as primary treatment, seeking a chemotherapy regimen to improve the results is natural. No controlled trials have shown any advantage for the drug-treated patients. In uncontrolled trials, both fluorouracil infusions and a three-drug combination of vincristine, bleomycin, and methotrexate with leucovorin rescue have been used as adjuvants to radiotherapy with apparent improvement in the median survival compared to what might have been achieved with radiotherapy alone.

No complications of therapy are unique to the treatment of advanced esophageal cancer. If chemotherapy is used as an adjuvant to radiotherapy, the clinician must be alert for synergistic mucosal toxicity of the combination.

II. Gastric carcinoma

A. General considerations and aims of therapy

1. **Epidemiology.** The incidence of stomach cancer is decreasing dramatically in this country, and it now ranks sixth as a cause of cancer deaths. No improvement has been seen, however, in 5-year survival rates, which range from 5 to 15 percent. (The only curative modality at present is surgery.) The male to female ratio is 1.5:1. Stomach cancer is still the leading cause of cancer death in Japanese males, and it is also common in China, Finland, Poland, and Chile.

2. **Clinical picture and evaluation.** The most common symptoms are weight loss, abdominal pain, vomiting, changes in bowel habits, anorexia, and early satiety. The diagnosis is generally made by barium swallow, endoscopy, and cytology, usually in combination. Metastases are to the liver, pancreas, omentum, esophagus, and bile ducts by direct extension and to regional and distant lymph nodes, such as those in the left axilla and supraclavicular area. Pulmonary and bone metastases are a late finding. Patients with suspected gastric cancer should have a careful evaluation of the liver, with liver function tests, liver scan, or ultrasound.

3. **Treatment and prognosis.** Most stomach cancers are adenocarcinomas. Important prognostic factors include tumor grade and gross appearance; diffusely infiltrating lesions are less likely to be cured than sharply circumscribed, nonulcerating ones. The presence of regional lymph node involvement and involvement of contiguous organs on the surgical specimen indicate an increased likelihood of recurrence, as does the presence of dysphagia at the time of diagnosis. Patients with proximal lesions or lesions requiring total, rather than distal subtotal, gastrectomy are also at greater risk.

B. Treatment of advanced disease

1. **Single agents** with activity include fluorouracil, semustine (methyl-CCNU), doxorubicin (Adriamycin™), and mitomycin.

2. **Combinations** of these agents appear more active than single drugs, and the use of combinations is associated with a higher response rate and longer duration of remission.

   a. **FAM.** The FAM (fluorouracil, Adriamycin™, and mitomycin) regimen, introduced by workers from Georgetown University, appears to be as active as any.

      (1) **Fluorouracil,** 600 mg/m^2 IV days 1, 8, 29, and 36

      (2) **Doxorubicin** (Adriamycin™), 30 mg/m^2 IV days 1 and 29

      (3) **Mitomycin,** 10 mg/m^2 IV day 1

      The cycle is repeated every 56 days. A gain of nearly a year in survival was associated with response in the initial studies.

   b. **Other active regimens** include fluorouracil and doxorubicin; fluorouracil and semustine; and fluorouracil, doxorubicin, and semustine. All of these regimens are associated with hematologic toxicity, sometimes severe, and patients must be carefully monitored.

C. **Adjuvant therapy.** The Gastrointestinal Tumor Study Group (GITSG) has completed a study of adjuvant chemotherapy in patients following surgical resection, which suggests that a combination of fluorouracil and semustine is associated with longer relapse-free survival than no chemotherapy.

1. **Fluorouracil,** 325 mg/m^2 IV on days 1 to 5

2. **Semustine,** 150 mg/m^2 orally on day 1

3. **Fluorouracil,** 375 mg/m^2 IV on days 36 to 40

The cycle is repeated every 10 weeks for 2 years. Semustine is stopped after a total cumulative dose of 1000 mg/m^2.

D. **Combined modality therapy.** A large number of patients have locally unresectable or incompletely resectable disease, and it has been known for some time that fluorouracil, used in conjunction with radiotherapy, adds to the survival of such patients so long as they have no evidence of metastatic disease and have disease that can be encompassed by a treatment port. Another GITSG program compared combination chemotherapy with fluorouracil and semustine in such patients with and without radiotherapy. The results are not definitive in that short-term results were better with the chemotherapy while long-term results were better with the combined modality treatment. It seems reasonable to use the combined modality treatment until more data are available.

1. The **local gastric lesion** is treated with two courses of 2500 rad each, given over a 3-week period with a 2-week rest period between courses.

2. **Fluorouracil,** 500 mg/m^2, is given IV for the first 3 days of each course of radiation.

3. Ten weeks after completion of the radiotherapy, chemotherapy with **fluorouracil** and **semustine** is begun on the schedule listed previously in **C** for adjuvant chemotherapy and continued until relapse.

E. **Complications.** Hematologic and gastrointestinal toxicities from the chemotherapy may be accentuated by concurrent radiotherapy. If sufficiently severe, chemotherapy, radiotherapy, or both should be held until improvement; consideration is given to treating at reduced doses.

F. **Treatment of refractory disease.** If the patient's disease recurs on the recommended regimens, it is reasonable to use as single agents any of the drugs noted in **B**, page 91, that have not been used previously. Thus, for FAM relapsers, semustine can be given in full doses, such as 200 to 250 mg/m^2. For relapsed patients on fluorouracil and semustine, the combination of mitomycin and doxorubicin (Adriamycin™) (FAM without fluorouracil) is a rational choice.

III. Cancer of the small intestine

A. General considerations and aims of therapy

1. **Carcinoid tumors.** Carcinoid tumors are the most common tumors of the appendix and ileum. They may develop in other parts of the GI tract, but much less commonly. The usual histologic criteria of malignancy may not always be applicable, and invasion and evidence of distant spread are more useful prognostic features.

In one series, the 60 percent of patients with intestinal carcinoids that were still confined to the wall of the gut had a 5-year survival of 85 percent while those with tumors invading the serosa or beyond had a 5 percent 5-year survival. Patients in the latter group were nearly always symptomatic, while patients in the former group were not; their tumors were discovered at surgery for "appendicitis" or other causes. Tumors of the appendix are usually "benign" by these criteria while those of the ileum are more often invasive. Surgical resection is the definitive therapy.

2. **Carcinoid syndrome.** About 10 percent of patients are afflicted with the carcinoid syndrome, which includes diarrhea, abdominal cramps, malabsorption, and flushing. With tumors of intestinal origin, liver metastases are nearly always present. Serotonin is thought to be responsible for the abdominal symptoms, and its metabolite 5-hydroxyindoleacetic acid (5-HIAA) is excreted in large quantities in the urine and is a useful marker of disease activity. The symptoms may respond to simple antidiarrheal therapy, but the serotonin antagonists cyproheptadine or methysergide are often helpful. *p*-Chlorophenylalanine has been used to inhibit the synthesis of serotonin by the tumor. The flushing caused by the syndrome has been attributed to the bradykinin, formed by the interaction of kallikrein made by the tumor with a plasma protein. Phenothiazines and steroids may be helpful in the control of flushing.

3. **Adenocarcinomas** of the small intestine are so uncommon that there is no large chemotherapy experience to recommend. It is reasonable to treat metastatic disease as recommended for gastric or colon cancer.

4. The treatment of small intestinal **sarcomas** and **lymphomas** will be described in Chapters 15 and 18.

B. Treatment of advanced carcinoid tumors

1. **Effective agents.** Doxorubicin (Adriamycin™), fluorouracil, and the investigational agent streptozocin have all been shown to have some activity in this disease. Responses have also been seen with melphalan, cyclophosphamide, and methotrexate. A major advantage of using streptozocin in combination is its lack of myelotoxicity. Response rates for combinations of fluorouracil and streptozocin or streptozocin and cyclophosphamide in treating carcinoids of various kinds are 25 to 35 percent with the overall response rate for patients with tumors of intestinal origin 41 percent. Median durations of response of 7 months may be expected, and patients with a good performance status have the greatest likelihood of response. Tumor response correlates well with 5-HIAA excretion.

2. **Recommended regimen**

   a. **Streptozocin,** 500 mg/m^2 IV days 1 to 5 *and*

   b. **Fluorouracil,** 400 mg/m^2 IV days 1 to 5

   Repeat the course every 6 weeks if the disease has responded or is stable.

   If the patient does not respond, doxorubicin, 60 to 75 mg/m^2 IV every 3 weeks, can be given, with appropriate monitoring of cardiac function and leukocyte count.

C. **Precautions.** Treatment of carcinoid tumors may precipitate or exacerbate the carcinoid syndrome during the first days of treatment, and serotonin antagonists should be available.

IV. Cancer of the large intestine

A. **General considerations and aims of therapy.** Taken together, cancers of the colon and rectum are by far the most frequent malignancies of the GI tract, and they account for the most deaths. Less than one half of patients found to have large bowel cancers are cured by surgery, although that modality is still the only curative one available. There have been some advances in early diagnosis and in techniques of surgery, but nationwide mortality figures have not really changed appreciably. In some institutions, the relative incidence of colon cancer is increasing while the incidence of rectal cancer is decreasing. Local recurrence is much more common in rectal cancer (40%–50%). About 50 percent of large bowel cancer recurrences are in the liver.

1. **Staging.** The most commonly used staging system is that of Dukes or its modifications. This system classifies the tumor in terms of the extent to which it penetrates the bowel wall and involves regional lymph nodes. Dukes A lesions are confined to the mucosa and submucosa and have a 5-year survival of more than 80 percent. B_1 lesions penetrate through the muscularis, but not yet to the serosa, with a survival of 60 to 80 percent. B_2 lesions penetrate to the serosa or through it into the pericolic fat, and survivals range from 40 to 70 percent. Dukes C lesions indicate node involvement. If the serosa has not been penetrated (in one system of classification), it is called a C_1 lesion with about 35 to 60 percent 5-year survival; the C_2 lesions are through the serosa, have positive nodes, and have a 15 to 30 percent survival. Dukes D lesions have distant metastases at the time of initial staging and have virtually no 5-year survivors. This staging method at surgery is helpful in selecting patients who are at sufficiently high risk to justify adjuvant therapy, such as chemotherapy or irradiation.

2. The **serum carcinoembryonic antigen** (CEA) level may parallel disease activity, although it is not increased in all patients with colon cancer. It is worth measuring preoperatively and, if elevated, postoperatively, since a failure of an elevated value to return to normal may signify incomplete removal of the tumor. Likewise, a return to elevated values after an initial fall to normal may indicate recurrence. CEA values may also be an indicator of response during chemotherapy treatment with a fall signifying improvement and a rise heralding regrowth of tumor.

B. **Treatment of advanced disease**

1. **Effective agents and combinations.** For nearly 25 years, fluorouracil has been the standard drug in the treatment of advanced colorectal disease that is not amenable to surgical or radiotherapeutic control. Response rates have varied widely, but a generally agreed on figure is 20 percent. Several institutions have reported response rates of about 40 percent when fluorouracil was combined with semustine and, in some instances, vincristine and dacarbazine. However, when these combinations were tested by large cooperative groups, these response

rates did not hold up. Increased toxicity, particularly myelosuppression, was often observed. It must be concluded reluctantly that no combination has as yet been shown to be clearly superior to fluorouracil alone with respect to survival, although the combination of semustine (methyl-CCNU), vincristine (Oncovin®), fluorouracil, and streptozocin (MOF-STREP) may be superior.

2. **Dose, schedule, and route of administration** of fluorouracil have been studied intensively. We prefer an IV loading dose for 5 days, then 1 month later initiate a weekly dose. However, repeating the 5-day course at monthly intervals is a reasonable alternative. It is likely that those patients with some degree of mild toxicity, such as leukopenia, will have a higher response rate than those without. Survivals on average are improved by about 6 months in responding patients.

3. **Liver metastasis.** If the patient's disease is primarily in the liver, the response rate with fluorouracil alone is only about 10 percent. Consideration should be given to MOF-STREP in such a patient, since the response rate may be higher (45%) than with fluorouracil alone. Intermittent hepatic artery infusion with fluorouracil, which has a response rate of about 50 percent, should also be considered. Continuous infusion with permanent catheters and a portable pump using floxuridine has been reported to have a 73 percent response rate.

4. **Recommended regimens**

   a. **Fluorouracil,** 500 mg/m^2 IV push days 1 to 5, then 500 mg/m^2 IV weekly beginning with day 28. Dose may be escalated by 50 mg/m^2 increments if there is no stomatitis or diarrhea and if there is minimal effect on the leukocyte count. Dose may be given PO, but absorption is erratic and this route is not preferred.

   b. **MOF-STREP**

      (1) **Semustine,** 30 mg/m^2 PO days 1 to 5 every 10 weeks

      (2) **Fluorouracil,** 300 mg/m^2 IV days 1 to 5 every 5 weeks

      (3) **Vincristine,** 1 mg IV every 5 weeks

      (4) **Streptozocin,** 500 mg/m^2 IV weekly in a 20- to 30-minute infusion

   c. **Hepatic artery infusion.** The catheter must be carefully positioned by an experienced angiographer through the axillary or femoral artery. A continuous infusion of 5000 units/day of heparin is given with 800 mg/m^2/day of fluorouracil for 4 days, then 600 mg/m^2 for a maximum of 17 days as tolerated. Weekly doses of 600 mg/m^2 IV can then be given to maintain whatever response has occurred or the hepatic artery infusion can be repeated in the hospital in 4 to 6 months if the IV therapy does not prevent relapse. The position of the catheter needs to be checked twice weekly.

C. **Combined modality treatment**

   1. **Colon cancer.** For many years, studies have been directed at improving the prognosis of surgically resected but relatively high-risk large-

bowel cancer (Dukes B_2 and C). A large body of data may be summarized by saying that no randomized controlled study of *colon* cancer has clearly shown a survival benefit of adjuvant chemotherapy or immunotherapy sufficient to warrant its routine use. The GITSG compared (1) immunotherapy with the methanol-extractable residue of BCG (MER), (2) combined fluorouracil and semustine chemotherapy, (3) combined chemotherapy and immunotherapy, or (4) a no-treatment control group. No significant difference in survival or recurrence rate between any of the four groups was found. A British study has shown some benefit for liver directed–portal vein infusion with fluorouracil postoperatively, but this is not yet recommended for routine use. Historically, controlled studies have sometimes shown a positive effect of fluorouracil, but they cannot be considered definitive enough to warrant therapy based on their conclusions.

2. Rectal cancer

a. Preoperative radiation.
Several studies have shown a benefit for preoperative radiation in rectal cancer although there are disadvantages in terms of accuracy of staging, delay before surgery, incomplete knowledge of extent of tumor for treatment planning, and inappropriate administration of radiation to patients with early (Dukes A or B_1) or advanced (Dukes D) lesions. Accordingly, major attention has been given to trials of postoperative radiation with and without chemotherapy.

b. Postoperative radiation, with and without chemotherapy.
A recently completed GITSG trial in Dukes B_2 and C rectal cancer has shown that treatments with chemotherapy alone, radiation therapy alone, or the combination are significantly better than no treatment in terms of recurrence rate, and that the best treatment to date is that which uses the combined modalities, although the differences from the other treatments are not yet significant. Survival benefits are not yet evident, but can be expected with a sufficient follow-up period. At present the radiation–chemotherapy from that trial is recommended:

(1) **Radiotherapy,** 4000 to 4400 rad in 5 weeks

(2) **Fluorouracil,** 500 mg/m^2 IV on each of the first 3 days and last 3 days of radiotherapy, *then*

(3) Five weeks later begin **fluorouracil,** 325 mg/m^2 IV days 1 to 5 and 375 mg/m^2 days 36 to 40 *and*

(4) **Semustine,** 130 mg/m^2 PO day 1

Repeat the chemotherapy cycle every 10 weeks for 18 months.

D. Complications of therapy or disease.
The complications of chemotherapy are those attributable to the individual drugs. In the adjuvant setting, it is possible that the combination of fluorouracil and semustine will be complicated by a few cases of acute nonlymphocytic leukemia; attempts to define the need for both drugs are important. Myelosuppression, nausea, vomiting, and diarrhea are common and require dose modification.

E. Treatment of refractory disease. No satisfactory treatment exists for the patient who fails treatment with fluorouracil. Some patients with liver disease failing IV therapy may respond to fluorouracil given as a hepatic artery infusion. The combination of cyclophosphamide, methotrexate, and vincristine has produced some responses but response rates are of the order of 10 percent and are usually quite brief. The regimen is

1. **Cyclophosphamide,** 300 mg/m^2 IV weekly

2. **Vincristine,** 1.4 mg/m^2 IV weekly (maximum dose 2.0), *and*

3. **Methotrexate,** 25 mg/m^2 IV weekly

Selected Reading

Bucholtz, T. W. et al. Clinical correlates of resectability and survival in gastric carcinoma. *Ann. Surg.* 188:711, 1978.

Carter, S. K., and Comis, R. L. Gastric cancer: Current status of treatment. *J.N.C.I.* 58:567, 1977.

Davis, H. L., and Kisner, D. L. Analysis of adjuvant therapy in large bowel cancer. *Cancer Clin. Trials* 1:273, 1978.

Ezdinli, E. Z. et al. Chemotherapy of advanced esophageal carcinoma: Eastern Cooperative Oncology Group experiences. *Cancer* 46:2149, 1980.

Kemeny, N. et al. Therapy for metastatic colorectal carcinoma with a combination of methyl-CCNU, 5-fluorouracil, vincristine and streptozotocin (MOF-STREP). *Cancer* 45:876, 1980.

Macdonald, J. S. et al. 5-Fluorouracil (5-FU), Adriamycin and mitomycin-C (FAM) combination chemotherapy in the treatment of advanced gastric cancer. *Cancer* 44:42, 1979.

Moertel, C. G. Chemotherapy of gastric and pancreatic carcinoma. *Surgery* 85:509, 1979.

Panettiere, F. J. et al. Cis-diamminedichloride platinum (II), an effective agent in the treatment of epidermoid carcinoma of the esophagus. *Cancer Clin. Trials* 4:29, 1981.

Reed, M. L. et al. The practicality of chronic hepatic artery infusion therapy of primary and metastatic hepatic malignancies. Ten-year results of 124 patients in a prospective protocol. *Cancer* 47:402, 1981.

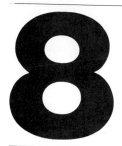

Carcinomas of the Pancreas, Liver, Gallbladder, and Bile Ducts

John C. Marsh

Cancers of the pancreas, liver, and biliary passages account for about 5 percent of all cancers and about 8 percent of all cancer deaths. Virtually all such patients die of their disease, although recent advances in diagnostic techniques allow for some cautious optimism. Surgery remains the only curative modality, but radiotherapy and chemotherapy are achieving increasingly important palliative roles. Controlled clinical trials have been useful in gathering knowledge of the natural history, prognostic features, and activity of various regimens.

I. Adenocarcinoma of the pancreas

A. General considerations and aims of therapy. This cancer has been increasing in incidence over the last several decades and is now the fourth leading cause of cancer death. Nearly all patients may be expected to die of their disease, primarily because the organ is not susceptible to easy evaluation and the disease is far advanced (i.e., not curable) by the time symptoms occur and the diagnosis is made. Cigarette smoking, chemical exposure, and more recently, coffee drinking have been implicated as possible etiologic factors. Pancreatic cancer is more common in men than in women and in blacks than in whites. This cancer is a disease of late middle age, with a peak age incidence of about 60.

The most common symptoms are weight loss and abdominal pain that often radiates to the back. Anorexia, nausea and vomiting, and jaundice are also common. Physical findings include hepatomegaly, jaundice, abdominal mass, and ascites. Ultrasonography and CT scans are useful techniques for visualizing the pancreas and allowing biopsy of suspicious areas; sometimes, laparotomy may be avoided if the lesion is clearly inoperable.

Carcinoembryonic antigen (CEA) is elevated in the serum of most patients with pancreatic cancer, and it can parallel the clinical progression or regression of the disease, although it is not specific.

Although surgery remains the only curative modality, the overall results are poor. Operative mortality is high, the proportion of explored patients having resectable disease is low, and the 5-year survival rate of resected patients is only about 5 percent. Earlier diagnosis and successful adjuvant therapy may improve this dismal outlook.

B. Chemotherapy of advanced disease. Careful evaluation of promising drugs for pancreatic cancer is still in the early stages. Patients with this disease are often in poor condition at diagnosis with weight loss, anorexia, and severe pain, so performance status is low. Such patients are

Table 8-1. Combination Chemotherapy of Carcinoma of Exocrine Pancreas

Regimens	Dosages
SMF	Streptozocin, 1 g/m^2 IV days 1, 8, 29, and 36 Mitomycin, 10 mg/m^2 IV day 1 Fluorouracil, 600 mg/m^2 IV days 1, 8, 29, and 36 Repeat cycle every 8 weeks
FAM	Fluorouracil, 600 mg/m^2 IV days 1, 8, 29, and 36 Doxorubicin (Adriamycin™), 30 mg/m^2 days 1 and 28 Mitomycin, 10 mg/m^2, IV day 1 Repeat cycle every 8 weeks

often treated reluctantly, since it is well known that patients with poor performance status usually have a poor response to chemotherapy. The frequent hepatic involvement by tumor or biliary obstruction compromises liver function and can complicate the use of some anticancer agents that are excreted and metabolized by the liver. Few drugs have had satisfactory evaluation, in part because this generally requires measurable disease, which is usually present only in patients with advanced disease.

1. **Single agents.** Fluorouracil has had the longest and most thorough evaluation in this disease, with response rates in the range of 20 percent. The IV route is superior to the oral route. Other drugs with some apparent activity include streptozocin (36% response rate in collected small series), mitomycin (27% response rate), and doxorubicin (Adriamycin™) (13% response rate). The nitrosoureas have been disappointing. Other agents that have been tested but found to be ineffective include dactinomycin and methotrexate. In addition, the Gastrointestinal Tumor Study Group (GITSG) has carefully evaluated the investigational agents hexamethylmelamine, galactitol, maytansine, and chlorozotocin, none of which has shown much evidence of activity.

2. **Combination chemotherapy.** Although the activity and number of single agents are not great, some data are available for combination chemotherapy, developed in part from active drugs. Perhaps the most promising regimens have come from the Georgetown group, using the combinations of streptozocin, mitomycin, and fluorouracil (SMF) or fluorouracil, doxorubicin (Adriamycin™), and mitomycin (FAM) (Table 8-1). The SMF regimen given in an 8-week cycle to patients with a good performance status has resulted in responses in 32 to 43 percent of patients. The responders had a 10-month survival compared to a 3-month survival for nonresponders. For best results, patients should be treated as early as possible while they still have a relatively good functional status.

Results from the FAM regimen are equally promising with 40 percent of patients responding. The survival of responders is 1 year.

3. **Complications.** The major toxicity of the SMF and FAM regimens is myelosuppression with both leukopenia and thrombocytopenia, which may lead to sepsis or bleeding in a minority of patients. Those receiv-

ing SMF may develop nephrotoxicity, manifested by proteinuria or impairment of glomerular filtration. These side effects can be expected to stabilize when streptozocin is stopped. Mild to moderate nausea and vomiting are universal, but usually well tolerated.

C. **Combined modality therapy.** Because the results of attempted surgical cure are so dismal, attempts are being made to improve them. The GITSG is conducting a study begun in 1974 that compares the effects of radiation therapy and fluorouracil given during radiotherapy and weekly therafter for 2 years postoperatively versus surgery alone. There is, as yet, no significant difference between these two treatment arms, and it is not yet possible to recommend adjuvant therapy on a routine basis.

A far larger group of patients is composed of those patients who are explored and found to have disease that is inoperable but is still localized to the area of the pancreas and neighboring structures. A controlled study by the GITSG has shown that radiation with 6000 rad plus fluorouracil is better than 4000 rad plus fluorouracil, and that both treatment arms are better than 6000 rad alone. The median survival of the best group was 39 weeks.

1. Three courses of 2000 rad in 2 weeks are given (6000 rad total), and each course is separated by 2 weeks.

2. Fluorouracil, 500 mg/m^2 IV is given on the first 3 days of each 2000 rad course.

3. Beginning 4 weeks after the last course, fluorouracil, 500 mg/m^2 IV is given weekly for 2 years or until there is progressive disease.

II. **Malignant islet-cell carcinomas of the pancreas**

A. **General considerations.** Islet-cell tumors of the pancreas occur with a frequency of about 1/100,000 people annually. They are capable of hypersecretion of insulin, glucagon, gastrin, and occasionally serotonin, ACTH, and secretin. From 10 to 25 percent are malignant. Most of these secrete insulin, either alone or in combination with glucagon or gastrin. About 20 percent of malignant islet-cell tumors are nonfunctioning. The median age is 52, with no particular racial or sex predilection. Fasting hypoglycemia is the usual clinical presentation, with a small number having the Zollinger-Ellison syndrome, composed of hypersecretion of gastric acid, diarrhea, and intractable peptic ulceration. Jaundice is rare since the tumors are usually in the body or tail of the pancreas without biliary tract obstruction. Ninety percent of patients have liver metastases at the time of diagnosis so that surgical cure, in contrast to benign tumors, is rare. Other areas of involvement include abdominal nodes and peritoneum with bone and lung metastases a late finding. The median survival in a 1950 series, without systemic therapy, was less than 1 year.

B. **Treatment of advanced disease.** Streptozocin, a nonmyelosuppressive nitrosourea showing diabetogenic effects in animal studies, is the cornerstone of therapy. A recent cooperative group study has shown that the survival is somewhat better when fluorouracil is added to streptozocin (26 months with fluorouracil versus 16.5 months without). The overall response rate was 63 percent versus 36 percent, and the complete response rate was 33 percent versus 12 percent. The two-drug combination is the current treatment of choice. The regimen is as follows:

1. **Streptozocin,** 500 mg/m^2 IV days 1 to 5 *and*

2. **Fluorouracil,** 400 mg/m^2 IV days 1 to 5

The treatment is repeated every 6 weeks.

C. **Complications.** Mild to moderate nausea, vomiting, or both occur in 60 percent of patients, and renal impairment is seen in 30 percent. About one third of these patients develop creatinine levels greater than 2 mg/100 ml. Leukopenia is seen in 75 percent of patients; 10 percent have a white count less than 1000/mm^3. Thrombocytopenia is seen in 25 percent of patients; one half have a platelet count of less than 50,000/mm^3. Stomatitis occurs in 5 percent. Liver function test abnormalities can also occur. Deaths caused by treatment are rare.

III. Primary carcinoma of the liver

A. **General considerations and aims of therapy.** Primary liver cancer is relatively rare in the United States, accounting for less than 1 percent of cancer deaths, but it is very common in certain parts of Asia and Africa, where it may be a leading cause of cancer death, especially in males. About 90 percent of hepatomas are hepatocellular; the remainder are cholangiocarcinomas or mixed. The disease is more common in men than in women, and it has a peak in the sixth decade. About one half of all patients have cirrhosis, which may be secondary to alcohol, viral hepatitis, or hemochromatosis. A large proportion of patients have had prior exposure to viral hepatitis. This exposure is indicated by the presence of the hepatitis B surface antigen (HB$_s$Ag), which is found in 15 to 80 percent of patients with hepatoma. In China, the incidence of hepatoma parallels the pattern of virus infections, and the availability of a vaccine in these endemic areas offers the hope of significant cancer prevention.

The majority (70%–80%) of patients with hepatocellular carcinoma have a significant elevation of serum alpha fetoprotein (AFP), which although not specific, may be a guide to progression or regression of disease.

Although cure is possible through surgical means, only 10 to 20 percent of patients have localized, resectable lesions in the absence of cirrhosis. Operative mortality is 10 to 30 percent. Long-term survival may be achieved in about 16 to 20 percent of those patients resected. Recurrence may be in the residual liver, regional nodes, lungs, or bone. Radiation therapy alone is of little benefit, since a tolerable, cancerocidal dose to the whole liver cannot be given.

Clinical staging of patients with hepatoma has shown that adverse prognostic factors include severe weight loss, ascites, portal hypertension, impending or overt liver failure, elevated AFP, and a serum bilirubin greater than 2 mg/100 ml. This conclusion was based on experience with African patients in whom it was suggested that the disease is more fulminating (median survival of 1 month) than that seen in the Orient or the United States. Such functional assessment and understanding of the clinical and geographic factors that determine the natural history of the disease are imperative for interpreting the results of therapy.

B. **Chemotherapy of advanced disease.** At present, the clinical factors, as described in **A,** probably play more of a role in determining survival than chemotherapy does. The response of African patients to chemotherapy may well be different from that of Americans. In the last 6 years a large number of chemotherapy experiences have been reported.

1. **Systemic therapy.** Systemic fluorouracil generally does not have much effect. Doxorubicin (Adriamycin™) has been reported to have response rates of 15 to 17 percent primarily for patients in the United States and 44 to 100 percent for patients in Uganda. A direct comparison of patient populations is available from a recent Eastern Cooperative Group (ECOG) study in which South African patients had a response rate of 22 percent (2/9), while patients in the United States had a response rate of 10 percent (3/29). Combinations of doxorubicin (Adriamycin™) with fluorouracil, streptozocin, or bleomycin have not been convincingly better. Fluorouracil and mitomycin and fluorouracil and carmustine have been reported to have 38 and 37 percent response rates respectively. Zinostatin (neocarcinostatin), a new agent, has been reported to have a 20 percent response rate. Because of the small number of patients involved in each series, the variable clinical states that determine response rates, and the possible geographic differences that may determine response and survival, it is not possible to select a "best" regimen. Doxorubicin (Adriamycin™) alone may be as useful as any other regimen.

2. **Intraarterial therapy.** Because cancer is apparently limited to the liver in many patients, and because intraarterial fluorouracil has been shown to have a higher response rate than systemic therapy in the treatment of metastatic liver disease, trials of intraarterial chemotherapy in liver cancer have been quite naturally of interest. Unfortunately, no regimen has as yet been proved to be definitively superior. Several regimens, including intraarterial fluorouracil and mitomycin, IV and intraarterial doxorubicin (Adriamycin™), and intraarterial doxorubicin (Adriamycin™) and fluorouracil combined with whole liver irradiation, have given response rates of about 50 percent.

   Hepatic artery ligation can reduce tumor size in both primary and metastatic liver disease, and this technique has been combined with intraarterial chemotherapy. It is not possible to judge how this combination of modalities compares to other studies.

3. **Recommended treatment.** At the present time, therefore, in the absence of clear evidence determining the best mode of therapy, it is reasonable to treat patients with doxorubicin (Adriamycin™), 60 mg/m^2 IV every 3 weeks. If controlled clinical trials are available, patients should be considered for them.

IV. **Angiosarcoma of the liver.** Although this is a rare tumor, it is reported that its incidence increases several hundredfold in patients with long-term industrial exposure to vinyl chloride. It is a diffuse process, nearly always fatal within 6 months of diagnosis. Doxorubicin (Adriamycin™), cyclophosphamide, and methotrexate every 3 to 4 weeks have been reported to be effective in a small number of patients with responses lasting 4 to 10 months and survivals of 11 to 53 months.

V. **Carcinomas of the gallbladder and bile ducts**

A. **General considerations.** Cancer of the gallbladder occurs predominantly in women who are late middle-aged or elderly. Its incidence closely parallels that of gallstones. Both conditions are very common among American Indians of the Southwest. Nearly all patients have gallstones. The surgical cure rate is in the range of 3 percent; the most successfully treated patients are those who are operated on for gallstones and the carcinoma is fortuitously found. Local invasion is to regional structures, including bile ducts, liver, pancreas, stomach, duodenum, and regional nodes.

Cancer of the extrahepatic bile ducts occurs as frequently as cancer of the gallbladder, affects males somewhat more often than women, and has an age distribution similar to that of gallbladder cancer. It is somewhat more common in patients with ulcerative colitis. Like gallbladder cancer, it is usually an adenocarcinoma. Most bile duct cancers are proximal rather than distal, which is unfortunate, because the distal variety are more easily treated surgically. Surgical cure is, like gallbladder cancer, in the range of 3 percent. Palliative bypass surgery may relieve jaundice and pruritus and decrease susceptibility to infection. Good palliation and long-term survival has been reported in some patients receiving radiotherapy.

B. Chemotherapy of advanced disease. Because of the relative rarity of this cancer, the difficulty of direct measurement of tumor, and a low activity of drugs, few data are available.

1. **In gallbladder cancer,** one series reported no responses to fluorouracil in 36 patients and another series reported 5 to 12 percent responses to oral fluorouracil alone or combined with streptozocin or semustine. Some improvement may be seen with the addition of doxorubicin (Adriamycin™) and a nitrosourea to fluorouracil: three of five patients were said to have a measurable (but minimal) response.

2. **Extrahepatic bile duct cancer** is reported to respond poorly (5%) to fluorouracil, but somewhat better (7/15, or 47%) to mitomycin. A 31 percent response rate to FAM (see Table 8-1) was reported in a series of 13 patients recently with an additional 46 percent achieving disease stabilization. These preliminary results are encouraging. A similar response rate has been seen to oral fluorouracil combined with semustine in another small group of 13 patients. More studies are needed, but FAM is a reasonable choice for biliary tract cancer and probably for gallbladder cancer as well, although there are no specific data for the latter disease.

Selected Reading

International meeting on pancreatic cancer of the National Pancreatic Cancer Project. *Cancer* 47:1451, 1981.

Katz, M. Primary cancer of the liver. In D. S. Fischer and J. C. Marsh (Eds.), *Cancer Therapy*. Boston: G. K. Hall, in press, 1982.

Lee, Y.-T. N. Systemic and regional treatment of primary carcinoma of the liver. *Cancer Treat. Rev.* 4:195, 1977.

Lena, H. F., Benton, R. P., and Fischer, D. S. Carcinoma of the gallbladder and bile ducts. In D. S. Fischer and J. C. Marsh (Eds.), *Cancer Therapy*. Boston: G. K. Hall, in press, 1982.

McBride, C. M. Primary carcinoma of the liver. *Surgery* 80:322, 1976.

Marsh, J. C. Endocrine Tumors. In D. S. Fischer and J. C. Marsh (Eds.), *Cancer Therapy*. Boston: G. K. Hall, in press, 1982.

Wiggins, R. G. Pancreatic Cancer—Diagnosis and Therapy. In D. S. Fischer and J. C. Marsh (Eds.), *Cancer Therapy*. Boston: G. K. Hall, in press, 1982.

Carcinoma of the Breast

Roland T. Skeel

I. Natural history, evaluation, and modes of treatment

A. Epidemiology and etiology. Carcinoma of the breast is the most common cause of cancer deaths among women. In 1981 approximately 110,000 new cases were diagnosed with more than 37,000 deaths. The incidence varies widely among different populations: women in Western Europe and the United States have a higher incidence than women in other parts of the world. Although discrete causes of breast cancer are not known, many factors increase a woman's risk for developing the disease. Among the strongest of the risk factors is family history, particularly if more than one family member has developed breast cancer at an early age. Other factors that increase the risk are early menarche, late age at first birth, and prior benign breast disease (particularly if there is a high degree of benign epithelial atypia). Lactation was once thought to protect from breast cancer, but it is now no longer believed to have that benefit. Although breast cancer may occur among men, it represents less than 1 percent of all breast cancers and is uncommonly seen in most hospitals.

B. Detection, diagnosis, and pretreatment evaluation

1. Screening. Because of the belief that more lives can be saved if breast cancer is diagnosed at an early stage, many programs have been designed to detect small early cancers. Monthly breast self-examination for all women after puberty, yearly breast examinations by a physician or other trained professional (particularly for women over the age of 40), and yearly mammography for women over the age of fifty (younger with certain high-risk factors) are the methods most commonly recommended. Each method appears to be of some help in detecting early lesions that can be successfully removed before metastasis has occurred. The exact contribution of each method to decreasing the mortality from breast cancer, however, has not been determined.

2. Presenting signs and symptoms. Breast cancer is most often discovered by a woman herself as an isolated, painless lump in the breast. If the mass has gone unnoticed or ignored for a time, there may be fixation to the skin or underlying chest wall, ulceration, pain, or inflammation. Some early lesions will present with discharge or bleeding from the nipple. At times, the primary lesion will not be discovered, and the woman will present with symptoms of metastatic disease, such as pleural effusion, nodal disease, or bony metastases. About one half of all lesions are in the upper outer quadrant of the breast (where most of the glandular tissue of the breast is). Twenty percent are central masses, and 10 percent are in each of the other quadrants. One half of all women will have axillary node metastasis unless the primary tumor has been detected by screening mammography or other screening method.

3. **Staging.** Carcinoma of the breast is staged according to the size and characteristics of the primary tumor (T), the involvement of regional lymph nodes (N), and the presence of metastatic disease (M). An abridged version of the commonly used TNM classification of breast cancer is shown in Table 9-1, and the stage grouping is shown in Table 9-2. Staging is commonly done prior to surgery, then again after surgery when the primary tumor size and the histologic involvement of the lymph nodes are known. It is important to note that in 30 percent of the patients without clinical evidence of axillary lymph node involvement, the histologic evaluation will show cancer; and in a somewhat smaller number, nodes that clinically appear positive contain no cancer when examined histologically.

4. **Diagnostic evaluation**

   a. **Prior to biopsy** the woman should have a careful **history,** during which attention should be paid to **risk factors,** and a **physical examination,** with a focus not only on the involved breast, but the opposite breast, all lymph node areas, the lungs, bones, and liver. This examination should be followed by bilateral mammography to help assess the extent of involvement and to look for additional homolateral or contralateral disease.

   b. **Excisional biopsy** of the primary lesion is performed, and the specimen is given intact (not in formalin) to the pathologist, who can divide the specimen for histologic examination, hormone receptor assays, or other tests. The tissue for receptor studies must be rapidly frozen with either dry ice or liquid nitrogen to preserve receptor activity.

   c. **Following confirmation of the histology** the patient is evaluated for possible metastatic disease.

      (1) **Mandatory studies** include a chest x-ray, a complete blood count, and a blood chemistry profile.

      (2) **Other studies,** including skeletal survey and radionuclide scans of the bones and liver, are optional unless the history, physical examination, or blood studies suggest a poor prognosis or point to specific organ involvement.

5. **Histology.** Seventy-five to 80 percent of all breast cancers are infiltrating ductal carcinomas and 10 percent are infiltrating lobular carcinomas, both of which have very similar biologic behavior. The remainder of the histologic types of invasive breast carcinoma may have a somewhat better prognosis, but are usually managed more according to the stage than the histologic type.

C. **Approach to therapy**

1. **Surgery** has been, and remains, the primary mode of therapy for most women with carcinoma of the breast. Although surgery has been used

Table 9-1. Abridged TNM Classification of Breast Cancer

Primary Tumor (T)	Description
T_1	Tumor $\leq$ 2 cm
T_{1a}	No pectoral fixation
T_{1b}	Pectoral fixation
T_2	Tumor 2–5 cm
T_{2a}	No pectoral fixation
T_{2b}	Pectoral fixation
T_3	Tumor > 5 cm
T_{3a}	No pectoral fixation
T_{3b}	Pectoral fixation
T_4	Any size tumor with extension to chest wall (not pectoral muscles)
T_{4a}	Chest wall fixation
T_{4b}	Skin fixation
T_{4c}	Chest wall and skin fixation
T_{4d}	Inflammatory carcinoma

Nodal Involvement (N)	
N_0	No nodes palpable
N_1	Movable homolateral axillary nodes
N_{1a}	Not considered malignant clinically or only histologic metastasis pathologically
N_{1b}	Considered malignant clinically or grossly positive pathologically
i	< 0.2 cm metastases pathologically
ii	1–3 nodes positive pathologically
iii	$\geq$ 4 nodes positive pathologically
iv	Beyond node capsule
v	> 2 cm diameter node
N_2	Fixed homolateral axillary nodes
N_3	Homolateral supraclavicular or infraclavicular malignant nodes or edema of arm

Distant Metastasis (M)	
M_0	None known
M_1	Metastases present

Table 9-2. Stage Grouping of Breast Cancer

Stage	T	N	M
I	T_1	N_0 or N_{1a}	M_0
II	T_2	N_{1b}	M_0
III	T_3	N_2	M_0
IV	T_4	N_3	M_1

Note: Patients are staged in the highest group possible for their composite TNM. For example, a patient with T_{1a} N_2 M_0 would be a Stage III because of the N_2 status.

for many years in the treatment of this disease, there is still controversy regarding the optimal surgical procedure for each stage of breast carcinoma. The operation that is probably most commonly performed is some version of the modified radical mastectomy in which the breast, the pectoralis fascia (with or without the pectoralis minor muscle), and lymph nodes are removed. For most women, more extensive operations are probably of no benefit and lesser operations, unless combined with some other form of therapy, may be insufficient, particularly in terms of providing important prognostic information regarding the status of the axillary lymph nodes.

2. **Radiotherapy's** role in the management of carcinoma of the breast has been expanding during the past 15 years. Radiotherapy may be used in conjunction with excisional biopsy of the cancer (leaving the remainder of the breast intact) as part of the primary therapy. In this circumstance the radiotherapy is commonly delivered using a combination of implantation of radioactive substances and external beam therapy. Radiotherapy may also be given after mastectomy in women who have a high likelihood of local recurrence, and it is highly effective in preventing the reappearance of disease in the treated fields. Local recurrences and distant metastasis also are frequently treated successfully with radiotherapy. This mode of treatment is particularly critical in the management of painful bony lesions or sites of impending pathologic fracture.

3. **Chemotherapy and endocrine therapy** are used both for the treatment of early disease when there is a high likelihood of recurrence and for the treatment of advanced disease with distant metastasis. **Endocrine therapy** may consist of surgical, chemical, or radiotherapeutic ablation of the ovaries, adrenal glands, or the anterior pituitary gland; or it may consist of additive therapy with estrogens, progestins, androgens, or antiestrogens. Endocrine therapy is generally ineffective in those patients with low levels of estrogen and progesterone receptors in their cancer and increasingly effective as the level of receptor rises. Chemotherapy is apparently equally effective regardless of the level of the hormone receptors in the cancer cell. While endocrine and cytotoxic chemotherapy are most commonly used sequentially, studies are now under way using both modalities in combination in an attempt to exploit their independent effects and nonoverlapping toxicities.

4. **Multimodal therapy** has had more of an impact on carcinoma of the breast than any other common cancer affecting adults.

   a. **Postoperative chemotherapy** for women with a high risk of recurrence owing to positive axillary nodes (i.e., nodes containing cancer) has unequivocally been shown to improve survival of premenopausal women and probably improves survival of postmenopausal women as well, providing they are given full doses of chemotherapy.

   b. **Radiotherapy** to the breast and nodal areas following excisional biopsy or quadrantectomy of the breast cancer appears in several series to be as effective a treatment as mastectomy, both in terms of local recurrence and of survival. The place of this mode of combined therapy in the management of carcinoma of the breast is not yet completedly defined, particularly with respect to long-term complications and recurrence rates, but for some patients it may be not only equivalent, but preferable treatment.

c. **Consultation** with a surgeon, radiotherapist, and medical oncologist is critical once the diagnosis of carcinoma is either highly suspected or histologically confirmed. It is important to have all of these oncology specialists see the patient before any decisions regarding therapy are made so that the primary physician and the patient can have opinions from several perspectives about the optimal management for the patient.

It is equally critical to have the patient (and her family if she desires) share in the therapy decisions after she has heard the options, the relative advantages and the disadvantages of each option, and the recommendations of the consultants. The patient should be given an opportunity to hear why the recommended treatment is thought by the physicians to be best and to decide whether that is acceptable to her.

D. **Prognosis.** There is a broad spectrum in the biologic behavior of breast carcinoma from the very aggressive, rapidly fatal, inflammatory carcinoma to the relatively indolent disease with late-appearing metastasis and survival of 10 to 15 years. At least two parameters are helpful in predicting the likelihood of relapse and survival: the stage of the disease and the estrogen receptor status at diagnosis.

1. **Stage.** Axillary node involvement and size of the primary tumor are both determinants of the likelihood of survival.

   a. **Nodes.** In one large National Surgical Adjuvant Breast Project study, 65 percent of all patients who had a radical mastectomy survived 5 years and 45 percent survived 10 years. If no axillary nodes were positive, the 5-year survival was nearly 80 percent, and the 10-year survival was 65 percent. If any axillary nodes were positive, the 5-year survival was less than 50 percent, and the 10-year survival was 25 percent. If four or more nodes were positive, the 5-year survival was 30 percent, and the 10-year survival was less than 15 percent.

   b. **Primary tumor.** Patients with large primary tumors do not do as well as women with small tumors, irrespective of the nodal status, although those patients with a large primary tumor are more likely to have node involvement. Inflammatory carcinomas (T_{4d}) have a particularly poor prognosis with a median survival of less than 2 years and a 5-year survival of less than 10 percent.

2. **Estrogen receptors.** It has recently been found that patients without estrogen receptors (or with very low levels) are twice as likely to relapse during the first 2 years from diagnosis as those who are receptor positive. This observation is true for both premenopausal and postmenopausal patients within each major node group (0, 1–3, $\geq$ 4).

3. **Other prognostic factors** have been less well studied or are inconclusive. One intriguing study carried out an immuno-histologic assessment of carcinoembryonic antigen (CEA) and found that patients who

had CEA-negative tumors had significantly higher 5- and 10-year survival rates. Presumably, the presence of the oncofetal antigen is reflective of a rapidly growing tumor that is able to escape host control. Pretreatment measures of the rate of disease progression are also being developed and may help to predict how well patients will do.

II. Chemotherapy and endocrine therapy

A. General considerations and aims of therapy. Carcinoma of the breast is responsive to many cytotoxic chemotherapeutic agents, hormonal agents, and other endocrine manipulations.

1. **Endocrine therapy** is presumed to be effective because the breast cancer tissue retains some of the endocrine sensitivity of the normal breast tissue. Thus, in the premenopausal woman, if the breast cancer growth is supported by estrogen production from the ovary, antiestrogen therapy or removal of endogenous estrogen by oophorectomy logically results in regression of the cancer, at least those tumor cells that are dependent on the estrogen. (The dependent cells seem to be those that have the estrogen receptors.) Not easily deduced is the reason that additive estrogen therapy may cause regression of breast cancer in postmenopausal women. Since we know, however, that the women who respond to additive estrogen therapy come from the same group of women who respond to antiestrogen therapy, it seems that the large doses of estrogens used in the treatment of breast cancer have an antihormonal effect, either directly on the tumor or through a feedback mechanism by way of other hormones.

2. **Chemotherapy.** As in other cancers, the basis for the effectiveness of cytotoxic drugs in the treatment of carcinoma of the breast is not well understood. It is clear, however, that combinations of drugs are considerably more effective than single agents (although how many is enough is not so clear), and nearly all treatment programs use the drugs in various combinations.

3. **The aims of therapy** differ depending on the stage of disease that is being treated.

   a. **In early disease** the aim is to eradicate micrometastases in order to render the patient free of disease and prevent recurrence of the disease. Coincident with this aim is the necessity to carry out this treatment with a minimum of drug-induced toxicity, both short- and long-term. Of particular concern is the possibility of second cancers arising several years after the completion of chemotherapy. Thus, a goal of investigational studies has been to try to determine the minimum therapy that is effective in preventing recurrences of disease.

   b. **In advanced disease** the aim is usually to temporarily reduce the tumor burden and the resultant disability in order to improve the patients symptoms and performance and to prolong meaningful survival. While long-term toxicity is not usually of great import, short-term toxicity is a major area of concern for both physician and patient, since the aim of therapy is to improve how the patient feels as much as it is to prolong the time of remaining life.

B. Effective agents for treating carcinoma of the breast can be found among the alkylating agents, antimetabolites, natural products (antibiotics and vinka alkaloids), hormones, and hormone antagonists.

1. Among the cytotoxic drugs, the most commonly used agents include doxorubicin (Adriamycin™), cyclophosphamide, methotrexate, fluorouracil, and vincristine. Each of these agents has response rates of 20 to 40 percent when used as a single agent. Since combinations are so much more effective (60–80% responses) than single agents, these drugs are rarely used alone.

2. Among the hormones and antihormones, the most commonly used agents are tamoxifen, diethylstilbestrol, fluoxymesterone, and prednisone. The first three may be used alone or in combination with cytotoxic drugs; prednisone is nearly always used together with cytotoxic agents.

C. Treatment of early disease. Treatment is recommended for all premenopausal women who have any positive axillary nodes. Treatment is recommended with caution for postmenopausal women who have positive axillary nodes. It may be of benefit, as well, to women with negative estrogen and progesterone receptors, a large primary tumor (> 3 cm), or both, although this benefit remains to be demonstrated.

1. Recommended regimen: CMF, a combination of:

a. Cyclophosphamide, 100 mg/m^2 PO days 1 to 14

b. Methotrexate, 40 mg/m^2 IV days 1 and 8

c. Fluorouracil, 600 mg/m^2 IV days 1 and 8

Repeat the cycle every 4 weeks for 12 cycles

2. Dose modification is outlined in Table 9-3.

3. Response to therapy. It is impossible to determine whether individual patients respond to treatment for micrometastatic disease, since there are no individual parameters to measure. The effectiveness of such treatment must therefore depend on population studies. Since breast cancer may have a very long natural history, and disease may recur after 5 and 10 years, it is critical to defer final conclusions until at least 5 and preferably 10 years have passed. It is possible to make some kinds of observations, however, regarding the benefits of this kind of multimodal therapy.

a. In premenopausal women, both disease-free survival and absolute survival are longer in women treated with CMF than in those women who receive no therapy following mastectomy. In the first 4 years, the failure rate for the treated patients is about one-half that of the untreated patients. Women who have one to three positive axillary nodes appear to derive somewhat greater benefit than those with four or more positive nodes.

b. In postmenopausal women, the benefit is less clear in the studies that have been reported thus far. It is apparent that there is a minimal effective dose and duration of drugs that are required for therapy of micrometastases to be effective. If women are arbi-

Table 9-3. Dose Modification for Chemotherapy of Breast Carcinoma

HEMATOLOGIC TOXICITY

WBC	Platelets	Percent Full Dose of All Myelosuppressive Drugs
$\geq$ 4000 and	$\geq$ 100,000	100
< 4000 or	< 100,000	50
< 2500 or	< 75,000	0*

*Wait one week and repeat count. If nadir WBC is < 1600 or platelet count is < 50,000, reduce subsequent doses by 25%. If nadir WBC is > 3500 and platelet count is > 125,000, increase dose by 25%.

RENAL DYSFUNCTION

Serum Creatinine	Percent Full Dose		
mg/100 ml	*M[1]*	*D,T*	*Others*
< 1.5	100	100	100
1.5–2	50	75	100
2–3.5	0	50	100
> 3.5	0*	0*	0*

*Safe guidelines cannot be given, and expert evaluation is required before therapy is given.

HEPATIC DYSFUNCTION

Bilirubin	Percent Full Dose	
	A, VLB, VCR	*C, M, F, D, T*
< 1.5	100	100
1.5–3	50	100
3.1–5	25	100
> 5	0*	0*

*Safe guidelines cannot be given, and expert evaluation is required before therapy is given.

Hemorrhagic cystitis. Discontinue cyclophosphamide and substitute melphalan, 4 mg/m^2 PO days 1–5 of each cycle.

Gastrointestinal toxicity. For debilitating vomiting or diarrhea, reduce doses of C, M, F, and A by 25% for one cycle. For severe mucositis (ulcerations that inhibit eating) reduce subsequent F, M, and A by 50%. Reescalate if possible.

Cardiotoxicity. Discontinue doxorubicin.

Hypercorticism. If side effects such as hypertension, severe insomnia, psychosis, or uncontrolled diabetes occur, reduce or stop prednisone.

Neurotoxicity. Reduce vincristine or vinblastine dose by 50% for moderate paresthesias or severe constipation. Discontinue for severe paresthesias, decreased strength, difficulty walking, cranial-nerve palsies, etc.

Note: Drug abbreviations are as follows: A = doxorubicin (Adriamycin™), C = cyclophosphamide, D = dibromodulcitol, F = fluorouracil, M = methotrexate, T = thiotepa, VCR = vincristine, VLB = vinblastine.

trarily given less therapy than they can tolerate, their likelihood of remaining disease free seems to be less than those women who are given full doses of the drugs. This observation has led to the recommendation that if postoperative chemotherapy is to be given, doses should be as high as the patient can tolerate and should be continued for the entire planned period (usually 1 year).

D. Treatment of advanced disease is undergoing continuing evolution with the aim of improving the quality and duration of remissions and survivals for women with advanced disease. For patients with local or regional recurrences of disease, with bony metastasis, or with cerebral metastasis, radiotherapy usually has an important role to play in their management, and a radiotherapist should participate in planning for the patients' treatment. Regardless of the role of radiotherapy, however, chemotherapy or endocrine therapy will be indicated in patients who have advanced disease.

1. **Endocrine therapy** is indicated in women who have positive estrogen or progesterone receptors in their tumor tissue. It is not recommended (particularly as the sole therapy) for treatment of women with low levels of receptors or as treatment of brain metastasis, lymphangitic pulmonary metastasis, or other dire visceral disease in which a slow response could jeopardize survival.

   a. **Premenopausal women**

      (1) Oophorectomy *or*

      (2) Tamoxifen*, 10 mg PO twice daily

   b. **Postmenopausal women**

      (1) Tamoxifen, 10 mg PO twice daily *or*

      (2) Diethylstilbestrol, 15 mg PO daily in 3 divided doses

      Starting doses of diethylstilbestrol may need to be as low as 3 mg daily because of nausea.

   c. **Secondary endocrine therapy** may be indicated in women who have had a good response to the primary endocrine manipulation and then relapsed. Choices for therapy in this circumstance include

      (1) Hypophysectomy *or*

      (2) Adrenalectomy—either surgically or with aminoglutethemide (see Chap. 4, p. 38, for details of administration) *or*

      (3) Androgens, such as fluoxymesterone, 20 to 30 mg PO daily

2. **Cytotoxic chemotherapy,** rather than endocrine therapy, is commonly used as the first treatment for advanced disease because the responses are more rapid, and the rate of response is greater when drugs are used in combination than when endocrine therapy is used alone.

---

*Tamoxifen is not approved by the Food and Drug Administration for treatment of premenopausal women.

a. Primary therapy is therapy used as the first nonendocrine therapy for patients with advanced disease. Although several regimens have been shown to be effective, two are recommended: the first for patients in whom doxorubicin (Adriamycin™) is not contraindicated, and the second for patients with recent myocardial infarction or congestive heart failure in whom the risk of any further myocardial compromise by doxorubicin would be too great.

(1) CAF, a combination of

   (a) Cyclophosphamide, 100 mg/m^2 PO days 1 to 14

   (b) Doxorubicin (Adriamycin™), 30 mg/m^2 IV days 1 and 8

   (c) Fluorouracil, 500 mg/m^2 IV days 1 and 8

Repeat the cycle every 4 weeks. When the cumulative doxorubicin (Adriamycin™) dose reaches 550 mg/m^2, substitute methotrexate, 40 mg/m^2.

(2) CMFP, a combination of

   (a) Cyclophosphamide, 100 mg/m^2 PO days 1 to 14

   (b) Methotrexate, 40 mg/m^2 IV days 1 and 8

   (c) Fluorouracil, 600 mg/m^2 IV days 1 and 8

   (d) Prednisone, 40 mg/m^2 PO days 1 to 14, in the first three cycles only

Repeat the cycle every 4 weeks.

b. Secondary therapy will depend on what treatment the patient has previously had. If the patient relapses while on a CMF or CMFP treatment or within 6 months after finishing CMF treatment for micrometastatic disease, it is not likely that these drugs used in combination will be helpful in achieving a second remission. Since doxorubicin (Adriamycin™) is among the most effective agents in breast carcinoma, it should be used in any combination in this situation. Two effective combinations are

(1) VATH, a combination of

   (a) Vinblastine, 4.5 mg/m^2 IV day 1

   (b) Doxorubicin (Adriamycin™), 45 mg/m^2 IV day 1 (maximum cumulative dose, 550 mg/m^2)

   (c) Thiotepa, 12 mg/m^2 IV day 1

   (d) Fluoxymesterone (Halotestin®), 20 mg PO daily

Repeat cycle every 3 weeks, if blood counts permit.

(2) DAVH, a combination of

   (a) Dibromodulcitol, 135 mg/m^2 PO days 2 to 11 as a single daily dose

   (b) Doxorubicin (Adriamycin™), 45 mg/m^2 IV day 1 (maximum cumulative dose, 550 mg/m^2)

   (c) Vincristine, 2 mg IV day 1

(d) Fluoxymesterone (Halotestin®), 20 mg PO daily as a single dose starting day 1

Repeat cycle every 4 weeks if counts permit.

3. **Dose modifications** are outlined in Table 9-3.

4. **Response to therapy**

   a. **Endocrine therapy.** Of patients who are estrogen receptor negative, less than 10 percent will have a response either to additive or ablative endocrine therapy. If the estrogen receptors are positive, about 60 percent of the women will have a partial, or better, response of their cancer to either additive or ablative endocrine therapy. Responses to endocrine therapy tend to last somewhat longer than responses to cytotoxic chemotherapy, frequently lasting 12 to 24 months.

   b. **Cytotoxic chemotherapy** produces responses in 60 to 80 percent of patients regardless of their estrogen receptor status. The responses to therapy at times may be quite durable, but the median duration in most studies is less than 1 year.

E. **Complications of therapy.** Acute toxicities are primarily hematologic and gastrointestinal. Subacute toxicities include alopecia, hemorrhagic cystitis, hypertension, edema, and psychoneurologic abnormalities. Chronic or long-term toxicities may be cardiac or neoplastic. Dose modifications for the more common problems are given in Table 9-3. These guidelines are designed to be helpful in selecting a course of therapy that will be effective with the least risk of life-threatening toxicity. Because of individual differences, toxicities that are worse than expected may occur, and the responsible physician must always be alert for special circumstances that may dictate further attenuation of the drug doses. The drug data lists in Chapter 4 should be consulted for the individual precautions and toxicities of each drug.

Selected Reading

Fisher, B. et al. Ten year follow-up results of patients with carcinoma of the breast in a cooperative clinical trial evaluating surgical adjuvant chemotherapy. *Surg. Gynecol. Obstet.* 140:528, 1975.

LiVolsi, V. A. et al. Fibrocystic disease in oral contraceptive users. *N. Engl. J. Med.* 299:381, 1978.

Moxley, J. H. et al. Primary treatment of breast cancer. Summary of the National Institutes of Health Concensus Development Conference. *J.A.M.A.* 244:797, 1980.

Osborne, C. K. et al. Review. Modern approaches to the treatment of breast cancer. *Blood* 56:745, 1980.

Veronesi, U. et al. Comparing radical mastectomy with quadrantectomy, axillary dissection, and radiotherapy in patients with small cancers of the breast. *N. Engl. J. Med.* 305:6, 1981.

Weiss, R. B., Henney, J. E., and DeVita, V. T. Multimodal treatment of primary breast carcinoma. *Am. J. Med.* 70:844, 1981.

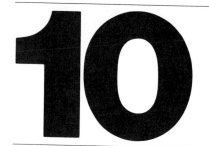

Gynecologic Cancer

Steven E. Vogl

The chemotherapy of gynecologic cancer presents a spectrum of efficacy and toxicity. Chemotherapy is of no established value in vulvar cancer. In cancers of the uterine cervix and endometrium, chemotherapy is of relatively minor palliative value. In epithelial ovarian cancer, chemotherapy is the mainstay in the treatment of advanced disease, with rates of response in excess of 70 percent. A small proportion of patients with metastatic ovarian cancer are even cured by chemotherapy. In germ cell ovarian tumors, systemic chemotherapy results in the cure of a substantial number of women when it is given after complete resection of local disease. Finally, chemotherapy has almost completely replaced surgery and radiation therapy for the treatment of gestational trophoblastic disease (hydatidiform mole and choriocarcinoma) because of its almost uniform curative ability in this disease.

Because the role of systemic drug treatment differs so markedly in the different gynecologic neoplasms, each type of cancer will be discussed separately with the appropriate treatment regimens.

I. Epithelial ovarian cancer

A. General considerations and aims of therapy.
In the United States, ovarian cancer causes more deaths in women than any other gynecologic neoplasm (estimated to be 11,600 in 1982). Approximately two thirds of women with ovarian cancer present with peritoneal metastases manifested by vague abdominal discomfort and abdominal distention from ascites. Since very few women with metastatic ovarian cancer are cured, a major thrust of research in this field has been an attempt to devise means of detecting early ovarian cancer before peritoneal spread has occurred. So far, no means are available to do this.

1. **Stage I** ovarian cancer is disease confined to one or both ovaries. The prognosis is quite good when the tumor is well differentiated and no rupture of the tumor has occurred. Such patients may be treated by surgery alone, with a 5-year disease-free survival rate in excess of 90 percent.

2. **Stage II** ovarian cancer is defined as disease that has spread beyond the ovaries but is confined to the pelvis. As surgical staging has become more sophisticated, and as more surgeons are doing routine biopsies of apparently uninvolved areas on the bowel serosa, the diaphragm, the peritoneal surfaces, and the paraaortic nodes, true stage II disease has become increasingly rare. The rarity of true stage II ovarian cancer makes sense, since there is no anatomic barrier at the top of the pelvis to confine metastatic disease to this area. While

randomized prospective trials are not available, historical comparisons strongly suggest that women with stage II ovarian cancer benefit from intensive treatment after initial hysterectomy and bilateral salpingo-oophorectomy. Five-year disease-free survival has been reported in 50 to 80 percent of patients treated with either single-agent chemotherapy (melphalan, see **B.1**) or whole abdominal radiation with boost radiation to the pelvis.

3. **Stage III** ovarian cancer is disease that has metastasized into the abdominal cavity or retroperitoneal lymph nodes.

4. In **stage IV** disease, there is either parenchymal involvement of the liver or metastases outside the abdominal cavity. The usual sites of involvement in stage IV disease are the pleural spaces and supraclavicular nodes. Skin involvement is rare except at sites of paracentesis where tumor cells have been implanted. Lung involvement is also unusual, and involvement of bones or brain is extremely rare. Stage IV disease was separated from stage III, since extra-abdominal disease precludes any attempt at encompassing the disease in a single radiation field.

B. Treatment of advanced ovarian cancer

1. **Single agent chemotherapy: melphalan.** Standard treatment of advanced ovarian cancer through the early 1970s consisted of using a single alkylating agent; of these, melphalan was preferred since it is orally administered and causes neither alopecia nor vomiting in the vast majority of women. Although it is no longer the treatment of choice for most women, melphalan alone is still used for some patients who either cannot tolerate or who refuse more effective, but more aggressive, combination chemotherapy.

   a. The **dose** of melphalan is 7 mg/m^2 PO days 1 to 5 every 4 weeks.

   b. **Response.** Approximately 40 percent of women with palpable tumors or ascites respond to melphalan therapy with shrinkage of tumor, reduction in ascites or pleural effusion, and improved sense of well-being. The median duration of response on melphalan is 7 months, and the median survival for women with stage III and IV disease is approximately 12 months. Melphalan cures approximately 35 percent of women with metastatic ovarian cancer provided their largest tumor nodule at the time of initiation of chemotherapy (after initial laparotomy) is less than 2 cm in diameter. In contrast, cure is almost unheard of in women who have tumor masses larger than 2 cm when they begin systemic chemotherapy. Histologic grade is also a prognostic factor for survival on melphalan chemotherapy, with most of the long-term survivors with metastatic ovarian cancer having well-differentiated tumors.

2. **Role of radiotherapy.** Melphalan is as efficient as whole abdominal radiation with a pelvic boost in curing women with metastatic ovarian cancer with minimal tumor burdens. Attempts to combine alkylating agent chemotherapy with whole abdominal irradiation have been unsuccessful because of convergent toxicity on the bone marrow. Pelvic irradiation is now thought to have little place in the treatment of ovarian cancer, since the field of spread is to the whole abdomen.

3. **New agents and combinations.** In the past 10 years, three agents have been demonstrated to be at least as effective as melphalan in the chemotherapy of ovarian cancer: cisplatin, hexamethylmelamine, and doxorubicin (Adriamycin™).

   a. **Alkylating agent failures.** In women who fail alkylating agent chemotherapy, the combination of cisplatin, 40 to 75 mg/m^2 IV day 1, and hexamethylmelamine, 200 mg/m^2 PO daily in divided doses days 8 to 21 every 3 weeks, produces responses in more than 50 percent of women, with a median response duration of 8 months.

   b. **CHAD as initial therapy.** The application of these new active agents in combination as part of initial chemotherapy has substantially improved the response rate over that observed with melphalan alone. The highest response rates have been reported with regimens containing cisplatin as part of initial therapy.

      (1) **CHAD,** a combination of

         (a) Cyclophosphamide, 600 mg/m^2 IV day 1

         (b) Doxorubicin (Adriamycin™), 25 mg/m^2 IV day 1

         (c) Cisplatin, 50 mg/m^2 IV day 1

         (d) Hexamethylmelamine, 150 mg/m^2 PO in divided doses daily on days 8 to 21

      This combination is given every 4 weeks.

      In the preliminary results of one randomized trial, patients treated with the CHAD regimen had a response rate of 67 percent with 40 percent complete remissions, compared to a response rate of 43 percent with only 20 percent complete remissions for patients treated with melphalan.

      (2) **Dose modifications.** For white blood counts of 3000 to 4000/μl or platelet counts of 75,000 to 100,000/μl, the dose is reduced to 67 percent. If counts are below these levels, therapy is withheld until they rise. The dose of hexamethylmelamine sometimes needs to be reduced in order to prevent the patient from being continually nauseated but need not be reduced in midcycle unless myelosuppression is profound.

      (3) **Prevention of nephrotoxicity.** Cisplatin can be safely given out of the hospital with a trivial incidence (3%) of mild and reversible nephrotoxicity by employing a program of hydration and diuresis. In this program, furosemide is first given in a dose of 40 mg as an IV bolus, and an infusion is begun of 2 liters of 5% dextrose and 0.45% saline with 10 mEq of potassium chloride/liter infused over 2 hours. After 30 minutes of infusion, the patient is given 12.5 g of mannitol IV to insure a brisk diuresis, followed immediately by 50 mg/m^2 of cisplatin as an IV bolus.

      (4) **Nausea and vomiting** from cisplatin may be managed by parenteral droperidol 2.5 mg combined with prochlorperazine 10 mg given IM at the start of the infusion and every 4 hours for two or three more doses. Hexamethylmelamine is not available

commercially (as of early 1982), but it is an investigational agent available from the National Cancer Institute to qualified cancer chemotherapists for the treatment of advanced ovarian cancer.

(5) **Other toxicities.** Forty percent of women treated with this four-drug regimen experienced white blood counts of less than 2000. Occasionally, a patient becomes infected and dies of septicemia (less than 2%). Doxorubicin (Adriamycin™) produces alopecia in all patients, and approximately 25 percent of patients develop mild paresthesias related to neurotoxicity from hexamethylmelamine and cisplatin. Paresthesias generally do not occur until the second 6 months of chemotherapy. Care must be taken during drug administration to avoid extravasation of doxorubicin (Adriamycin™), since a severe ulcer may result. Because of cumulative cardiotoxicity, doxorubicin (Adriamycin™) should be discontinued after a cumulative dose of 450 to 550 mg/m^2.

C. Duration of therapy. The optimal duration of systemic chemotherapy is not clear. For those women beginning chemotherapy with palpable masses greater than 2 cm in diameter, treatment should probably continue until time of relapse since few are cured. For those women beginning chemotherapy with tumor masses less than 2 cm in diameter, consideration should be given to stopping chemotherapy after 6 to 12 months of treatment. Many gynecologists advise a second laparotomy and multiple biopsies of apparently uninvolved areas as a means of assuring the physician that the patient is indeed disease free before stopping effective treatment.

D. An alternate regimen with efficacy in approximately 70 percent of women with advanced ovarian cancer consists of 50 mg/m^2 of cisplatin and 50 mg/m^2 of doxorubicin (Adriamycin™) given once every 3 weeks. After a cumulative dose of doxorubicin (Adriamycin™) of 500 to 550 mg/m^2, the drug should be stopped to avoid a high incidence of cardiac toxicity. These women may then be maintained on cyclophosphamide and hexamethylmelamine with or without cisplatin.

Once ovarian cancer has progressed in spite of chemotherapy with cyclophosphamide, hexamethylmelamine, and cisplatin, there is no treatment of established value, and radiation therapy should be reserved for those women with symptomatic masses in one area of the abdomen or pelvis.

II. Endometrial cancer

A. Approach to therapy: stages I to III. Approximately 80 percent of women with endometrial cancer have their disease confined to the uterine cavity without cervical involvement (stage I). The cure rate for such patients is generally in excess of 75 percent, and chemotherapy has no place in their management. Women with deep myometrial invasion or with poorly differentiated endometrial cancers have a worse prognosis, and they are often treated with surgery plus either preoperative or postoperative pelvic irradiation to encompass node-bearing areas. The efficacy of such radiation has not been proved, however.

When endometrial cancer involves the cervix (stage II), there is a high incidence of spread to parametrial tissues, and radiation therapy has an important role in the treatment of these patients. Cure rates of approximately 50 to 70 percent have been reported with combined surgery and radiation. If the cancer is clearly outside the uterus (stage III), the 5-year survival with surgery plus radiotherapy is about 25 percent.

B. Role of chemotherapy in recurrent and metastatic disease (stage IV). Chemotherapy has its place in the palliative management of patients with pelvic recurrence after failure of radiation therapy or with distant metastases.

    1. Cytotoxic chemotherapy. While some response has been reported with a number of agents, activity is best documented for doxorubicin (Adriamycin™) in a dose of 60 mg/m^2 every 3 weeks, with approximately 20 to 40 percent of patients responding. Combinations of doxorubicin (Adriamycin™) with an alkylating agent and fluorouracil have produced high response rates in a few small series of patients, but these rates have not been confirmed in larger studies. Cisplatin is reported to have had significant activity in two small trials, but none in a third.

    2. Progestational agents have been known for approximately 30 years to produce responses in 30 percent of women with metastatic endometrial cancer. The response rate with progestational agents is poor in women with pelvic recurrence or those with poorly differentiated tumors. Megestrol acetate (Megace®) is the most easily administered progestational agent, given in a dose of 40 mg PO qid.

III. Cancer of the uterine cervix. While approximately 7200 women in the United States die annually of cancer of the uterine cervix, only a few of these women are treated with chemotherapy, as cervical cancer has traditionally been considered a neoplasm resistant to chemotherapeutic agents. This conclusion has resulted from the lack of activity of alkylating agents, doxorubicin (Adriamycin™), and fluorouracil against this tumor. Cisplatin, in a dose of 50 mg/m^2 every 3 weeks, produces responses in 30 to 50 percent of patients, as does a combination of mitomycin, 10 mg/m^2 every 6 weeks, with vincristine and bleomycin. A combination of all four drugs, with vincristine, 1 mg/m^2 IV every 3 weeks, and bleomycin, 10 units/week IM, produced responses in 11 of 14 patients. The median response duration was only 3 months, and the longest response was 7 months. Remissions are often dramatic, and occur within a few days of starting chemotherapy. Chemotherapy has, as yet, no established role in the management of other than recurrent or metastatic disease.

IV. Gestational trophoblastic disease. The availability of curative chemotherapy with either methotrexate or dactinomycin has revolutionized the treatment of gestational trophoblastic disease. This term has replaced the former ones: *hydatidiform mole, chorioadenoma destruens,* and *choriocarcinoma* since the pathologic terms are of little significance when simple drug treatment can cure almost all patients.

A. HCG in diagnosis of gestational trophoblastic disease. Choriocarcinoma is unusual among human neoplasms in that a sensitive and specific marker is available, the beta subunit of human chorionic gonadotropin (HCG). When the levels of the beta subunit are elevated (above 5 mIU/ml in most laboratories), the diagnosis is either trophoblastic disease or pregnancy until proved otherwise. Thus, patients with molar pregnancies can be followed after evacuation with serial serum measurements of the beta subunit of chorionic gonadotropin. Chemotherapy with either methotrexate or dactinomycin should be administered if the level falls and then begins to rise on weekly follow-up blood tests. Only 20 percent of women with molar pregnancies, if followed in this fashion, will require chemotherapy for titers that cease to fall or begin to rise in the first 8 weeks of follow-up.

B. Chemotherapy regimens

1. **Dactinomycin,** when given alone, is administered in a dose of 0.4 to 0.45 mg/m^2 IV days 1 to 5 every 2 to 3 weeks.

2. **Methotrexate,** when given alone, can be administered in doses of 11 to 19 mg/m^2 IV or IM days 1 to 5 every 2 to 3 weeks.

C. Duration of therapy. Chemotherapy should be continued for one cycle beyond undetectable titers of chorionic gonadotropin in the peripheral blood.

D. High-risk criteria. Single-agent chemotherapy is effective in nearly 100 percent of patients with metastatic trophoblastic disease unless (1) the urinary titer of gonadotropin is greater than 100,000 IU/24 hr, (2) the time from the antecedent event (term pregnancy or evacuation of the mole) is more than 4 months before initiation of treatment, or (3) there are metastases to either the brain or the liver.

E. Treatment of high-risk patients. If any of these high-risk criteria apply, then patients are generally treated with "triple therapy" consisting of methotrexate, 11 mg/m^2 IV days 1 to 5, dactinomycin, 0.37 mg/m^2 IV days 1 to 5, and cyclophosphamide, 110 mg/m^2 IV days 1 to 5, repeated in 3 weeks if the blood counts permit. This therapy is quite toxic and causes considerable myelosuppression and major risk of infection and bleeding.

F. Role of radiotherapy. In patients with brain metastases, whole brain irradiation is imperative *immediately* to control the tumor and to reduce the risk of sudden intracranial hemorrhage. The dose of brain radiation should be 2000 to 3000 rad in 2 weeks. Radiation has also been used to treat hepatic lesions, and surgical excision has been used to treat nonresponding pulmonary nodules. Even in high-risk patients, cures have been reported in excess of 75 percent and even 46 percent of patients with brain metastases have been cured.

V. Vulvar cancer. Available literature on vulvar cancer chemotherapy consists largely of anecdotal reports of small numbers of patients. Response to chemotherapy has been reported with doxorubicin (Adriamycin™), bleomycin, and cisplatin. Chemotherapy should be reserved for recurrent or metastatic disease and must be administered with caution to this elderly and debilitated patient population.

VI. Germ cell and gonadal stromal tumors of the ovary

A. Germ cell tumors. Localized malignant teratomas, embryonal carcinomas, and endodermal sinus tumors of the ovary have a poor prognosis, with fewer than one half of patients surviving. Most of the survivors have had adjuvant chemotherapy. The most commonly used regimen with established activity in metastatic disease is a combination of vincristine, dactinomycin (actinomycin-D), and cyclophosphamide (VAC). Vincristine is given every 2 weeks in a dose of 1.2 mg/m^2 (maximum dose 2 mg) for 12 doses; dactinomycin is given in a dose of 0.3 to 0.4 mg/m^2 IV days 1 to 5; and cyclophosphamide is given in a dose of 150 mg/m^2 IV days 1 to 5. Cycles are repeated every 4 weeks. A single report has documented major activity with 50 percent complete remissions using the combination of vinblastine, bleomycin, and cisplatin (VBP) developed for testicular cancer (see Chap. 11). This report strongly suggests that VBP is now the chemotherapy of choice for these tumors.

B. Stromal tumors. Literature is limited on the chemotherapy of tumors of the gonadal stroma. Dysgerminoma in the female is the equivalent of seminoma in the male, and it is extraordinarily sensitive to radiation therapy, which should be administered whenever all evident disease can be encompassed in a tolerable radiation field. Granulosa cell cancers have been reported to respond to alkylating agents, as well as to combinations of dactinomycin, fluorouracil, and cyclophosphamide. So far, there is little experience with cisplatin-based combination chemotherapy in these tumors. Granulosa cell tumors are often indolently progressive even when recurrent or metastatic, so that chemotherapy should be given only when the patient has significant symptoms.

Selected Reading

DeVita, V. T. (Ed.). Ovarian carcinoma. *Semin. Oncol.* 2:3, 1975.

Keller, A. (Ed.). Proceedings of the National Cancer Institute mini-symposium on ovarian cancer. *Cancer Treat. Rep.* 63:235, 1979.

Lewis, J. L. Current status of treatment of gestational trophoblastic disease. *Cancer* 38:620, 1979.

Vogl, S. et al. Chemotherapy for advanced cervical cancer with bleomycin, vincristine, mitomycin C, and cis-diamminedichloroplatinum (II) (BOMP). *Cancer Treat. Rep.* 64:1005, 1980.

Vogl, S., Zaravinos, T., and Kaplan, B. Toxicity of cis-diamminedichloroplatinum II given in a two-hour outpatient regimen of diuresis and hydration. *Cancer* 45:11, 1980.

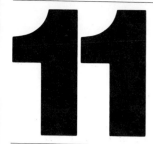

Urologic and Male Genital Malignancies

William D. DeWys

Cancers arising in the urinary and male genital systems represent a broad spectrum of biologic behavior and responsiveness to therapy. In some cancers, such as those arising in the bladder, a major objective is how to best manage local recurrence and invasion. In others, such as testicular or prostatic cancer, the major challenge is treatment of metastatic disease that has spread by way of the lymphatic system or the blood circulation to nodes, lungs, and bone.

The spectrum of response to therapy ranges from a low likelihood of, at best, partial responses in cancer of the kidney to a good chance of complete remission and cure of metastatic disease from testicular cancer. In some cancers, chemotherapy has no impact on average survival, although it may benefit the limited number of patients who respond to therapy. In other cancers, such as testicular cancer, benefits can be expressed in terms of improved average survival and probable cures.

I. Carcinoma of the kidney

A. General considerations and aims of therapy. Carcinoma may arise from either the parenchyma of the kidney or from the transitional cell lining of the collecting system. (These latter carcinomas behave and respond more like carcinomas of the bladder than carcinomas of the kidney. See section II.) Carcinomas arising from the parenchyma are adenocarcinomas or undifferentiated carcinomas. The term *hypernephroma* is sometimes used because their structure resembles the cortical tissue of the adrenal gland, but this term is a misnomer. Localized cancers are best treated by radical (perinephric fat, etc.) nephrectomy. Metastatic disease, if localized, may also be surgically resected. These tumors are relatively radioresistant; postoperative radiation is discouraged but palliative radiation of painful metastases may sometimes be worthwhile. Patients with inoperable metastatic disease should be considered as candidates for palliative hormonal therapy or chemotherapy.

B. Treatment regimens. Treatment options include hormonal therapy or cytotoxic chemotherapy.

1. Hormonal therapy. Progesterone was initially reported to give partial remissions in 15 percent of patients but subsequent studies suggest that the response rate is lower. Tamoxifen, an antiestrogen, has also been studied, and about 5 percent of patients may achieve a partial remission, and an additional 20 percent may have temporary stabilization of disease. Some renal cancers contain estrogen receptors. Although the correlation between receptor and response to therapy is not well established, we would suggest that those patients whose tumor contains estrogen receptors be treated with either

   a. Medroxyprogesterone acetate (Depo-Provera®), 800 mg IM weekly, *or*

   b. Megestrol acetate (Megace®), 160 mg PO daily, *or*

   c. Tamoxifen, 10 mg PO, bid

   2. **Cytotoxic chemotherapy.** The choices of cytotoxic chemotherapy include

   a. Vinblastine, 5 mg/m^2 IV weekly, *or*

   b. Lomustine 130 mg/m^2 PO every 6 weeks

   The major dose-limiting toxicity of either of these drugs is hematologic, and if the WBC is less than 4000/µl or the platelet count is less than 100,000/µl, treatment should be delayed until recovery to these values.

C. **Complications of therapy.** Hormonal therapy is generally free of side effects other than the occasional fluid retention that occurs with progestins. In tumors of other sites, tamoxifen has precipitated endocrine manifestations of malignancy, and these manifestations may possibly occur with renal cell carcinoma. If an endocrine manifestation, such as hypercalcemia, develops, hormonal therapy should be discontinued, and the endocrine manifestation should be managed symptomatically.

Complications of cytotoxic therapy include nausea, which can usually be controlled with antiemetics. Vinblastine may cause mucosal toxicity or myalgias, such as jaw pain, both of which can be managed with dose adjustments. Lomustine may cause pulmonary fibrosis related to cumulative doses in the range of 1 g/m^2. If this cumulative dose is reached, periodic monitoring of the pulmonary diffusing capacity is suggested.

II. Bladder cancer

A. **General considerations and aims of therapy.** Cancer of the bladder is usually transitional cell carcinoma. Rarely, squamous cell carcinoma or adenocarcinoma may develop, but these rare cell types are outside the scope of this text. Planning of treatment for bladder cancer must take into account the anatomic stage (A to D), the histologic grade (I to IV), and the tumor location within the bladder.

   1. **Superficial stage, low-grade tumors.** At one end of the spectrum is well-differentiated carcinoma (grades I and II) confined to the mucosa (stage A) or superficial muscle layer (stage B$_1$), which can usually be treated with transurethral resection. However, these patients are at risk of developing additional primary tumors in their bladder, and this risk may be reduced by administration of intravesical chemotherapy. In some patients, there may be diffuse carcinoma in situ, and this may also be treated with intravesical chemotherapy.

   2. **Deep stage, high-grade tumors.** Patients with tumors with deeper invasion (more than one half of the muscle layer = stage B$_2$, or into perivesical fat = stage C) are usually best managed with a combination of radiation therapy and surgery. The role of adjuvant chemo-

therapy in these patients, especially those with undifferentiated tumors (grades III and IV) is currently under investigation, and we have no recommendation at present.

3. **Metastatic tumors.** Patients with local recurrence beyond the scope of surgery or radiation therapy and patients with metastases are candidates for systemic chemotherapy. This therapy may achieve complete remission and prolongation of survival, or partial remission (30%) with less clear-cut effect on duration of survival.

B. Treatment regimens and evaluation of response

1. Intravesical chemotherapy

a. **Method of administration and follow-up.** This therapy is administered through a Foley catheter; the catheter is clamped for 1 hour and then emptied. This procedure delivers a high local concentration to the tumor area. The effectiveness of therapy cannot be measured individually when the objective of treatment is to prevent recurrence of bladder cancer, but an effect can be demonstrated on a population basis. These patients, however, require life-long surveillance with periodic cystoscopic examinations (initially every 3 months, then every 6 months, then annually) because even with intravesical chemotherapy, an increased risk of developing new primary tumors persists. Patients being treated for diffuse in situ carcinoma should have biopsy confirmation of a return of normal mucosa after several instillations of chemotherapy. They also require life-long cystoscopic surveillance.

b. **Specific therapeutic regimens** include

(1) Thiotepa, 30 mg intravesically weekly for 3 weeks, then every 3 weeks for 5 cycles *or*

(2) Mitomycin, 30 to 40 mg intravesically weekly for 8 weeks

2. Systemic chemotherapy

a. **Active drugs.** Drugs that have definite activity against bladder cancer include fluorouracil, cyclophosphamide, doxorubicin (Adriamycin™), and cisplatin. Of these, cisplatin is probably the most active and would be considered the drug of choice if there are no contraindications to its use.

b. **Specific regimens** to consider are

(1) Cisplatin, 40 to 60 mg/m^2 IV every 3 weeks with vigorous diuresis (see diuresis regimen in Chapter 4, Cisplatin), *or*

(2) Doxorubicin (Adriamycin™), 60 mg/m^2 IV every 3 weeks, *or*

(3) Cyclophosphamide, 1 g/m^2 IV every 3 weeks, *or*

(4) Fluorouracil, 500 mg/m^2 IV weekly, *or*

(5) Cisplatin, 60 mg/m^2 IV, doxorubicin (Adriamycin™), 40 mg/m^2 IV, and cyclophosphamide, 400 mg/m^2 IV. Repeat every 3 weeks.

c. **Response to therapy.** The combination of cyclophosphamide, doxorubicin (Adriamycin™), and cisplatin may produce a higher complete response rate than the single agents, but its overall response rate (complete plus partial) is about 35 percent, which is not significantly better than cisplatin alone.

Response to any of the regimens is monitored by periodic measurement of tumor masses with the expectation that most patients who respond will show improvement by 6 weeks of therapy. If a patient fails to respond to one therapeutic trial, a second trial using one of the other drugs listed should be considered. However, if a patient has two successive failures, a response to any subsequent therapy becomes quite unlikely.

C. Complications of therapy

1. **Intravesical therapy.** Some patients experience local discomfort, but this discomfort does not usually limit therapy. Local fibrosis may develop after repeated instillations of thiotepa, but fibrosis is infrequent with the eight instillations recommended above. There is less experience in this regard for mitomycin. Some of the administered thiotepa may be absorbed systemically and may cause bone marrow toxicity. Blood counts should be monitored before each instillation, and treatment should be delayed if the counts have decreased. Since mitomycin is a large molecule, systemic absorption has not been a problem. Alkylating agents, such as thiotepa, are known to increase the risk of second malignancies. This risk is another reason for limiting the number of instillations as outlined above.

2. **Systemic therapy.** The major dose-limiting toxicity of cisplatin is renal damage. This damage can usually be prevented by vigorous hydration and chloride diuresis, but serum creatinine should be checked before each dose. The other drugs listed have marrow toxicity requiring periodic blood counts and dose adjustments. Doxorubicin (Adriamycin™) may cause cardiac damage, but the incidence of a clinically important degree of this effect will be less than 10 percent if the total cumulative dose is less than 550 mg/m^2.

III. Prostatic cancer

A. **General considerations and aims of therapy.** Selection of therapy for prostatic cancer is based on the extent of disease and the patient's general medical condition, since this tumor is predominantly a disease of aged men. In some patients, cancer is an incidental histologic finding in a specimen removed by transurethral resection for what was clinically thought to be benign hypertrophy. If only a few chips are involved and the tumor is well differentiated, no further therapy is needed since this may represent complete removal of an occult malignancy. If multiple chips are involved and/or the tumor is poorly differentiated, there is a high likelihood of residual cancer and additional therapy, such as radical prostatectomy, should be considered. For patients with a palpable nodule but no extension outside of the prostate (stage B), radical prostatectomy is generally the preferred treatment. Patients with extension beyond the prostate are usually best treated with high-dose (7000 rad) radiation therapy. Patients with metastases may be treated with palliative radiation therapy, hormonal therapy, or chemotherapy. The aim is maximum relief of symptoms with the least toxicity. Asymptomatic patients with metastases can have treatment delayed until symptoms develop with no decrease in likelihood of benefiting from therapy.

B. Treatment of symptomatic metastatic disease

1. **Hormonal therapy** is usually the first therapy for symptomatic metastatic prostatic cancer, and 75 percent of patients treated with either orchiectomy or estrogen administration experience subjective response lasting an average of more than 1 year. Most of these responders will also have objective evidence of response. The choice between these two options can be based on patient preference and existing medical conditions that would favor one or the other. Patients who have had previous thromboembolic disease or congestive heart failure probably should not receive estrogens, which may exacerbate these conditions. If the patient is to receive estrogens, we recommend 500 rad to the breast area to prevent the development of painful gynecomastia. The usual regimen for estrogen administration is diethylstilbestrol (DES), 1 mg PO daily. Higher doses are occasionally used because of the variable suppression of plasma testosterone levels with daily 1 mg DES doses, but the increased risk of cardiovascular problems at DES doses of 5 mg daily have made the 1 mg daily dose the most commonly used.

2. **Cytotoxic chemotherapy.** If patients relapse or fail to respond to hormonal therapy, they are not likely to respond to secondary hormonal therapy and should be considered for cytotoxic chemotherapy.

   a. **The drug of choice** is doxorubicin (Adriamycin™), 60 mg/m^2 IV every 3 weeks. Patients who have received extensive radiation therapy should initially receive 40 mg/m^2 with subsequent escalation to 60 mg/m^2 if the initial dose is well tolerated.

   b. **Evaluation of response** is often difficult because easily measured disease is frequently not present. However, a marker is usually present (acid phosphatase, alkaline phosphatase, lactic dehydrogenase, or carcinoembryonic antigen) that may provide an early indicator of response. Later, reduction in the extent of disease may be seen on a bone scan or chest x-ray film. The alkaline phosphatase level may be difficult to interpret since an increasing level may reflect either increasing disease or healing of bone in response to tumor regression.

   c. **Alternate regimens.** If the patient fails on doxorubicin (Adriamycin™) or if there is a contraindication to its use, alternate regimens include

   (1) Cyclophosphamide, 1 g/m^2 IV every 3 weeks, *or*

   (2) Fluorouracil, 500 mg/m^2 IV weekly, *or*

   (3) Methotrexate, 40 mg/m^2 IV weekly, *or*

   (4) Cisplatin, 40 mg/m^2 IV every 3 weeks

   Combinations of drugs have been studied but none is clearly better than doxorubicin (Adriamycin™) as a single drug.

C. **Complications of therapy.** The complications of orchiectomy include local surgical complications, such as hematoma, and loss of libido. The complications of estrogen therapy include fluid retention and an increased risk of thromboembolic events.

Table 11-1. Clinical and Surgical Staging of Testicular Cancer

Stage	Definition	Clinical	Surgical
I	Limited to testis	Lymphangiogram, CT scan, etc., negative	Retroperitoneal nodes histologically negative
II	Spread to nodes below diaphragm	Lymphangiogram and/or CT scan positive	Nodes histologically positive
III	Spread beyond retroperitoneal nodes	Positive chest x-ray, liver scan, etc.	Same as clinical, or serum markers positive after testis and retroperitoneal nodes removed

The side effects of doxorubicin (Adriamycin™) include mucositis, marrow suppression, and cardiotoxicity.

IV. Testicular cancer

A. General considerations and aims of therapy. Because testicular cancer occurs most frequently in the third and fourth decades of life, its impact on society is perhaps greater than other more common cancers that occur primarily in older people. It is thus fortunate that curative therapy is possible even in advanced disease. The strategy for cure must take into account the histology and the stage of disease. It is useful for discussion to divide staging into clinical and surgical stages (Table 11-1).

This distinction between clinical and surgical staging is necessary because the sensitivity and specificity of the noninvasive staging procedures are only 80 to 85 percent. Thus, a patient may be clinically judged to have stage I disease but on surgical staging be found to have histologic involvement of retroperitoneal lymph nodes. The following discussion on adjuvant therapy for nonseminomatous tumors is based on surgical staging.

B. Treatment regimens. Selection of therapy for testicular cancer after inguinal orchiectomy and appropriate staging is based both on histologic type and stage.

1. Seminoma is usually not staged surgically, and both stages I and II are treated with radiation therapy. For clinical stage I, radiation therapy is directed to the retroperitoneal nodes because the risk of involvement of nodes is 20 percent, even when the lymphangiogram is negative. For clinical stage II, radiation is extended to encompass the mediastinum and supraclavicular nodes, since these areas are at risk for metastases when the retroperitoneal nodes are involved. Stage III seminoma is usually best treated with combination chemotherapy (see **IV.C.1**).

2. Pure choriocarcinoma has a very high risk of distant metastases, and it is best treated with combination chemotherapy for all stages.

3. **Other cell types** (embryonal carcinoma, teratocarcinoma, and mixed types). For these cell types, the therapeutic plan is based on surgical staging.

   a. For **stage I,** we recommend close monitoring (every month for 1 year then every 2 months for 1 year) of the chest x-ray film and serum markers (beta subunit of human chorionic gonadotropin [βHCG], alpha fetoprotein, and lactic dehydrogenase) with institution of chemotherapy should any of these become abnormal.

   b. The treatment of **stage II** disease is currently under investigation in a cooperative international study to which patients should be referred. If patients are unable to participate in this study, two cycles of combination chemotherapy (see **IV.C.1**) are recommended. This recommendation is based on evidence that 40 percent of these patients have clinically undetectable metastases that will progress if not treated, and estimates that two cycles of combination chemotherapy will kill more than 10^9 tumor cells.

C. **Combination chemotherapy.** For patients with **stage III** disease of any cell type or choriocarcinoma of any stage, combination chemotherapy is recommended.

1. **Treatment regimens.** Two combinations have evolved that have equivalent efficacy. The therapist should use the one with which he is most familiar. The combinations are the following:

   a. **VBP**

      (1) Vinblastine, 6 mg/m^2 IV days 1 and 2

      (2) Bleomycin, 30 units IV weekly

      (3) Cisplatin, 20 mg/m^2 IV daily days 1 to 5

      Repeat every 3 weeks.

   b. **VAB**

      (1) Vinblastine, 4 mg/m^2 IV day 1

      (2) Dactinomycin (actinomycin-D), 1 mg/m^2 IV day 1

      (3) Bleomycin, 30 units IV push, then 20 mg/m^2 IV as a constant infusion days 1 to 3

      (4) Cisplatin, 120 mg/m^2 IV day 4 with mannitol diuresis

      (5) Cyclophosphamide, 600 mg/m^2 IV day 1

      Repeat every 3 weeks.

2. **Follow-up.** The current recommendation is for four cycles of chemotherapy (omitting bleomycin in the fourth cycle of VAB). Patients who are in complete remission at the conclusion of four cycles receive no further chemotherapy and are followed at monthly intervals for 1 year, then every 2 months for 1 year with serum markers and chest x-ray. Patients who are in partial remission should undergo surgical resection of residual disease. If this surgery reveals fibrous tissue or mature teratoma, no further chemotherapy is given and follow-up is as above. Patients who have resection of viable tumor, who have

unresectable residual tumor, or who fail to respond to initial therapy should receive second-line chemotherapy.

3. **Second-line chemotherapy.** At the present time, etoposide (VP-16) is thought to be the best second-line drug, but it is not yet marketed. As a single agent it will produce at least partial response in more than one half of previously treated patients. When combined with cisplatin and bleomycin about one quarter of patients will experience a complete response and an additional one quarter will experience a partial remission that can be converted to a complete clearing with surgery. The dose of etoposide is 100 mg/m^2 IV days 1 to 5, repeated every 3 weeks.

D. **Prognosis.** With the strategy given, we can summarize progress in the therapy of nonseminomatous testicular cancer as follows:

	Cure Rate (%)	
Stage	**1970**	**1980**
I	90	98
II	50	98
III	10	70

E. **Complications.** The toxicity from the combinations listed in **IV.C.1** is formidable but generally acceptable because of the young age of the patients treated (mean is 25 years) and the clear-cut benefits. Toxicities include nausea and vomiting, mucositis, granulocytopenic fevers, and pulmonary fibrosis.

Selected Reading

DeWys, W. D. Management of testicular cancer. *Curr. Concepts Oncol.* 2:10, 1980.

Einhorn, L. H. and Williams, S. D. Chemotherapy of disseminated testicular cancer: a random prospective study. *Cancer* 46:1339, 1980.

Vulgrin, D. et al. VAB-6 combination chemotherapy in disseminated cancer of the testis. *Ann. Intern. Med.* 95:59, 1981.

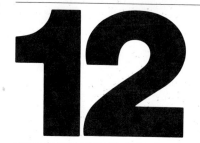

Thyroid and Adrenocortical Carcinomas

Roland T. Skeel

Endocrine cancers account for 1.5 percent of all cancers diagnosed and 0.4 percent of cancer deaths. Thyroid cancer, which is by far the most common endocrine malignancy, accounts for 90 percent of endocrine cancers and 60 to 70 percent of the deaths from this group of diseases. Although the role of cytotoxic chemotherapy is limited in endocrine cancers, it does have benefit in selected cases of carcinoma of the pancreatic islet cells, the thyroid, and the adrenal cortex. The treatment of pancreatic islet cell carcinomas and other pancreatic malignancies is discussed in Chapter 8. In this chapter we consider the chemotherapy of advanced refractory metastatic thyroid cancer and adrenocortical carcinomas.

I. Thyroid carcinoma

A. Background

1. **Incidence and etiology.** About 10,000 new cases of thyroid carcinoma are diagnosed yearly in the United States. It is 2 to 3 times more common in females than in males, and males tend to get the disease at a later age. Some cases of thyroid cancer appear to be related to radiation of the neck in childhood. The cause in most instances is unknown, although experimentally prolonged stimulation by thyroid stimulating hormone (TSH) may lead to the development of thyroid carcinomas.

2. **Cell types and prognosis.** The most common histologic types of thyroid carcinoma are papillary adenocarcinoma (40%–50%), follicular adenocarcinoma (25%), mixed papillary/follicular adenocarcinoma (20%), medullary carcinoma (1%–5%), and anaplastic carcinoma (15%–20%). For those patients with papillary or mixed histology, the prognosis is excellent with less than 15 percent mortality at 20 years. Patients with pure follicular carcinoma do not do as well as those patients with papillary elements, while those with anaplastic carcinoma have a dismal prognosis, with a median survival of less than 1 year and virtually all patients dying within 5 years. Prognosis is also related to the size of the primary tumor, age at diagnosis, and sex. For all intervals from diagnosis, females survive longer than males. This may be related in part to the fact that males tend to be older than women at the time of diagnosis, which also confers a poorer prognosis, and are more likely to have a worse histologic type than are females. Lymph-node metastasis is associated with a somewhat poorer outcome although it does not carry the dire consequences of nodal metastasis in other neoplasms.

B. Diagnosis and staging. Any solitary nonfunctioning thyroid nodule should be considered a possible malignant tumor until proved otherwise.

While toxic goiters are less likely to contain carcinoma, a hyperfunctioning thyroid nodule does not automatically confer benignity. As most thyroid tumors spread primarily by local extension and regional nodal metastasis, assessment of the extent of disease is concentrated on the neck. Presurgical studies include inspection and palpation, indirect laryngoscopy, radionuclide scanning, esophagogram, computed tomography or soft tissue tomograms of the neck, and needle aspiration cytology. Chest x-ray should be performed before surgery, and if there is any clinical or laboratory suggestion of bone metastasis, a radionuclide bone scan should be performed.

C. Treatment

1. **Surgery.** Surgery is the only definitive therapy for carcinoma of the thyroid. Although some controversy persists regarding the extent of surgery required, many surgeons prefer a bilateral subtotal thyroidectomy. If cancer is present in cervical lymph nodes, a total thyroidectomy with a dissection of all involved nodes seems to result in an improved survival.

2. **Radiotherapy.** Treatment with radioiodine (^{131}I) can be effective in patients with known incompletely resected thyroid carcinoma and possibly as an adjuvant in patients who have had potentially curative surgery. Effective radioiodine treatment requires (a) a functioning tumor capable of accumulating the iodine and (b) appropriate preparation by withholding thyroid hormone and administering TSH to assure maximum uptake by any remaining carcinoma. External radiation is reserved for anaplastic carcinoma, which does not take up iodine.

3. **Thyroid hormone** is used to replace the hormone lost after thyroidectomy. It is also used to suppress TSH with the hope that this will help prevent recurrence of the thyroid cancer. Thyroxine, 200 to 250 μg daily is usually necessary to obliterate the TSH response to thyrotropin releasing hormone. The dose must be adjusted in each patient to obtain maximal suppression of TSH without thyrotoxicosis.

4. **Cytotoxic chemotherapy**

   a. **Doxorubicin** (Adriamycin™), 60 to 75 mg/m^2 IV every 3 weeks has resulted in objective responses in one third of patients with advanced refractory metastatic thyroid carcinoma. The duration of response may be several months and, as with many cancers, patients who respond objectively to the doxorubicin (Adriamycin™) survive a few months longer than those who do not.

   b. Cisplatin has shown some activity as a single agent in advanced carcinoma and is being studied in combination with doxorubicin (Adriamycin™).

II. Adrenocortical carcinoma

A. Background

1. **Incidence, etiology, and prognosis.** Adrenocortical carcinoma is a very rare tumor with less than 200 new cases occurring yearly in the United States. There is no family predilection, and no etiologic factors have been established. Although some reports have shown a higher

incidence in females, population-based registries indicate a somewhat higher incidence in males. It is a highly malignant cancer with a 5-year mortality of 75 to 90 percent.

2. Clinical features and pathology. Many patients with adrenocortical carcinoma will present with endocrine signs and symptoms of Cushing's syndrome, virilization, or feminization owing to an increase in the production of a wide variety of steroid hormones. Hormonal manifestations are more common in children and females than in males because the adult male is already fully virilized. Other frequent presenting symptoms are upper abdominal pain, weight loss, loss of appetite, and malaise. Nearly one half of all patients will have a palpable abdominal mass at the time of diagnosis. Pathologic patterns vary with respect to cellular arrangement and pleomorphism, and occasionally there may be some difficulty in separating adenomas from carcinomas. The histologic pattern does not correlate with the functional characteristics of the tumor. There is discrepancy of opinion whether functioning carcinomas have a better prognosis than nonfunctioning carcinomas. Size, invasion of the capsule and surrounding structures (including blood vessels), degree of anaplasia, and mitotic activity are important pathologic criteria in establishing a diagnosis of malignancy.

B. Treatment

1. Surgery. Up to one half of adrenocortical carcinomas can be resected (although incompletely in some patients); the remainder have either too extensive local invasion or metastasis to other sites in the abdomen, liver, lungs, or other locations. Of those patients resected *for cure* 40 percent will remain disease-free. The remainder of the patients will die, usually with extensive metastatic disease, in an average of less than 1 year.

2. Radiotherapy is successful in giving symptomatic relief from pain owing to local or metastatic lesions in one half of the patients treated. It has also been used to prevent local recurrence following surgical resection (4000–5500 rad over 4 weeks), but the benefit is uncertain.

3. Chemotherapy

a. Mitotane (o,p′-DDD), a close chemical relative of the insecticide DDT, has been used to treat inoperable and metastatic adrenocortical carcinoma since 1960. Objective tumor regression is seen in 34 to 60 percent of patients and is most often accompanied by a decrease in excessive hormone production. A reduction in hormone production, however, is not as regularly accompanied by an objective tumor response.

(1) Dose and administration. Treatment is started with mitotane, 2 to 6 g daily in 3 divided doses. If this dose is not tolerated because of side effects, the dose is reduced by one half, then gradually increased until full doses are achieved. If symptoms are not seen at 6 g daily, the dose may be increased in monthly 1-g increments, but usually no higher than 10 g daily.

(2) Glucocorticoid and mineralocorticoid replacement during mitotane therapy is necessary to prevent hypoadrenalism:

      (a) Cortisone acetate, 25 mg PO in AM and 12.5 mg PO in PM

      (b) Fludrocortisone acetate, 0.1 mg PO in AM

    (3) Side effects. Nausea and vomiting occur in 80 percent of patients, somnolence and weakness in 60 percent, adrenal insufficiency in 50 percent (without replacement), and dermatitis in 20 percent. As the maximal doses are often limited by the severity of and the patient's tolerance to the side effects, the total daily dose may have a wide range from patient to patient.

    (4) Other drugs. Very few other drugs have been used in more than an occasional patient. Cisplatin has been used alone and together with mitotane in a small number of patients and has resulted in objective tumor and hormone responses.

Selected Reading

Gottlieb, J. A., and Hill, C. S. Chemotherapy of thyroid cancer with Adriamycin™. *N. Engl. J. Med.* 290:193, 1974.

Harwood, J., Clark, O. H., and Dunphy, J. E. Significance of lymph node metastasis in differentiated thyroid cancer. *Am. J. Surg.* 136:107, 1978.

King, D. R., and Lack, E. E. Adrenal cortical carcinoma. A clinical and pathologic study of 49 cases. *Cancer* 44:239, 1979.

Richie, J. P., and Gittes, R. F. Carcinoma of the adrenal cortex. *Cancer* 45:1957, 1980.

Shields, J. A., and Farringer, J. L. Thyroid cancer. Twenty-three years' experience at Baptist and St. Thomas Hospitals. *Am. J. Surg.* 133:211, 1977.

Tattersal, M. H. N. et al. Cis-platinum treatment of metastatic adrenal carcinoma. *Med. J. Aust.* 1:419, 1980.

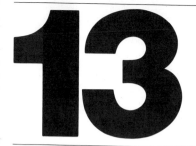

Melanoma and Other Skin Malignancies

Larry Nathanson

I. Melanoma

A. Introduction

1. Natural history

a. **Origin and occurrence.** Melanoma is a malignancy originating in the melanocytes of the skin. These cells, in embryologic development, originate in the neural crest, migrate to the skin and eye, and in adult life are responsible for the formation of skin pigment. About 10 percent of melanomas originate in some extradermal site, primarily in the eye, mucous membrane, anus, or external genitalia. The disease has doubled its incidence in the last decade, possibly because of increased exposure to actinic radiation, particularly in the ultraviolet-B spectrum. Melanoma is equally prevalent in men and women and has a peak age of incidence in the sixth decade. Early recognition and early diagnosis of this disease result in prompt and curative surgical management.

b. **Types of primary lesions.** There are three major types of cutaneous lesions. In order of increasing aggressiveness, they are lentigo maligna melanoma, superficial spreading melanoma, and nodular melanoma. These lesions vary in size from the lentigos (5 cm or greater) to the smaller, palpable, nodular melanoma. Symptomatically, they all share characteristic history of growth and one or more of the following symptoms: change in pigmentation, ulceration, itching, or bleeding when the lesions become actively malignant. On examination, they share a tendency to have irregular margins, and variegated coloring of hues of blue, red, or white; these signs help distinguish them from benign nevi.

c. **Metastasis.** At initial presentation, up to 30 percent of patients will have disease spread beyond the local lesion. In about one half, disease has spread no further than regional nodes; in the other half, there will be evidence of distant metastasis. Of those with only local disease initially, about one third will subsequently develop metastasis. In 20 percent, metastasis appears first in soft tissues alone (lymph nodes, skin, or subcutaneous tissue), and in 80 percent, it appears in other tissues and organs (particularly liver, lung, brain, or bone) alone or together with soft tissue disease.

2. Staging

of melanomas is often difficult because of the poor resolution of diagnostic radiologic studies. However, in patients at high risk for advanced disease, in addition to the usual conventional roentgenograms and radionuclide scans, CT scanning of the head and body may be helpful in staging procedures. Gallium scanning and lymphangiography are occasionally useful, as is full lung tomography.

3. **Surgical treatment.** Primary disease is conventionally treated with wide excision of the primary lesion, but routine prophylactic regional lymph node dissection has not been proven to increase survival. The prognosis of an excised primary lesion varies inversely according to the thickness of the lesion.

B. Chemotherapeutic interventions

1. Systemic therapy

a. **Patient selection.** In selecting patients with metastatic melanomas as candidates for chemotherapy, favorable clinical factors predicting the likelihood of chemotherapeutic response must be kept in mind. These include patients who have

   (1) Good performance status (initially ambulatory)

   (2) Soft tissue disease or a relatively small number of visceral sites (pulmonary metastasis are most sensitive)

   (3) Youth (less than 65 years of age)

   (4) Not had prior chemotherapy

   (5) A normal hemogram, hepatic, and renal function

   (6) No CNS metastases (or at least no unstable disease)

   (7) Female gender

b. **Single agent chemotherapy.** A number of single agents have been found to have antitumor activity in melanoma. These agents vary widely in response rates as reported by differing authors.

   (1) **Dacarbazine** (DTIC) has been the standard single agent for treatment of this disease, and is usually given at a dose of 200 mg/m^2 IV days 1 to 5 every 3 weeks or 750 mg/m^2 IV day 1 every 6 weeks. Response rate is 20 to 25 percent.

   (2) The **nitrosoureas** have each been used in melanoma and probably have similar efficacy.

      (a) Carmustine, 150 mg/m^2 IV every 6 weeks *or*

      (b) Semustine, 200 mg/m^2 PO every 6 weeks *or*

      (c) Lomustine, 100 to 130 mg/m^2 PO every 3 weeks

      These regimens are the most commonly used, and each has a response rate of 15 to 20 percent.

   (3) Dactinomycin, alkylating agents, vinca alkaloids, and procarbazine all have response rates of 10 to 15 percent.

c. **Multiple agent chemotherapy.** A number of chemotherapeutic combinations have been used in melanoma, and some regimens with data on significant numbers of patients are listed in Table 13-1. These combinations include the use of carmustine (or semustine or lomustine), hydroxyurea, and dacarbazine in the BHD or MHD regimen. This drug combination is associated with a 30 to 40

Table 13-1. Combination Chemotherapy of Malignant Melanoma

Regimen	Dosage
BHD or MHD	Carmustine (BCNU), 100–150 mg/m² IV day 1 (or Lomustine, 100–150 mg/m² PO day 1 or Semustine, 100–150 mg/m² PO day 1) Hydroxyurea, 800–1200 mg/m² PO days 1–5 and 22–26 Dacarbazine, 100–150 mg/m² IV days 1–5 and 22–26 **or** days 2–5 and 23–26 Repeat cycle every 6 weeks
BOLD	Bleomycin, 7.5 units 1st course, 15 units subsequent courses SC days 1 and 4 Vincristine (Oncovin®), 1 mg/m² IV days 1 and 5 Lomustine, 80 mg/m² PO day 1 Dacarbazine, 200 mg/m² IV days 1–5 Repeat cycle every 4–6 weeks
VBD	Vinblastine, 6 mg/m² IV days 1 and 2 Bleomycin, 15 mg/m² IV (24-hr infusion) days 1–5 Cisplatin, 50 mg/m² IV day 5
DTIC-ACT-D	Dacarbazine (DTIC), 750 mg/m² IV day 1 Dactinomycin (Actinomycin-D), 1 mg/m² day 1 Repeat cycle every 4 weeks

percent objective response rate and a median survival of 7 to 10 months. Another recently employed combination includes the use of dactinomycin and dacarbazine together in large single pulse doses given approximately once every 3 to 4 weeks. This combination has been reported by the Southwest Oncology Group to have a response rate approximately of 30 to 40 percent but to have a slightly longer median survival time. A program employing bleomycin, vincristine (Oncovin®), lomustine, and dacarbazine, the BOLD regimen, has recently been reported to have a 45 percent response rate. Median survival for all evaluable patients was 31 weeks.

The first non-dacarbazine-containing combination that has been reported to have a significant objective response rate in advanced disease is that employing vinblastine, bleomycin by 24-hour infusion, and cisplatin. Possibly the most toxic of the combination chemotherapy programs mentioned, it nonetheless has achieved a 45 to 50 percent objective response rate in previously treated patients with advanced disease. Median survival does not appear to have increased markedly over those programs previously mentioned. One of the major problems with this program, as with others, has been the high incidence of relapse in the CNS, a metastatic site that tends to respond poorly to chemotherapy. Any of the regimens in Table 13-1 are reasonable if the patient has a good performance status and can be expected to tolerate an intensive chemotherapy regimen.

d. **Adjuvant chemotherapy.** A variety of chemotherapy programs have been used in patients with high-risk primary melanoma (lesion thickness > 1.5 mm) or in patients with node metastasis. The efficacy of adjuvant chemotherapy in this setting is as yet controversial. Although several studies have suggested that either chemotherapy or a combination of chemotherapy and immunotherapy may be beneficial to patients with a high risk of recurrence, no study has unequivocally proven the usefulness of adjuvant therapy.

2. Regional chemotherapy

a. Infusion and perfusion. Arteriovenous isolation with perfusion chemotherapy has long been used in patients with regional melanoma, particularly that of the lower extremities. A variety of drugs has been employed including the alkylating agents (especially melphalan), and more recently, dacarbazine, and carmustine. Although, in some cases, this treatment appears to produce long disease-free survivals, it is not known whether this kind of treatment, with its attendant expense and hazards, is more effective than other less toxic treatments, such as intraarterial infusion. The use of heated perfusion may also represent an advance, but it is as yet untested in any careful prospective comparative study.

Intraarterial infusion has been carried out with the previously mentioned drugs, as well as with cisplatin. This treatment is technically much easier than perfusion. It may represent optimal treatment of patients with regional recurrent disease, especially when used with external tourniquet control.

b. Intracavitary chemotherapy. The use of intracavitary thiotepa, dacarbazine, or bleomycin may be of benefit in reducing the rate of development of pleural or peritoneal effusions. Colloidal gold (^{198} Au), or chromic phosphate (^{32}P) is occasionally helpful for this complication, as is tetracycline, a sclerotogenic agent. All of these drugs should be administered through an indwelling chest tube as described in Chapter 23 (p. 224).

c. Brain metastases. Melanoma of the CNS has been a particularly difficult problem because of the relatively common occurrence of such lesions. The standard approach is radiotherapy to the whole brain in one of several dose schedules accompanied initially by corticosteroids. No chemotherapeutic regimen, including nitrosoureas, which are known to cross the blood-brain barrier, has been effective in the control of CNS metastases. However, some patients may respond for long periods of time to CNS radiotherapy, particularly if no other visceral site is involved.

d. Intralesional immunotherapy. Intralesional immunotherapy, particularly with bacillus Calmette-Guérin (BCG) has been shown in a number of reports to control both injected and uninjected regional intradermal metastases (satellitosis). Although this treatment is not applicable to patients who have distant disease or extremely bulky regional disease, in patients with early recurrence it may produce long disease-free survivals. Occasional cases of systemic BCG infection occurring with this treatment are usually easy to control with antituberculous chemotherapy.

3. New treatment approaches.
Specific immunotherapy utilizing tumor cell extracts together with some nonspecific adjuvants such as BCG or Freunds Complete Adjuvant (FCA) has not been adequately

studied in this disease. Its use and apparent efficacy in lung cancer, however, suggests this approach in the future.

Antipigmentary chemotherapy, particularly with drugs that are tyrosinase inhibitors or that may inhibit cysteine incorporation into nucleic acid polymerases, has antitumor effects in experimental melanomas. These drugs include alpha-methyltyrosine, 6-hydroxy-dopa and isopropylcatechol. Their efficacy has not yet been demonstrated in any clinical study.

The use of hormones in treatment of melanoma has been suggested by the discovery that some melanoma patients have tumor cells that contain estrogen-binding protein. Although there are reported antitumor effects, the use of tamoxifen, diethylstilbestrol, phenestrin, or estracyte has not demonstrated a high enough response rate to justify routine use of any of these hormonal preparations in melanoma.

The retinoids have been used in a variety of experimental melanomas and appear to have effect both on inhibition of pigment formation as well as slowing tumor growth. This is as yet an experimental technique.

Radiopotentiating agents may have a place in the treatment of melanoma. For example, the use of cisplatin may potentiate the antitumor effects of radiation. Hyperthermia either alone or as a radiopotentiator has been shown to have antitumor effects in superficial lesions of metastatic melanomas.

II. Nonmelanoma skin cancer

A. Etiology and epidemiology.
Nonmelanoma skin cancer is the most common type of malignancy in the United States, and it has been estimated that there will be in excess of 400,000 new cases in the United States in 1982.

The most common types of skin cancer are basal cell carcinoma (BCC) and squamous cell carcinoma (SCC). This summary will exclude other types of skin tumors such as mycosis fungoides and tumors of the skin appendages.

BCC and SCC are more common in males than in females. The most frequent etiologic factor is that of exposure to actinic radiation. Accordingly individuals with fair skin and light hair and eyes tend to have a high incidence of the diseases. In addition, it is more common on the lower extremities of the female than male. Individuals with chronic sun exposure are at a particular risk for this disease. Whites have a greater incidence than Orientals who in turn have a greater incidence than blacks. BCC is more common than SCC in whites and SCC is more common than BCC in blacks. Multiple primary skin cancers can be seen in affected individuals.

Other etiologic factors include exposure to x-rays, chronic scarring (especially that occurring with burns), chronic inflammatory states, and exposure to arsenic.

B. Actinic keratosis

1. Natural history.
Actinic keratoses (solar keratosis, senile keratosis) are lesions found in the exposed areas of the skin and are assumed to

be precancerous since SCC may arise from them. In the patient predisposed to the development of such lesions, use of sun protective creams (*p*-aminobenzoic acid etc.) may be an important preventive medical practice.

2. **Topical chemotherapy.** Fluorouracil is used as a 1% solution or cream on the face, and up to a 5% concentration on the arms, applied twice daily for 2 to 4 weeks by the patient rubbing it in with fingertips. Care must be taken around the eyes but individuals may be treated in the periorbital skin. Fluorouracil must be applied smoothly with avoidance of accumulated ointment in the nasal–labial folds. After application, the hands must be washed. Erythema begins 3 to 7 days after treatment and progresses to scaling, erosion, and tenderness, at which time the application should be stopped. The reaction subsides rapidly and lesions on the face heal within 2 to 6 weeks and somewhat longer on the arms. Repeated courses of fluorouracil may be used and an overly brisk reaction may be treated locally with topical steroids. Because topical steroids protect against the inflammatory effect of fluorouracil but do not diminish its antitumor effect, it seems likely that fluorouracil exerts its effects by a cytotoxic mechanism, rather than a nonspecific inflammatory sloughing of superficial skin layers. This sloughing may in part be due to a local delayed hypersensitivity reaction.

C. Basal cell carcinoma (BCC)

1. **Natural history.** The most common type of BCC is the nodulo-ulcerative or "rodent ulcer" form. It presents as a well-defined nodule that has rolled pearly or translucent borders with telangiectases running across it, and a central concave area that is often ulcerated. A variety of histologic subtypes of this tumor may exist including solid, keratotic, cystic, and adenoid varieties. Pigmented types, which may resemble malignant melanoma (pigmented basal cell epithelioma), are important because of this differential diagnosis. These lesions have a low metastatic potential, and 85 percent of them are present on the skin of the head and neck. In neglected cases (1%–2% of total patients) metastases may occur; when seen, such metastases occur an average of 11 years after the primary lesion was first noted. Lymph nodes, lung, and bone may be involved in decreasing order of likelihood.

2. **Topical treatment.** Superficial surgery, electrodesiccation, chemosurgery, or radiation therapy may be used on these lesions. The cure rate should be above 95 percent regardless of the technique employed. Chemosurgery usually employs the use of zinc-chloride fixative paste (Mohs' technique).

The use of fluorouracil in a topical solution or ointment, as described under the treatment of actinic keratosis (**II.B.2**), is usually reserved for patients with multiple or widespread lesions because of the efficacy of the nonchemotherapeutic techniques. Deeply invasive tumors are not appropriately treated with fluorouracil because the drug only penetrates a few millimeters into the skin.

D. Squamous cell carcinoma (SCC)

1. **Natural history.** Squamous cell carcinoma may occur at any site on the skin as well as on mucous membranes—particularly on the lips, vulva, penis, and anus. The area from which it arises rarely appears normal, but usually has the changes we associate with actinic keratosis. The latter process may be considered an in situ stage of SCC. A rough, scaly surface with thickening of the skin and often well circumscribed macular changes are frequently present. A reddish, brownish, or grayish cast to the skin may also be present. Crusting, thickening, or ulceration strongly suggest malignant change. An indurated border also is suggestive of malignancy. The primary lesion histopathologically is in the epidermis, with cells penetrating into the dermis often with keratinization and epidermal pearl formation. The degree of cellular differentiation, atypicality of cells, and depth of penetration of the tumor are all prognostic factors. About 2 percent of patients develop metastatic tumors and 90 percent of these metastases are to the lymph nodes only. One half of patients with lymph node metastases and 60 percent of patients with distant metastases die within 5 years.

   The exceptional lesions that arise in normal-appearing skin or in other pre-existing lesions (scars of thermal, chemical, or radiation injury) tend to be more aggressive than those that arise in actinically damaged skin. Surgery by a variety of different means is the conventional treatment of SCC, as it is of BCC. This includes curettage or desiccation. Radiation therapy, cryotherapy, and chemosurgery have all been used. All produce cure rates in excess of 94 percent. Treatment of locally recurrent tumors is less satisfactory, and the importance of patients receiving prompt and adequate treatment early in the disease must be emphasized. As in BCC, the use of Mohs' chemosurgery with zinc-chloride fixative paste may be highly effective in SCC.

2. **Topical chemotherapy.** Superficial SCCs may be effectively treated with 5% topical fluorouracil with relatively little toxicity and an essentially 100 percent cure rate. However, it is important with more invasive lesions to avoid the possibility that fluorouracil may fail to control microscopic islands of invasive SCC and therefore may delay appropriate therapy. When treatment of more invasive or noduloulcerative SCC is contemplated, 20% fluorouracil under occlusive dressings may be employed if standard therapy is refused or contraindicated. As a rule, at least 3 weeks of treatment are required, but at times it may be necessary to treat for up to 12 weeks.

   In patients who have widespread multifocal superficial tumors developing, as in xeroderma pigmentosum, chronic arsenic exposure, extensive radiation dermatitis, or long-term extensive actinic changes, the use of surgical techniques may be impossible. In these patients, applications of dinitrochlorobenzene (DNCB), purified protein derivative of tuberculin (PPD), streptokinase-streptodornase (SKSD), or other agents may be clinically useful. These medications are applied in topical fashion to a large area of the skin in increasing concentrations and can produce selective lytic effects on malignant epidermal cells even when the cells are present in microscopic foci that otherwise would not be readily detectable. The allergic contact dermatitis that results from the application of these immunoadjuvants appears to destroy the great majority of microscopic basal cell carcinomas. Whether these allergic reactions are directly responsible for tumor lysis or whether they simply result from an attraction of sensitized "killer" lymphocytes to the areas where microscopic deposits of epidermoid neoplastic epidermal cells are present is not yet known. The fact that neoplastic epidermal cells are selectively killed has an important clinical implication. Scarring rarely develops from this type of treatment because normal epidermal cells remain viable and are not replaced by proliferating fibroblasts.

Selected Reading

Andrade, R. et al. (Eds.) *Cancer of the Skin: Biology, Diagnosis, Management.* Philadelphia: Saunders, 1976.

Bellet, R. E. et al. Chemotherapy of Metastatic Malignant Melanoma. In W. H. Clark, L. I. Goldman, and M. J. Mastrangelo (Eds.), *Human Malignant Melanoma.* New York: Grune & Stratton, 1979.

Constanza, M. et al. Metastatic basal cell carcinoma. *Cancer* 34:230, 1974.

Levene, M. B., Haynes, H. A., and Goldwyn, R. M. Cancers of the Skin. In *Cancer: Principles and Practice of Oncology.* V. T. DeVita, S. Hellman, and S. A. Rosenberg (Eds.). Philadelphia: Lippincott, 1982.

Nathanson, L. Epidemiologic and Etiologic Considerations in Malignant Melanoma. In J. Costanzi (Ed.), *Melanoma.* The Hague, The Netherlands: Martinus Nijhoff, 1982.

Nathanson, L. Malignant Melanoma. In P. R. Bergevin, J. Blom, and D. C. Tormey (Eds.), *A Guide to Therapeutic Oncology.* Baltimore: Williams & Wilkins, 1979.

Nathanson, L., Kaufman, S. D., and Carey, R. W. Vinblastine, infusion bleomycin, and cis-dichlorodiammine-platinum chemotherapy in metastatic melanoma. *Cancer* 48:1290–1294, 1981.

Strauss, A., Dritschilo, A., Nathanson, L., and Piro, A. J. Radiation therapy of malignant melanomas: an evaluation of clinically used fractionation schemes. *Cancer* 47:1262–1266, 1981.

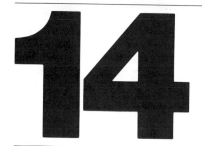

Primary Tumors of the Brain

Roland T. Skeel

I. Occurrence, tumor characteristics, and approach to treatment

A. Incidence. Primary tumors of the brain result in 2 to 3 percent of all deaths caused by cancer. This relatively low overall frequency belies their importance, however, for in persons under the age of 35 they are the second most common cause of cancer death. Although the total incidence of metastatic brain tumors is probably several times higher than that of primary brain tumors (up to 18% of patients who have cancer are found to have brain metastasis at autopsy), patients who first present with signs of an intracranial lesion are more likely to have a primary than a metastatic tumor.

B. Tissues from which primary brain tumors arise. The great majority of the primary intracranial neoplasms arise from either meningeal or neuroepithelial tissue. Meningiomas, the principal tumor type arising from meningeal tissue, constitute about one third of all primary intracranial tumors. Their behavior is generally benign, and surgical removal is most often curative. As chemotherapy has no role in the treatment of these tumors, meningiomas will not be considered further in this chapter.

C. Common primary malignant tumors. The major tumors arising from neuroepithelial tissue are the *astrocytoma,* the *oligodendroglioma,* and the *ependymoma,* which are all derived from glial cells, and the *medulloblastoma,* which appears to arise from more primitive neuroepithelial tissue and may have both glial and neuronal components.

D. Histologic grading. The glial-derived tumors all occur with a broad range of histologic differentiation, which ranges from slightly anaplastic to highly anaplastic. The potential curability and survival of patients with this group of tumors are highly dependent on the degree of anaplasia, and accurate histologic grading of the gliomas is critical in their evaluation and treatment planning.

E. Approach to therapy. With all four of the primary tumor types, the general approach to therapy is to surgically debulk the tumor (when possible) and then to follow surgery with radiotherapy with or without the addition of chemotherapy.

1. Surgery. How much tumor can be removed by surgery, or whether it can be removed at all, depends on the location of the lesion and how extensive and grossly infiltrating it is. Because even the least anaplastic gliomas tend to infiltrate normal brain tissue surrounding the obvious tumor mass, it is unusual to cure patients with surgery alone without resultant unacceptable neurologic deficits.

2. **Radiotherapy** has a major role as part of a combined modality treatment program for gliomas in even the less anaplastic, prognostically favorable lesions. Radiotherapy has an additional function in medulloblastomas, which have the greatest tendency of the CNS tumors to metastasize within the cranial spinal axis by shedding cells that form secondary implants. To treat patients with medulloblastomas, radiotherapy to the entire neuroaxis must follow surgical reduction or removal of the primary lesion.

3. **Chemotherapy** is used to treat patients with the more malignant gliomas. This group includes the more anaplastic neoplasms from any of the three glial tumors, which have variously been called glioblastoma multiforme, malignant astrocytoma, anaplastic astrocytoma, or Kernohan Grade III–IV astrocytoma, ependymoma, or oligodendroglioma. Because of the highly malignant features of medulloblastoma, and its tendency to spread through the neuroaxis, chemotherapy is also used to treat this tumor.

II. Chemotherapy of primary intracranial neoplasms

A. General considerations and aims of therapy

1. **Reduce cerebral edema and tumor mass.** Because of their location in the CNS, intracranial tumors, even while relatively small, may cause serious neurologic dysfunction including seizures, headache, and impairment of mental, motor, and sensory function. This dysfunction is the result of a combined effect of the tumor and a variable degree of surrounding cerebral edema. Therapy is therefore directed toward reducing the edema and the irritation of the normal brain (manifested as seizures) as well as reducing the size of the malignant tumor mass.

2. **Selection of chemotherapy.** The choice of chemotherapeutic agents for the treatment of malignant gliomas and other primary brain tumors must take into account physicochemical and pharmacokinetic considerations.

   a. **Physicochemical factors** that favor penetration of the blood-brain barrier include

   (1) High lipid solubility

   (2) Low degree of ionization at physiologic pH

   (3) Molecular weight of less than 500 daltons

   b. **Pharmacokinetic factors** including blood flow, peak serum levels, half life, and tissue distribution of the drug play an important role in determining effectiveness and drug scheduling.

   c. **Tumor factors.** Tumor-related factors are also important in the choice of appropriate agents. Despite their high degree of anaplasia, a large percentage of cells in gliomas appears to be in a resting state (G_0) and thus relatively insensitive to cycle active agents. Tumor heterogeneity is also characteristic of the gliomas and subpopulations may exist within a given tumor that are differentially resistant to a specific chemotherapeutic agent. Taken together, these factors are all likely to contribute to the difficulty in finding chemotherapeutic programs that will benefit a majority of the patients with gliomas.

3. **Aims of treatment.** The two major aims of therapy in gliomas are to reduce the neurologic deficit and consequent disability and to prolong useful and comfortable life by the reduction of the tumor mass and associated edema.

B. **Malignant gliomas.** Of all the chemotherapeutic agents that have been used in the treatment of malignant gliomas, the nitrosoureas are clearly the most effective, resulting in response rates of 40 to 50 percent when used alone and modest increases in survival when used together with radiotherapy. Regardless of the therapy, however, in the more malignant group of gliomas (those with marked anaplasia) the median survival is just 35 to 45 weeks from the time of first therapy. While the addition of chemotherapy to radiotherapy does not make a great difference in the median survival in patients with marked anaplasia, some evidence suggests that there is a small cohort that lives longer if multimodal therapy is given at the outset. In one study, the 18-month survival was 8 percent with radiotherapy alone and 18 percent with radiotherapy plus a nitrosourea. It thus seems warranted to treat the more malignant gliomas from the outset with combined radiotherapy and a nitrosourea.

Other agents that have some activity when administered systemically include hydroxyurea, procarbazine, dacarbazine, and mithramycin. Although several drug combinations have been tried, none yet shows any clear advantage.

1. **Nitrosourea treatment**

   a. The most effective agent that has been widely tested is carmustine given at a dose of 80 mg/m^2 IV days 1 to 3 every 6 to 8 weeks.

   b. Alternatives if oral therapy is desired or necessary are these:

      (1) Semustine, 220 mg/m^2 PO once every 6 to 8 weeks *or*

      (2) Lomustine, 130 mg/m^2 PO once every 6 to 8 weeks

   c. With each of the nitrosoureas, a second cycle should not be started until there is evidence of adequate marrow recovery.

2. **When to treat.** These drugs may be used

   a. Concomitantly with radiotherapy, beginning during the first few days of radiotherapy *or*

   b. After the radiotherapy treatments have been completed, *or*

   c. When the patient has evidence of recurrence following radiotherapy

3. **Duration and subsequent treatment.** Therapy should be continued as long as the patient does not progress, and the marrow function, as evidenced by blood counts, remains adequate.

Once the patient has relapsed from the initial chemotherapy regimen, it is not likely that a second regimen will be effective, and further chemotherapy is generally not recommended unless the patient wishes to participate as a subject in the clinical investigation of new drugs.

C. **Medulloblastomas.** There has been much less experience with chemo-therapy of medulloblastomas than with malignant gliomas, and no firm recommendation can be made. Because of the tendency for cerebrospinal fluid seeding to take place, intrathecal therapy with methotrexate as well as systemic chemotherapy has been used.

1. **Chemotherapy regimens** that have been effective include

   a. Carmustine, 80 mg/m^2 IV days 1 to 3 every 6 to 8 weeks as determined by bone marrow recovery *or*

   b. Vincristine, 1 to 2 mg/m^2 (maximum 2 mg) IV weekly up to 4 weeks. Subsequent frequency and dose may need to be reduced because of neurotoxicity to once every 3 to 4 weeks, *or*

   c. Methotrexate, 10 to 15 mg/m^2 intrathecally twice weekly for 2 to 3 weeks, then as determined by marrow and patient tolerance

2. **Toxicity** of all of the drugs may be enhanced by previous radiotherapy. Whether combinations will be more effective than single agents, or whether the addition of chemotherapy to the initial treatment with surgery and radiotherapy will be beneficial, must await further investigation.

III. **Treatment of cerebral edema and the prevention of seizures**

A. **Cerebral edema.** Reduction of cerebral edema may be accomplished either with high-dose corticosteroids, osmotic diuresis, or both.

1. **Corticosteroids: initial therapy.** The most commonly used steroid for the treatment of cerebral edema is dexamethasone. Therapy may be given as follows:

   a. Give dexamethasone 8 to 12 mg PO or IV

   b. Follow with 4 to 8 mg every 6 hours for as long as needed

   The need for continued dexamethasone may be determined by the patient's objective or subjective response to therapy directed at the tumor itself.

2. **Selection of maintenance treatment.** Following improvement with specific antitumor therapy, the steroid dose may be tapered over 1 to 3 weeks, watching for a return of symptoms. If symptoms do return, the dose should be returned to a level that maximizes therapeutic benefit and minimizes unwanted side effects, such as gastric irritation, peptic ulcer, increased appetite, sleeplessness, cushingoid features, and psychological disturbances. Patients should be told of the possible side effects of the steroid therapy so that they do not interpret them as an indication of tumor activity. It is also advisable to suggest that patients take an antacid with the steroid and that they watch for the occurrence of oral and vaginal thrush, which can be effectively treated with mycostatin suspension or suppositories.

3. **Treatment of refractory cerebral edema**

   a. **High-dose dexamethasone.** Occasionally 16 to 32 mg of dexamethasone daily is not effective in controlling cerebral edema. In such circumstances it may be helpful to increase the dose as follows:

(1) Dexamethasone: 40 mg IV every 4 to 6 hours, usually for no longer than 48 to 72 hours. Particular attention must be paid to the possible induction of peptic ulceration with this high dose of corticosteroid. If symptoms have been controlled with the higher dose, tapering should begin within the first 2 to 3 days.

(2) If the high dose is not effective in alleviating the signs and symptoms of cerebral edema, treatment may be abruptly reduced to the previous maintenance level of 16 to 32 mg daily and then cautiously tapered down from that level.

b. Mannitol diuresis. An alternative to administering high-dose steroid in an urgent situation is to use an osmotic diuretic.

(1) Mannitol, 75 to 100 g (as a 15–25% solution) is given by a rapid infusion (20–30 min) to be repeated in 12 hours as needed. (These doses are recommended for a 70–100 kg person. For persons weighing more or less, the doses should be increased or reduced appropriately.)

(2) Cautions. Careful monitoring of electrolytes, intake and output, and body weight is essential to avoid dehydration.

(3) Duration. The osmotic diuresis may be discontinued when there is an improvement in the signs and symptoms of the cerebral edema and the corticosteroids or other measures to reduce cerebral edema have taken effect.

B. Seizures. As the occurrence of seizures is quite common in patients with cerebral neoplasms, many physicians recommend starting all such patients on *anticonvulsant therapy* with phenytoin, 300 mg/day, regardless of whether the patient has already experienced a seizure.

Selected Reading

Burger, P. C., and Vollmer, R. T. Histologic factors of prognostic significance in the glioblastoma multiforme. *Cancer* 46:1179, 1980.

Edwards, M. S., Levin, V. A., and Wilson, C. B. Brain tumor chemotherapy. An evaluation of agents in current use for phases II and III trials. *Cancer Treat. Rep.* 64:1179, 1980.

Goldsmith, M. A., and Carter, S. R. Glioblastoma multiforme. A review of therapy. *Cancer Treat. Rev.* 1:153, 1974.

Mellett, L. B. Physicochemical considerations and pharmacokinetic behavior in delivery of drugs to the central nervous system. *Cancer Treat. Rep.* 61:527, 1977.

Shapiro, W. R. Chemotherapy of primary malignant brain tumors in children. *Cancer* 35:965, 1975.

Walker, M. D. et al. Evaluation of BCNU and/or radiotherapy in the treatment of anaplastic gliomas. *J. Neurosurg.* 49:333, 1978.

Soft Tissue Sarcomas

Robert S. Benjamin

I. Classification and approach to treatment

A. Types of soft tissue sarcomas. The soft tissue sarcomas are a group of diseases characterized by neoplastic proliferation of tissue of mesenchymal origin. Thus, they differ from the more common carcinomas, which arise from epithelial tissue. Sarcomas can arise in any area of the body and from any organ; however, they most commonly arise in soft tissue of the extremities, trunk, retroperitoneum, or head and neck area. There are at least 21 different types of sarcomas, classified according to lines of differentiation toward normal tissue. For example, rhabdomyosarcoma shows evidence of skeletal muscle fibers with cross-striations; liposarcoma shows fat production; and angiosarcoma shows vessel formation. Precise characterization of the types of sarcoma is often impossible, and these tumors are called *unclassified sarcomas*. All of the primary bony sarcomas may arise from soft tissue leading to such diagnoses as extraskeletal osteosarcoma, extraskeletal Ewing's sarcoma, and extraskeletal chondrosarcoma. An increasingly common diagnosis at present is malignant fibrous histiocytoma. This tumor is characterized by a mixture of spindle, or fibrous, cells and round, or histiocytic, cells arranged in a storiform pattern with frequent areas of pleomorphic appearance and frequent giant cells.

B. Metastatic spread of all sarcomas tends to be through the blood rather than through the lymphatic system. The lungs are by far the most frequent site of metastatic disease, and local recurrence by direct invasion is the second most common area of involvement followed by bone and liver. CNS metastases are extraordinarily rare.

C. Staging of sarcomas is complex and demands an expert sarcoma pathologist.

1. **The primary determinant of stage is tumor grade:** grade 1 tumors are stage I, grade 2 tumors are stage II, and grade 3 tumors are stage III. Any tumor with lymph node metastasis is automatically stage III, and any tumor with gross invasion of bone, major vessel, or major nerve is stage IV.

2. **Further division of stages** I to III into A and B are made based on *tumor size:* A = tumor size less than 5 cm, and B = tumor size 5 cm or greater. In stage III, lymph node metastases are classified as III_C, and in stage IV, local invasion as noted in **I.C.1** is called IV_A, and IV_B represents distant metastases.

D. Primary treatment

1. **Surgery and radiotherapy.** Treatment of the primary tumor involves surgery with or without radiation therapy. If radiation therapy is not used, surgery must be radical. While this may often involve amputation, more and more frequently at present, complete excision of the involved muscle group from origin to insertion is performed.

2. **Adjuvant chemotherapy.** The role of adjuvant chemotherapy is unclear. Several studies are currently underway to investigate the use of adjuvant chemotherapy, while other investigators believe that adjuvant therapy is clearly indicated for patients whose histologic type, grade, or location is known to convey a poor prognosis.

E. Prognosis

is related to stage with a 5-year survival rate of 75 percent for stage I, 55 percent for stage II, and 29 percent for stage III. The survival rate for stage IV disease is less than 10 percent; however, a definite fraction of patients in this category can be cured. The majority of patients with stage IV disease, if left untreated, die within 6 to 12 months; however, there is great variation in actual survival and patients may go on with slowly progressive disease for many years.

F. Response to treatment

is measured in the standard fashion for solid tumors.

1. **Complete remission** implies complete disappearance of all signs and symptoms of disease.

2. **Partial remission** is a 50 percent or greater decrease in measurable disease, calculated by comparing the sum of the products of perpendicular diameters of all lesions before and after therapy. When disease is not measurable in two dimensions but can be followed objectively by angiogram, x-ray, ultrasound, or computerized tomography, a definite decrease in the amount of metastatic disease confirmed by two independent investigators is the equivalent of a partial response as calculated by a 50 percent decrease in measurable tumor.

3. **Lesser degrees of tumor shrinkage** are categorized by some physicians as stable disease and by others as improvement. Stable disease implies a less than 25 percent increase in disease for at least 8 weeks. For all response categories, no new disease must appear during response.

4. **Progression.** New disease in any area or a 25 percent or more increase in measurable disease constitutes progressive disease.

5. **Survival.** In all cases, patients whose disease responds objectively to chemotherapy survive longer than patients with progressive disease, and the degree of prolongation of survival is directly proportional to the degree of antitumor response that can be measured.

II. Chemotherapy of soft tissue sarcomas

A. General considerations and aims of therapy.

Although there are numerous types of soft tissue sarcomas, there is essentially no difference among them regarding responsiveness to a standard soft tissue sarcoma regimen. Two tumors, Ewing's sarcoma and rhabdomyosarcoma, particularly in the pediatric age group, are responsive in a fraction of cases to dactinomycin, vincristine, or both. The other tumors are not. The goal of therapy for patients with advanced disease is primarily palliative, although a small fraction, about 20 percent, of patients who achieve complete remission are, in fact, cured. The first aim, therefore, is to achieve complete remission, and we have demonstrated that the prognoses are the same whether complete remission is obtained by chemotherapy alone or chemotherapy with adjuvant surgery, that is, surgical removal of all residual disease. Thereafter, chemotherapy is continued. Short of complete remission, partial remission causes some palliation with relief of symptoms and prolongation of survival by approximately 1 year. Any degree of improvement or stabilization of previously advancing disease will likewise increase survival.

B. **Effective drugs.** The most important chemotherapeutic agent is doxorubicin (Adriamycin™), which forms the backbone of all combination chemotherapy regimens. Dacarbazine (DTIC®), a marginal agent by itself, adds significantly to doxorubicin (Adriamycin™) in prolonging remission duration and survival as well as increasing the response rate. Cyclophosphamide adds marginally, if at all, but is included in the most effective regimens.

The key to effective sarcoma chemotherapy is the steep dose-response curve for doxorubicin (Adriamycin™). At a dose of 45 mg/m^2, the response rate is less than 20 percent compared with a 37 percent response rate at a dose of 75 mg/m^2. A similar dose-response relationship exists within combination chemotherapy, and the regimens with the best reported results are those utilizing the highest doses.

C. **Primary chemotherapy regimen.** The most effective primary chemotherapy regimen is cyclophosphamide, doxorubicin (Adriamycin™), and dacarbazine (DTIC®) (CyADIC). This regimen is a modification of the standard CyVADIC regimen, which includes vincristine. Since analysis has shown that vincristine makes no significant contribution and produces neurotoxicity, its addition at a dose of 2 mg maximum or 1.4 mg/m^2 weekly for 6 weeks and then once every 3 to 4 weeks is recommended only for rhabdomyosarcoma and Ewing's sarcoma.

1. The **standard CyADIC regimen** is as follows:

   a. Cyclophosphamide, 600 mg/m^2 IV day 1

   b. Doxorubicin (Adriamycin™), 60 mg/m^2 IV day 1

   c. Dacarbazine (DTIC®), 250 mg/m^2 IV days 1 to 5

   Repeat cycle every 3 to 4 weeks.

2. **Dose modification.** Doses of doxorubicin (Adriamycin™) and cyclophosphamide should be increased or decreased by 25 percent each course of therapy in order to achieve a lowest absolute granulocyte count of approximately 500/μl. Maximum doxorubicin (Adriamycin™) dose is limited to 450 mg/m^2, at which point therapy should be discontinued. With Ewing's sarcoma and rhabdomyosarcoma, therapy is continued and dactinomycin, 2 mg/m^2 single dose or 0.5 mg/m^2 daily for 5 days, may be substituted for the doxorubicin (Adriamycin™) with continuation of the regimen for a total of 18 months.

3. An **alternative regimen for children with rhabdomyosarcoma** is the so-called pulse VAC regimen. Dactinomycin is given at a total dose of 2.0 to 2.5 mg/m^2 by divided daily injections over 5 to 7 days (e.g. 0.5

mg/m^2 daily for 5 days) repeated every 3 months for a total of 5 courses. Cyclophosphamide pulses of 275 to 330 mg/m^2/day for 7 days are given every 6 weeks with vincristine, 2 mg/m^2 on days 1 and 8 of each cyclophosphamide cycle. Cyclophosphamide cycles are terminated prematurely if the white blood count falls below 1500/μl. Chemotherapy continues for 2 years.

D. Secondary chemotherapy. Secondary chemotherapy for patients with sarcoma is uniformly unrewarding with response rates less than 10 percent for almost all drugs or regimens tested. When patients fail primary chemotherapy, therefore, they should be entered on a phase II study of a new agent to see if some activity can be established although reasonably good alternatives do not exist.

E. Complications of chemotherapy. Side effects of sarcoma chemotherapy can be classified in three categories: life-threatening, potentially dangerous, and unpleasant.

  1. **Life-threatening complications** of chemotherapy are infection or bleeding. Since thrombocytopenia of less than 20,000/μl rarely occurs with this type of chemotherapy, bleeding is rare. Approximately 20 percent of patients will have documented or suspected infection related to drug-induced neutropenia at some time during their treatment course. These infections are rarely fatal if treated promptly at the onset of the febrile neutropenic episode with broad spectrum, bactericidal antibiotics.

  2. **Potentially dangerous** side effects of chemotherapy include the following:

     a. Mucositis in less than 25 percent of patients, which may interfere with oral intake or may act as a source of infection

     b. Granulocytopenia, which predisposes the patient to infection but because of its brevity, rarely causes infection

     c. Thrombocytopenia, which is usually insignificant

     d. Cardiac damage from doxorubicin (Adriamycin™) rarely causes clinical problems at the doses recommended, with usually reversible congestive heart failure occurring in less than 5 percent of patients.

  3. **Unpleasant** but rarely serious problems include nausea and vomiting, primarily from dacarbazine, and alopecia, from doxorubicin (Adriamycin™) and cyclophosphamide.

Selected Reading

Benjamin, R. S. et al. The Chemotherapy of Soft Tissue Sarcomas in Adults. In *Management of Primary Bone and Soft Tissue Tumors.* Chicago: Year Book, 1977. Pp. 309–316.

Lindberg, R. D. et al. Conservative Surgery and Radiation Therapy for Soft Tissue Sarcomas. In *Management of Primary Bone and Soft Tissue Tumors.* Chicago: Year Book, 1977. Pp. 289–298.

Russell, W. O. et al. A clinical and pathological staging system for soft tissue sarcomas. *Cancer* 40:1562, 1977.

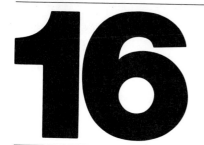

Bony Sarcomas

Robert S. Benjamin

There are four major sarcomas of bone, each differing somewhat in clinical behavior, chemotherapy responsiveness, and prognosis. All present as painful bony lesions, and all metastasize preferentially to lung and then to other bones.

Untreated prognosis is inversely proportional to chemotherapeutic responsiveness. The sarcomas will be considered in order of chemotherapeutic responsiveness, which is as follows: (1) Ewing's sarcoma, (2) malignant fibrous histiocytoma of bone, (3) osteosarcoma, and (4) chondrosarcoma.

Response to treatment is evaluated according to the usual criteria used for solid tumors and identical to that reported in Chapter 15 on soft tissue sarcomas. Angiography is particularly helpful in defining response of primary bone tumors to chemotherapy, and angiographic response correlates well with pathologic tumor destruction. Often, needle biopsy or complete resection and examination of the total specimen is required to follow response to therapy in a primary lesion and to confirm complete remission.

I. Ewing's sarcoma

A. General considerations and aims of therapy

1. **Tumor characteristics.** Ewing's sarcoma is a highly malignant small round cell tumor of bone. It occurs most commonly in the second decade with 90 percent of patients under age 30. There is a slight predominance of males. The most common locations are in the pelvis or the diaphysis of long tubular bones of the extremities. Often systemic symptoms of fever and leukocytosis suggest infection. Radiographically, the predominant feature is osteolysis, although sclerosis does occur. Frequently, the periosteal reaction has the so-called onion skin pattern with layering of subperiosteal new bone, frequently with spicules radiating out from the cortex. Prognosis, until recently, was extremely poor with a less than 10 percent 5-year survival and almost one half of the patients dead within 1 year of diagnosis.

2. **Primary treatment.** For this reason and because of the multilative surgery involved in resection of the primary lesion, radiotherapy has been the primary modality for local tumor control with adjuvant chemotherapy employed. As chemotherapy has improved and as techniques for limb salvage surgery have become more widely practiced, attempts to utilize surgery rather than radiation therapy are again increasing.

B. Chemotherapy

1. **CyVADIC regimen.** Perhaps the best chemotherapeutic regimen for Ewing's sarcoma is the CyVADIC regimen outlined in Chapter 15 (see p. 153) for soft tissue sarcomas.

   a. Cyclophosphamide, 600 mg/m^2 IV day 1

   b. Vincristine, 1.4 mg/m^2 (2 mg maximum) IV weekly for 6 weeks, then day 1 of each cycle

   c. Doxorubicin (Adriamycin™), 60 mg/m^2 IV day 1

   d. Dacarbazine (DTIC®), 250 mg/m^2 IV days 1 to 5

   Repeat cycle every 3 to 4 weeks.

2. **Dose modifications.** Courses are repeated with a 25 percent increase or decrease in dose of cyclophosphamide, depending on morbidity. Courses are repeated in 3 to 4 weeks as soon as recovery to 1500 granulocytes and 100,000 platelets occurs. Complications are as described in Chapter 15 (see p. 154), with the addition of peripheral neuropathy from vincristine. When the cumulative dose of doxorubicin (Adriamycin™) has reached 450 mg/m^2, dactinomycin is substituted at a dose of 2 mg/m^2 day 1 or 0.5 mg/m^2 daily for 5 days for a total of 18 months of chemotherapy.

3. **Alternative regimens** omit dacarbazine; vary doses of cyclophosphamide up to 1500 mg/m^2; give dactinomycin with, or in place of, doxorubicin (Adriamycin™); and in some cases, add high-dose methotrexate. Direct comparison of the various approaches has not shown marked superiority of one regimen over another.

4. **Responses.** The majority of patients with metastatic disease will obtain complete remission; however, almost all patients will relapse and ultimately die of disease. When chemotherapy is used in the therapy of primary disease with surgery or radiation, prognosis depends on the size and location of the primary tumor. Patients with large flat-bone lesions have a less than 30 percent cure rate compared with a 60 to 70 percent cure rate for those patients with round-bone lesions, which are generally smaller. An alarming complication of the chemotherapy–radiation therapy combination is a high frequency of second malignancies in cured patients, with 4 of 10 patients in one series developing secondary sarcomas within their radiated fields. This complication is another reason for considering surgical intervention rather than radiation, since chemotherapy is required for cure whether or not the primary lesion can be controlled with radiation.

5. **Secondary chemotherapy.** Occasional responses have been seen with etoposide (VP-16), other alkylating agents, nitrosoureas, and cisplatin. Nonetheless, secondary responses are extremely poor and the survival of a relapsed patient with Ewing's sarcoma is measured in weeks.

II. Malignant fibrous histiocytoma of bone. This recently reported entity, characterized by a purely lytic lesion in bone, has an exceptionally poor prognosis when treated with surgery alone, although numbers of reported patients are small. The tumor responds well to the CyADIC regimen for soft tissue sarcomas with more than one half of patients showing at least partial remission. In addition, cisplatin at a dose of 120 mg/m^2 every 4 weeks has caused remissions, even in patients who have failed primary therapy. A particularly attractive approach for patients with large, unresectable primary tumors is the use of cisplatin given by the intraarterial route. Complete tumor destruction in one patient and a good partial remission in a second patient have been reported among three patients so treated. After local tumor destruction, surgery may be employed to remove residual disease. Because of the primary poor prognosis, adjuvant chemotherapy with the CyADIC regimen is recommended until a 450 mg/m^2 cumulative doxorubicin (Adriamycin™) dose has been reached.

III. Osteosarcoma

A. General considerations. Osteosarcoma is a tumor with a poor prognosis in the absence of effective chemotherapy. It is the most common primary bone sarcoma. Frequently, it affects patients 10 to 25 years old and tends to be located around the knee in about two thirds of patients, with two thirds of those tumors involving the distal femur. As with other sarcomas of bone, pulmonary metastases are most common, followed by bony metastases.

B. Role of chemotherapy. Chemotherapy is usually employed in the adjuvant situation and its value in this regard has been conclusively demonstrated by the use of preoperative chemotherapy. Patients who demonstrate response to preoperative chemotherapy with complete or total tumor destruction have significantly improved survival. Response rates in evaluable tumors range from 30 to 80 percent. Cure of primary disease with adjuvant chemotherapy is 50 to 80 percent.

C. Effective agents. The three major single agents in the treatment of osteosarcoma are methotrexate, doxorubicin (Adriamycin™), and cisplatin. In addition, the combination of bleomycin, cyclophosphamide, and dactinomycin (BCD) has been effective.

D. Recommended regimen. A variety of regimens may be recommended based on preliminary, or more extensive, evaluation. These are as follows:

1. Doxorubicin (Adriamycin™) and cisplatin

  a. Doxorubicin, 75 to 90 mg/m^2 IV day 1

  b. Cisplatin, 90 to 120 mg/m^2 IV day 1

  Repeat every 4 weeks. Discontinue both drugs after 450 mg/m^2 cumulative doxorubicin (Adriamycin™) dose. If cisplatin must be discontinued earlier, substitute dacarbazine, 250 mg/m^2 IV days 1 to 5 or 1 g/m^2 IV day 1 as a single dose.

2. Alternating cyclic chemotherapy is as follows:

  a. High-dose methotrexate, 8 to 12 g/m^2 IV weekly for 4 weeks with leucovorin rescue (see **III.E.2**)

  b. Three weeks later start BCD

  (1) Bleomycin, 12 mg/m^2 IM daily days 1 and 2

(2) Cyclophosphamide, 600 mg/m^2 IV days 1 and 2

(3) Dactinomycin, 450 μg/m^2 IV days 1 and 2

c. Three weeks later repeat high-dose methotrexate weekly for 2 weeks

d. One week later give doxorubicin (Adriamycin™), 35 mg/m^2 IV days 1 and 2

e. Three weeks later repeat high-dose methotrexate weekly for 2 weeks. Recycle using the sequence of BCD, high-dose methotrexate, doxorubicin (Adriamycin™), and high-dose methotrexate for 5 courses.

E. Special precautions in administration

1. Cisplatin. Prehydration is necessary, either with overnight infusion of IV fluids at 150 ml/hr for an adult or 1 liter over 2 hours, followed by at least 6 liters of fluid for the first day following cisplatin administration. The addition of mannitol, 50 ml of a 20% solution prior to cisplatin followed by 200 ml of a 20% solution mixed with normal saline in a total volume of 1 liter to run simultaneously with the cisplatin over 2 to 3 hours is preferred by many investigators. Particular care in electrolyte balance, including frequent determinations of magnesium, is necessary. In the presence of severe hypomagnesemia, magnesium sulfate, 1 to 2 mEq/kg, may be infused over 4 hours.

2. High-dose methotrexate. Pretreatment creatinine clearance should be greater than 70 ml/min.

a. Methotrexate administration and alkalinization of urine. Before administration of high-dose methotrexate, ½ mEq/kg sodium bicarbonate is infused IV over 15 to 30 minutes in an attempt to create an alkaline urine. Allopurinol, 300 mg daily for 3 days, is given before starting methotrexate infusion. Methotrexate is dissolved in no more than 1000 ml of 5% dextrose in water with a final concentration of approximately 1 g/100 ml. The total dose ranges from 8 g/m^2 for fully grown patients to 12 g/m^2 for children. Fifty mEq of sodium bicarbonate is added per liter. Methotrexate is infused over 4 hours. Following completion of the methotrexate, 10 ml/kg of an IV infusion of 5% dextrose in water with 50 mEq/liter of bicarbonate is given over 2 hours, if the patient is unable to drink or if the 24-hour methotrexate levels of the previous high-dose methotrexate treatment have been greater than 1.5 × 10^{-5}M. The IV is then discontinued and the patient is encouraged to drink sufficient fluid to produce approximately 1600 ml/m^2 of alkaline urine for the first 24 hours, and 1900 ml/m^2 daily for the next 3 days. Sodium bicarbonate, 14 to 28 mEq every 6 hours PO, is administered to encourage alkaline urine. The pH of the urine is measured and if it is less than 7, an extra dose of bicarbonate is administered.

b. Leucovorin rescue. Twenty-four hours after the start of the methotrexate infusion, leucovorin, 10 to 15 mg PO is administered q6h for at least 10 doses, or IM if the oral medication is not tolerated.

c. **Serum methotrexate levels** should be followed daily and should fall approximately 1 log/day. When methotrexate concentration falls below 5×10^{-8}M, leucovorin may be safely discontinued. IV hydration is required whenever oral intake is insufficient to produce sufficient urine output as previously defined, for abnormal serum methotrexate concentration, for persistent vomiting, or for early toxicity.

F. **Complications.** Complications of chemotherapy depend on the drugs. For doxorubicin (Adriamycin™) and cyclophosphamide, the major complication is infection from neutropenia. Other complications include stomatitis, nausea and vomiting, and delayed cardiac toxicity, as discussed in the management of soft tissue sarcomas (Chap. 15, p. 154). Dactinomycin causes similar non-cardiac side effects. Methotrexate predominantly causes stomatitis, but it may cause myelosuppression and renal and hepatic abnormalities. Cisplatin and dacarbazine cause severe nausea and vomiting. In addition, cisplatin nephrotoxicity is primarily a tubular defect with hypomagnesemia as the most prominent manifestation, but hypocalcemia, hypokalemia, and hyponatremia also occur. Delayed cumulative nephrotoxicity can cause impaired glomerular function as well. Ototoxicity may also occur but is less common. Delayed neurotoxicity also occurs. Both cisplatin and methotrexate can, by causing renal toxicity, exacerbate their other side effects.

G. **Recurrence and treatment of refractory disease.** Patients refractory to a combination of doxorubicin (Adriamycin™) and cisplatin may respond to high-dose methotrexate; patients refractory to high-dose methotrexate may respond to doxorubicin (Adriamycin™)–cisplatin; and patients refractory to both may respond to BCD. However, treatment of refractory disease is usually disappointing, and participation in studies of new agents are indicated for patients whose disease cannot be resected. Surgical resection of pulmonary metastases remains the only viable secondary therapy for the majority of patients. For this reason, careful follow-up for detection of metastases while they are still at the stage of resectability is indicated.

IV. **Chondrosarcoma.** The chemotherapy for chondrosarcoma is totally inadequate and no regimen can be recommended except for the rare patient with mesenchymal chondrosarcoma, a subtype that may respond to CyADIC chemotherapy or cisplatin. The vast majority of patients are candidates only for surgical management. Metastatic disease should be treated on phase II protocols in an attempt to determine some effective type of chemotherapy that may be recommended in the future.

Selected Reading

Benjamin, R. S. et al. Chemotherapy for metastatic osteosarcoma. Studies by the M. D. Anderson Hospital and the Southwest Oncology Group. *Cancer Treat. Rep.* 62:237, 1978.

Ettinger, I. J. et al. Adriamycin™ and cis-diamminedichloroplatinum as adjuvant therapy in primary osteosarcoma. *Proc. Am. Assoc. Cancer Res. and Am. Soc. Clin. Oncol.* 20:438, 1979.

Gehan, E. A. et al. Osteosarcoma: The M. D. Anderson Experience, 1950–1974. In W. D. Terry and D. Windhorst (Eds.), *Immunotherapy of Cancer: Present Status of Trials in Man.* New York: Raven, 1978.

Rosen, G. Past Experiences and Future Considerations with T-2 Chemotherapy in the Treatment of Ewing's Sarcoma. In *Management of Primary Bone & Soft Tissue Tumors.* Chicago: Year Book, 1977. Pp. 187–204.

Rosen, G., Caparros, B., and Nirenberg, A. The Successful Management of Metastatic Osteogenic Sarcoma: A Model for the Treatment of Primary Osteogenic Sarcoma. In A. T. van Oosterom, F. M. Muggia, and F. J. Cleton (Eds.), *Therapeutic Progress in Ovarian Cancer, Testicular Cancer and the Sarcomas.* Hingham: Leiden University Press, 1980. Pp. 349–365.

Leukemias

Roland T. Skeel

I. **Types of leukemia and response criteria.** The leukemias are a group of neoplastic diseases characterized by an abnormal proliferation of blood cells and their immature precursors. Leukemia may involve either lymphocytic or nonlymphocytic cell lines, and within each group the characteristic cell may be either relatively mature or immature in appearance. The leukemias with immature appearing cells are termed *acute* because of their short natural history (1–5 months) when untreated, and those leukemias with cells having a more mature appearance are called *chronic* because of their more slow, progressive course (2–5 years).

A. **Leukemia categories**

1. **The four major groups** of leukemia are as follows:

    a. Acute lymphocytic leukemia (ALL)

    b. Acute nonlymphocytic leukemia (ANLL)

    c. Chronic lymphocytic leukemia (CLL)

    d. Chronic granulocytic (nonlymphocytic) leukemia (CGL)

2. **Subgroups.** ANLL includes several discernible subcategories that will be discussed **III.A.1.** CGL may also be referred to as *chronic myelocytic leukemia* or *chronic myelogenous leukemia* (both CML).

B. **Response to treatment** of leukemia is determined by the degree of reduction in the number of neoplastic cells in the blood, marrow, and extramedullary sites; and the return of the patient's functional status.

1. **Complete remission (CR)** indicates that the neoplastic cells have been reduced to undetectable levels, the marrow appearance and function have returned to normal (unless continually suppressed by chemotherapy), and the patient has regained essentially normal functional status.

2. **Lesser degrees of response** are called *partial response* or *improvement.* In the acute leukemias, CR is generally necessary for the patient to derive benefit from therapy, while in the chronic leukemias CR is difficult to achieve, and partial response or improvement may provide clinically significant improvement in the patient's symptoms.

II. **Acute lymphocytic leukemia (ALL)**

A. **General considerations and aims of therapy.** ALL is a disease found predominantly in childhood between ages 2 and 10.

1. **Morphologic types.** There are three morphologic variants.

   a. L1—Homogeneous cell population commonly seen in childhood

   b. L2—Heterogeneous cell population commonly seen in adults

   c. L3—Rare Burkitt-type homogeneous cell population

2. **The aim of treatment** in ALL is complete eradication of all leukemia cells from the body so that cure may be achieved. ALL is quite responsive to chemotherapy and upwards of 50 percent of all children without high-risk factors and who are treated for this disease may have long-term disease-free survival with permanent cure being likely. In contrast to this, a long-term disease-free survival is likely in less than 25 percent of children with high-risk factors. The following are factors associated with a poor prognosis in ALL:

   a. High white blood count

   b. Extramedullary infiltrate (including meningeal leukemia)

   c. Age of less than 2 or greater than 9

   d. Mediastinal mass

   e. T-cell markers on leukemia cells

   f. Black (race)

3. **Treatment of ALL** is comprised of three parts:

   a. Remission induction

   b. CNS prophylaxis

   c. Treatment during remission

   Although the treatment of ALL is relatively standardized, successful treatment is not guaranteed by following any standard protocol. Because the stakes are high, and seemingly minor differences in management may be critical, it is advised that all children and adults with ALL be evaluated and have their therapy directed by an experienced oncologist or hematologist. Most oncologists and hematologists look forward to having the primary care physician share in the care of the patient, as the latter can contribute greatly to the optimal management of this disease.

B. **Remission induction.** Remission induction therapy of ALL is probably more "standard" than most other chemotherapy regimens, although, as with treatment for other neoplasms, the treatment for ALL is not static but undergoing refinements to improve on the long-term benefits of treatment.

   1. **Prophylaxis of hyperuricemia and infection.** Before remission induction is begun, all patients must be started on allopurinol, 200 mg/m^2 PO daily to avert hyperuricemia that results in renal complications. Some oncologists recommend the use of trimethoprim 160 mg and sulfamethoxazole 800 mg bid (adult dose) to decrease the likelihood of severe infections.

2. Standard remission induction therapy consists of

  a. Vincristine, 2 mg/m^2 (up to 2 mg) IV weekly for 4 weeks *and*

  b. Prednisone, 40 mg/m^2 PO daily for 28 days, then taper over 1 week

  Additional therapy during induction is probably helpful in getting a few additional patients into remission and may obviate any need for cyclic "reinduction." Therapy may be *either* asparaginase or daunorubicin:

  c. Asparaginase

   (1) 1000 IU/kg IV days 1 to 10 *or*

   (2) 10,000 IU/m^2 IV days 1 and 8 *or*

   (3) 5000 IU/kg IV days 1, 8, and 15

  d. Daunorubicin, 25 mg/m^2 IV weekly for 4 weeks

  The L-asparaginase and daunorubicin are commonly used in patients in the high-risk categories although this use does not always prevent the subsequent recurrence of their leukemia.

C. CNS prophylaxis. Despite the effectiveness of vincristine and prednisone induction therapy in reducing the leukemia blast cells in the peripheral blood and marrow, more than 50 percent of patients will experience relapse in the CNS unless some therapy is directed toward eradicating cells in this sanctuary site. CNS prophylaxis is begun within 2 weeks after the achievement of complete remission. The most widely used program involves

1. Cranial irradiation, 2400 rad (less for children under 3 years old) in 150 to 200 rad fractions, *and simultaneously*

2. Intrathecal methotrexate, 12 mg/m^2 twice a week for five doses

The cranial irradiation is given down to the level of C-2 and anteriorly to include the posterior pole of the eye. The intrathecal methotrexate is given in the lumbar area using preservative-free saline or Elliot's B solution (artificial spinal fluid) as the vehicle. The volume of diluent should be large—at least 5 cc/m^2—to assure sufficient volume to reach the higher spinal meninges and to prevent a high local concentration of methotrexate.

D. Treatment during remission. Following CNS prophylaxis, treatment is continued during remission for at least 2 years and up to 5 years. Standard maintenance therapy is as follows:

1. Mercaptopurine, 50 mg/m^2 PO daily, *and*

2. Methotrexate, 20 mg/m^2 PO or IV weekly

Each agent is to be given continuously with adjustments for cytopenias as shown in Table 17-1. If leukocyte count is persistently above 3500 cells/μl, increase dosages by 25 percent.

3. The addition of cyclic reinduction with

  a. Vincristine, 1.5 mg/m^2 (up to 2 mg) IV weekly for 2 weeks *and*

Table 17-1. Dosage Adjustment for Hematologic Toxicity in ALL in Remission (Fraction of Full Dose of Mercaptopurine and Methotrexate)

Platelet Count (cells/μl)	White Blood Count (cells/μl)			
	>2500	2000–2500	1500–2000	<1500
>100,000	1	⅔	⅓	0
75,000–100,000	⅔	⅔	⅓	0
50,000–75,000	⅓	⅓	⅓	0
<50,000	0	0	0	0

Note: The aim in maintenance therapy is to keep the WBC between 2000 and 3500 and to keep the platelets above 75,000.

    b. Prednisone, 40 mg/m^2 PO daily for 14 days. Given every 10 to 12 weeks during remission therapy probably does not add to the overall result if the remission induction regimen contains asparaginase or an anthracycline.

E. Complications

1. **Complications arising during induction or maintenance chemotherapy** may result from the leukemia, its treatment, or a combination of both. Bleeding or infection may arise during the induction or maintenance phase and may be due to myelophthisis from the leukemia, drug-induced cytopenia, or drug-induced immunosuppression. The management of these problems is discussed in Chapter 25. Other possible side effects caused by the drugs include mucositis, anaphylaxis, neurotoxicity, cardiotoxicity, hepatic or pulmonary fibrosis, impaired fertility and second neoplasms.

2. **Complications from CNS prophylaxis** include a postradiation syndrome characterized by fatigue, lack of appetite, and somnolence. This syndrome usually abates without specific therapy. There have also been some reports of long-term psychological dysfunction and minor degrees of cerebral atrophy in some patients. The relative contributions of radiotherapy, intrathecal therapy, and systemic chemotherapy have not been clearly ascertained, although a demyelinating leukoencephalopathy has resulted from the parenteral administration of large doses of methotrexate to patients who have previously had cranial irradiation.

F. Recurrence and treatment of refractory disease. Patients who fail to respond to initial therapy or who relapse after initial response may be difficult to treat.

An effective regimen for the treatment of relapse is

1. Asparaginase, 15,000 IU/m^2 IV days 1 to 5, 8 to 12, 15 to 19, and 22 to 26, *and*

2. Vincristine, 2 mg/m^2 (up to 2 mg) IV days 8, 15, and 22, *and*

3. Daunorubicin, 30 to 60 mg/m^2 IV days 8, 15, and 22, *and*

4. Prednisone, 40 mg/m^2 PO days 8 to 12, 15 to 19, and 22 to 26

Additional available drugs of some value in ALL include cyclophosphamide, hydroxyurea, carmustine, and cytarabine, as well as a few investigational drugs.

III. Acute nonlymphocytic leukemia (ANLL)

A. General considerations and aims of therapy

1. **Morphologic types.** *ANLL* is a term used for a group of related leukemias that are primarily seen in adults. As a group, they are not nearly so responsive to chemotherapy as is ALL using either remission induction or survival as the measure. There are six morphologic variants, three showing predominantly granulocytic differentiation, two monocytic differentiation, and one erythrocytic differentiation.

   a. M1—Minimal myeloid differentiation without maturation

   b. M2—Myeloid differentiation with maturation to promyelocyte and beyond

   c. M3—Myeloid differentiation with highly abnormal cells packed with abnormal azurophilic granules or numerous Auer rods (hypergranular promyelocytic leukemia)

   d. M4—Heterogeneous, mixed myelomonocytic leukemia

   e. M5—Homogeneous monocytic leukemia

   f. M6—Erythroleukemia

   Some evidence suggests that those variants with a monocytic component (M4 and M5) respond better to treatment than those variants without one.

2. **The aim of treatment** in ANLL is CR, which can be expected in 55 to 80 percent of patients. Five to 10 percent of patients may have long-term disease-free survival. The likelihood of CR in patients over the age of 60 used to be poorer than in younger patients, but with more effective regimens and better support, the remission rate in the elderly now seems just as good. Treatment for ANLL is separated into two phases:

   a. Remission induction

   b. Treatment during remission

B. Remission induction.
Before remission induction therapy is begun, allopurinol must be started at a dose of 200 mg/m^2 PO daily. We also recommend the use of trimethoprim 160 mg and sulfamethoxazole 800 mg bid (adult dose) to decrease the likelihood of severe infection.

1. **A standard regimen** used for remission induction of ANLL consists of three drugs given in combination:

   a. Daunorubicin, 60 mg/m^2 IV push days 1 to 3

   b. Cytarabine, 200 mg/m^2 IV as a continuous infusion, days 1 to 5

   c. Thioguanine, 100 mg/m^2 PO q12h, days 1 to 5

2. **A bone marrow examination** is done sometime between the 12th and 14th days; if the marrow still has a significant infiltration of leukemia

cells, the cycle is repeated. The drugs are then stopped and the marrow is allowed to recover. When the cellularity has returned to normal, an assessment of the morphology is made to determine whether a marrow remission has been attained. If a CR has been achieved, the patient is given consolidation or maintenance therapy. If a CR has not been achieved, re-induction may be attempted. Marked marrow hypoplasia is anticipated with this regimen, and drug doses are neither held nor attenuated because of cytopenias. Facilities to support the patient through 3 to 5 weeks of profound leukopenia and thrombocytopenia must be available before therapy for ANLL is initiated.

C. **Treatment during remission.** There are a variety of opinions regarding what therapy should be used following the attainment of CR in ANLL, and even some question as to whether therapy during remission prolongs remission duration and survival. It clearly results in morbidity and some mortality. The objective of treatment during remission is to prevent recurrence of the leukemia. The alternatives to achieve this objective include (a) consolidation followed by maintenance, (b) consolidation followed by no therapy, and (c) maintenance alone.

1. **Consolidation** consists of one or two intensive cycles of chemotherapy designed to "consolidate" the gains made during remission induction. Doses are such to give an anticipated marrow hypoplasia from which the patient will recover in 7 to 14 days.

   a. Daunorubicin, 45 mg/m^2 IV days 1 and 2, *and*

   b. Cytarabine, 100 mg/m^2 as a 30-minute infusion q12h for 10 doses (days 1 to 5), *and*

   c. Thioguanine, 100 mg/m^2 PO q12h days 1 to 5

2. **Maintenance therapy** begins when the marrow and peripheral blood have recovered following either induction or consolidation therapy. Anthracyclines are generally not used because of cumulative cardiac toxicity. Drug doses are chosen to cause significant, but not life-threatening, cytopenias.

   a. Thioguanine, 40 mg/m^2 PO q12h for 8 doses (days 1–4), *and*

   b. Cytarabine, 60 mg/m^2 SC day 5 only

3. **Immunotherapy** during remission of ANLL remains an experimental, although promising means of therapy. While it does not appear to prolong remission duration, it may increase survival time by virtue of increasing the rate of second remissions and postrelapse survival.

4. **Bone marrow transplantation** is offered at a few centers for patients in their first or second remission of ANLL, and in selected patients under 30 years of age it results in a 60 percent disease-free survival for more than 1 year. It should not be undertaken by persons or centers without extensive experience.

D. **Complications.** Supportive care of patients undergoing remission induction therapy for ANLL is a major undertaking. Infection and bleeding are much more common in ANLL than in ALL because the induction therapy regularly produces temporary marrow aplasia, which may last from 14 to 35 days. During that period, death owing to infection, bleeding, or both are common, and measures to prevent and to treat them are a critical part of any treatment program. The management of these problems is discussed in Chapter 25. Additional complications caused by the chemotherapeutic agents include cardiotoxicity, mucositis, alopecia, nausea, and vomiting.

E. **Recurrence and treatment of refractory disease.** Second remissions may be achieved in 25 to 30 percent of patients who relapse. As noted above, second remissions may be more easily obtained in patients who have undergone maintenance therapy with immunotherapy, with or without chemotherapy, than in patients who have had maintenance therapy with chemotherapy alone. Regimens used include initial induction therapy or one of several investigational drugs, including 5-azacytidine, acridinyl anisidide (m-AMSA), rubidazone, high-dose methotrexate, and high-dose cytarabine.

IV. Chronic lymphocytic leukemia (CLL)

A. **General considerations and aims of therapy.** CLL is seen primarily in the older adult. In many patients the course is quite indolent and survivals of 5 to 10 years are not unusual. In other patients the course is more rapidly progressive, leading to death within a few years. It is doubtful whether treatment results in significant prolongation of life in CLL except perhaps when the disease has entered the active, more aggressive phase. Many oncologists and hematologists, therefore, recommend that therapy be reserved for those patients in whom the disease has become active as manifested by anemia, thrombocytopenia, granulocytopenia, rapid rise in peripheral lymphocytes, progressive painful enlargement of lymph nodes, liver, or spleen, and associated fatigue, weakness, and malaise, weight loss, or fever. The primary aim of therapy is to reduce the symptoms resulting from CLL, although in some patients treatment may prolong life for a few months to years.

B. **Treatment**

1. **Indolent Phase.** No therapy, or chlorambucil, 4 mg/m^2 PO daily until the peripheral lymphocyte count falls to 10,000, then reduce to 2 mg/day or stop until WBC is greater than 50,000.

2. **Active Phase**

   a. Chlorambucil, 3 to 6 mg/m^2 PO daily until the WBC falls to 10,000, then maintain with 1 to 2 mg/m^2 PO daily, *or*

   b. Chlorambucil, 30 mg/m^2 PO day 1 *and* prednisone, 80 mg/m^2 PO days 1 to 5, repeated every 2 weeks *or*

   c. CVP

      (1) Cyclophosphamide, 300 mg/m^2 PO days 1 to 5

      (2) Vincristine, 1.4 mg/m^2 (maximum 2 mg) IV day 1

      (3) Prednisone, 100 mg/m^2 PO days 1 to 5

      Repeat CVP every 21 days.

      If CR is achieved by 9 months, continue therapy for 6 months after CR is achieved, then discontinue. If PR, continue therapy for a total of 18 months.

d. Dose modifications are based on treatment-induced cytopenias.

(1) If the neutrophils are greater than 1000/µl and the platelets are greater than 75,000/µl, full doses of all drugs are given.

(2) If the neutrophils are 500 to 1000/µl or the platelets 50,000 to 75,000/µl, then chlorambucil and cyclophosphamide are reduced to 50 percent of full dose.

(3) If the neutrophils are less than 500 or the platelets are less than 50,000, all drugs are held until the counts rise above this level.

(4) Any other severe toxicity such as steroid-induced psychosis or severe diabetes would be cause for dose modification of the appropriate drug.

C. Complications. Anemia, granulocytopenia, and thrombocytopenia may result from the leukemia or the alkylating agent therapy. Infection may also result from hypogammaglobulinemia. The chlorambucil may rarely result in mild gastrointestinal upset, hepatotoxicity, and exfoliative dermatitis. Cyclophosphamide may cause hemorrhagic cystitis, but its likelihood is reduced by keeping fluid intake high. Short-term prednisone may cause peptic irritation and ulceration, diabetes mellitus, and fluid retention, but other complications are unusual when it is given only for a 5-day course.

V. Chronic granulocytic leukemia (CGL)

A. General considerations and aims of therapy. Chronic granulocytic leukemia (CGL) is a disorder that is seen primarily in patients between the ages of 30 and 60, although it may occur in children and older adults as well. It is characterized by two distinct phases—an early chronic period and a late acute blastic crisis. Treatment during the chronic phase is directed toward diminishing the symptoms of fatigue, weakness, abdominal discomfort from splenomegaly, and shortness of breath. During the acute phase, the aim of treatment is complete remission, for unless it is achieved, the functional marrow will become rapidly obliterated by leukemia cells.

B. Treatment of the chronic phase. There is a choice of two drugs that are commonly employed in the treatment of the chronic phase of CGL.

1. Busulfan, 3 to 4 mg/m^2 PO daily until the WBC is 50 percent of the original level, then 1 to 2 mg/m^2 daily, *or*

2. Hydroxyurea, 1 to 2 g/m^2 PO daily until the WBC is 50 percent of the original level, then 0.5 to 1.0 g/m^2 PO daily

Because symptoms tend to parallel the WBC, therapy should be aimed at keeping the count at less than 50,000/µl. If the cell count falls to less than 15,000 to 20,000/µl, all therapy is usually stopped, as the counts may continue to fall when therapy is discontinued. Intermittent and continuous therapy are equally effective as maintenance.

C. Treatment of the acute phase. The acute phase or *blastic crisis* of CGL may morphologically resemble ALL or ANLL. There is some evidence that those leukemias that resemble ALL or that have terminal deoxynucleotidyl transferase (TdT) in their cells will respond to vincristine and prednisone, while leukemias that resemble ANLL and that do not have

TdT in their cells will not. Therapy is thus selected on the basis of morphology and biochemical markers: blastic crisis resembling ALL is treated with a regimen such as the regimen used for ALL, and blastic crisis resembling ANLL is treated with one of the treatment programs used in that disease. In either case, the patient is often refractory to the drugs, and complete remissions are achieved in less than 25 percent of all cases treated.

D. Complications of treatment. Busulfan may result in bone marrow depression, wasting, amenorrhea, and pulmonary fibrosis. Gastrointestinal symptoms and alopecia may also be seen. Hydroxyurea may cause mild gastrointestinal distress, drowsiness, marrow depression, and dermatologic reactions.

VI. Other leukemias

A. Leukemic reticuloendotheliosis or hairy cell leukemia. This leukemia, which is characterized by cells that morphologically resemble "hairy" lymphocytes under phase microscopy, responds poorly to chemotherapy. In patients with progressive disease, splenectomy is the treatment of choice.

B. Smouldering ANLL. Some patients are seen in whom the peripheral blood is characterized by pancytopenia and the marrow by 20 to 50 percent blasts, with dyspoiesis of other marrow elements, but some normal marrow function. Such patients frequently survive 1 to 3 years without cytotoxic chemotherapy. They are likely to require frequent RBC transfusions, but only rarely have bleeding or infection problems early in the course of the disease. Because of the need for frequent blood transfusions, the RBCs should be washed free of leukocytes and platelets prior to transfusion to avoid the stimulation of HLA antibodies. Cytotoxic chemotherapy is notoriously unsuccessful and should be considered only when the leukemia has converted from a smouldering to an acute stage and the marrow has begun to be replaced by leukemia cells.

C. Hypergranular acute promyelocytic leukemia (M3 type). This leukemia is characterized by disseminated intravascular coagulation, which is exacerbated during remission induction therapy. This complication frequently can be averted by prophylactic administration of heparin in the first week of therapy. This type of leukemia seems to respond well to the regimens for ANLL that contain anthracyclines.

VII. Polycythemia vera

A. Aims of therapy. Polycythemia vera is a malignant-behaving disorder of blood cells characterized by an overproduction of all cellular elements in the marrow. This overproduction results in a sustained elevation in the red cell mass and, to a lesser extent, an increase in the number of white blood cells and platelets. Symptoms of headache, weakness, itching, dyspnea, visual disturbances, and signs of plethora and organomegaly are related to the overproduction of blood cells in the marrow or extramedullary sites. Treatment is therefore directed at controlling the overproduction, reducing the circulating red cell mass, or both.

B. Treatment regimens

1. Phlebotomy is performed as often as necessary to maintain the hematocrit at 45% or less. It must be used at the outset with ^{32}P or chlorambucil treatments.

2. **Radioactive phosphorus** (^{32}P), 2.3 mCi/m^2 (limit 5 mCi) IV. Repeat in 12 weeks if necessary to further reduce the blood counts.

3. **Chlorambucil,** 10 mg PO daily for 6 weeks, rest 1 month, then alternate 1 month on and 1 month off, adjusting the dose to avoid leukopenia or thrombocytopenia.

C. **Results and complications of therapy.** Each treatment is equally effective in terms of patient survival with a median life expectancy of 8 to 10 years from the time of diagnosis. There is significantly increased risk of acute leukemia developing in patients treated with chlorambucil, however, and for this reason it is no longer recommended by many hematologists. Other frequent causes of death, including thrombosis and hemorrhage, are similar in each treatment group. The optimal treatment of this disease remains undetermined.

Selected Reading

Beck, P. D. et al. Increased incidence of acute leukemia in polycythemia vera associated with chlorambucil therapy. *N. Engl. J. Med.* 304:441, 1981.

Gale, R. P. High remission-induction rate in acute myeloid leukemia. *Lancet* 1:497, 1977.

Koeffler, H. P., and Golde, D. W. Chronic myelogenous leukemia. New concepts. *N. Engl. J. Med.* 304:1201, 1981.

Mauer, A. M. Therapy of acute lymphoblastic leukemia in childhood. *Blood* 56:1, 1980.

Rai, K. R. et al. Clinical staging of chronic lymphocytic leukemia. *Blood* 46:219, 1975.

18

Lymphomas

Richard S. Stein

Hodgkin's disease and the non-Hodgkin's lymphomas constitute a diverse spectrum of lymphoproliferative malignancies. However, the disorders share a number of important clinical features: both are commonly present as solitary or generalized adenopathy, and for both diseases accurate clinical staging is the basis for rational therapeutic planning. Nevertheless, important clinical differences exist. In Hodgkin's disease, contiguous spread of tumor from node to node is the rule, and most patients present with disease limited to the lymph nodes (or to the lymph nodes and spleen) and are, therefore, candidates for curative radiation therapy. In contrast, the majority of patients with non-Hodgkin's lymphomas present with advanced disease. Furthermore, while Hodgkin's disease is curable regardless of stage (advanced Hodgkin's disease is curable by chemotherapy), only certain histologic types of non-Hodgkin's lymphoma—primarily those lymphomas included in the category of diffuse histiocytic lymphoma (DHL)—are curable when disseminated. For this reason, Hodgkin's disease and the major histologic types of non-Hodgkin's lymphoma must be considered separately.

I. Hodgkin's disease

A. Incidence and histologic types.
Hodgkin's disease accounts for approximately 1 percent of newly diagnosed malignancies in the United States. The average age of new cases is 32 years, and a bimodal incidence curve exists: one peak occurs near age 25 and another at age 55. Four major histologic types of Hodgkin's disease exist: lymphocyte predominance (10% of cases), nodular sclerosis (60% of cases), mixed cellularity (20% of cases), and lymphocyte depletion (10% of cases). Nodular sclerosis Hodgkin's disease is commonly seen in young adults, and is frequently associated with a large mediastinal mass. Lymphocyte depleted Hodgkin's disease is usually associated with symptomatic disease (section **I.B**) and frequent involvement of the bone marrow. Nevertheless, the critical variable with respect to the therapy of Hodgkin's disease is not the histologic type but the stage of the disease.

B. Staging

1. Modified Ann Arbor staging system.
The modified Ann Arbor staging system is used for patients with Hodgkin's disease. Classically, patients are placed in one of four stages and are further classified as to the presence or absence of symptoms: A denotes that no symptoms are present; B denotes that any or all of the following are present: (1) fever, (2) night sweats, and (3) unexplained weight loss of 10 percent or more of body weight. In addition, the subscript E (e.g., II_E) may be used to denote involvement of an extralymphatic site primarily or by direct extension, rather than hematogenous spread, as in the case of

mediastinal mass extending to involve the lung. Stage III Hodgkin's disease is subdivided into stages III_1 and III_2, based on recent evidence that the clinical approaches to these two substages should be greatly different. The modified Ann Arbor staging system is as follows:

a. **Stage I** is the involvement of a single lymph node region.

b. **Stage II** is the involvement of two or more lymph node regions on the same side of the diaphragm.

c. **Stage III_1** is the involvement of lymph node regions on both sides of the diaphragm. Abdominal disease is limited to the upper abdomen: spleen, splenic hilar, celiac, or porta hepatis nodes.

d. **Stage III_2** is the involvement of lymph node regions on both sides of the diaphragm. Abdominal disease includes paraaortic, mesenteric, iliac, or inguinal nodes, with or without disease in the upper abdomen.

e. **Stage IV** is the diffuse or disseminated involvement of one or more extralymphatic tissues or organs, with or without associated lymph node involvement.

2. **Staging tests.** Staging must be performed with consideration of therapeutic options and not just as a completion of a "checklist." In performing staging tests, one should remember that Hodgkin's disease tends to spread in a contiguous manner. Considering that the thoracic duct makes the left supraclavicular area and the abdomen contiguous sites, it should not be surprising that abdominal disease is found in 40 percent of patients with left supraclavicular presentations, and only 8 percent of patients with presentations in the right supraclavicular nodes. Procedures used for the staging of Hodgkin's disease are as follows:

a. **History taking.** Symptoms to watch for are fever, night sweats, and weight loss.

b. **Complete physical examination.** Attention must be paid to lymph nodes and spleen.

c. **Laboratory tests.** Complete blood count, platelet count, sedimentation rate, serum alkaline phosphatase, and tests of liver and kidney function must be made.

d. **Chest x-ray.** Tomograms must be considered if chest x-ray film is abnormal.

e. **Lymphangiogram.**

f. **Liver and spleen isotope scan.**

g. **Bone marrow biopsy.** May be omitted in patients who are in clinical stage IA or IIA after the above staging procedures have been performed.

h. **Staging laparotomy** should be done in selected patients only. If performed, laparotomy should include inspection, splenectomy, liver biopsies (wedge biopsy of left lobe with needle biopsy of both lobes), and lymph node biopsies of splenic hilar, celiac, porta hepatis, mesenteric, paraaortic, and iliac nodes.

Table 18-1. Hodgkin's Disease: Incidence of Stages and Results of Therapy

Stage	Incidence (%)	Potential Cure Rate (%)
IA	10	95
IIA	30	85
IB, IIB	10	70
III_1A	15	85
III_2A	10	65
IIIB	15	60
IVA, IVB	10	50

C. Therapy of Hodgkin's disease

1. **General considerations.** Therapy of Hodgkin's disease must be considered on a stage-by-stage basis. The incidence of the various stages of Hodgkin's disease is presented in Table 18-1 with an estimated cure rate for each stage. In general, limited stages of Hodgkin's disease are treated with radiation therapy (stages IA and IIA) and advanced stages (IVA and IVB) are treated with combination chemotherapy. For the intermediate stages, controversy exists regarding the nature of optimal therapy.

   Prior to initiating chemotherapy, patients should be placed on allopurinol, 300 mg/day to avert the hyperuricemia that may follow tumor lysis.

2. **Radiotherapy.** With respect to radiation therapy, studies have shown that the optimal dose for local control is 3600 to 4000 rad given in $3\frac{1}{2}$ to 4 weeks. With modern equipment, adequate radiation can be administered to involved areas while shielding adjacent tissues. Nevertheless, radiation injury, such as radiation pneumonitis or pericarditis, can occur infrequently. Similarly, inappropriate overlapping of radiation ports can result in damage to the overtreated area. If this damage involves radiation myelitis, the results can be disastrous owing to resultant paraplegia. Other potential side effects of radiation include hypothyroidism (often subclinical) and sterility (unless the ovaries are moved at the time of staging laparotomy, prior to pelvic irradiation). See Figure 18-1 (page 179) for standard radiation therapy ports.

3. **Stages IA and IIA.** Patients with stage IA disease are most commonly treated with mantle irradiation when the disease occurs above the diaphragm (as it does in 90% of cases), or with pelvic radiotherapy when the disease presents in an inguinal node. Patients with stage IIA disease are most commonly treated with mantle plus paraaortic–splenic radiotherapy. There is no firm evidence that adding chemotherapy or modifying the ports leads to either improved results or significantly decreased toxicity in these patients. Although patients with stage II_EA disease are generally treated like patients with stage IIA disease, numerous recent studies have shown that patients with large mediastinal masses are best treated with combined modality therapy, that is, combination chemotherapy as well as radiotherapy.

4. **Stages IB and IIB.** In view of the limited number of patients with these stages of disease, available data do not allow firm treatment

Table 18-2. Sliding Scale of MOPP Dose Adjustment for Myelotoxicity

WBC Count		Platelet Count	Dose (%)			
			M	O	P	P
>4000/mm^3	*and*	>100,000/mm^3	100	100	100	100
3000–4000/mm^3	*and*	>100,000/mm^3	50	100	50	100
2000–3000/mm^3	*or*	50,000-100,000/mm^3	25	100	25	100
1000–2000/mm^3	*and/or*	<50,000/mm^3	25	50	25	100
<1000/mm^3	*and*	<50,000/mm^3	0	0	0	0

recommendations to be made. These patients are most commonly treated with extended field radiotherapy or combined modality therapy, that is, radiation therapy plus 3 to 6 cycles of a combination regimen such as MOPP. Dose adjustments appear in Table 18-2.

  a. Mechlorethamine, 6 mg/m^2 IV days 1 and 8

  b. Vincristine (Oncovin®), 1.4 mg/m^2 (not to exceed 2.5 mg) IV days 1 and 8

  c. Procarbazine, 100 mg/m^2 PO days 1 to 14

  d. Prednisone, 40 mg/m^2 PO days 1 to 14, cycles 1 and 4 only

Repeat the cycle every 4 weeks for 6 cycles, minimum. Complete remission should be documented prior to discontinuing therapy.

5. **Stage IIIA.** Therapy of stage IIIA is still a matter of controversy. The two options that are most commonly considered are total nodal radiotherapy alone, or total nodal radiotherapy with combination chemotherapy, such as mechlorethamine, vincristine (Oncovin®), procarbazine, and prednisone (MOPP). While combined modality therapy may appear to be optimal, such therapy exposes all stage III patients to considerable toxicity—toxicity that may not be necessary in all patients. Also, recent studies have shown that combined modality therapy is associated with an increased risk (about 4% at 7 yr) of acute nonlymphocytic leukemia, which is generally refractory to chemotherapy. So, combined modality therapy should best be limited to patients in whom radiotherapy alone cannot produce adequate cure rates.

Recent studies have suggested that the extent of abdominal disease may be a rational basis for determining therapy in patients with stage IIIA Hodgkin's disease. Patients with stage III$_1$A disease appear to achieve optimal results when treated with radiotherapy alone, leaving chemotherapy for salvage treatment at the time of relapse. For patients with stage III$_2$A, the results of radiotherapy alone are inadequate, and either radiotherapy with chemotherapy or chemotherapy alone appears to be appropriate.

6. **Stage IIIB.** Patients with stage IIIB are commonly treated with combination chemotherapy alone, although they may be treated with combinations of radiotherapy and chemotherapy. The available studies have not established which of these approaches is superior.

7. **Stage IVA and IVB.** Therapy of these stages is generally combination chemotherapy. The standard chemotherapy regimen for the treatment of stage IV Hodgkin's disease is the MOPP regimen. The demonstration that MOPP chemotherapy could cure advanced Hodgkin's disease represents one of the major advances in modern cancer chemotherapy and has been one of the major rationales for the use of combination chemotherapy in other malignancies.

   a. **Critical dose and duration of MOPP therapy.** Several factors are critical to the success of the MOPP regimen. First, it is important to administer the drugs in accordance with prescribed schedules and not to modify drugs for toxicities such as nausea and vomiting, which should be controlled symptomatically with phenothiazines. Doses of vincristine should be cut by 50 percent only if ileus develops or if motor weakness occurs. Also, six cycles of MOPP constitute standard therapy, and MOPP therapy should be administered for at least six cycles and discontinued only if there is adequate documentation that a complete remission has occurred. If tests are equivocal, it is better to give additional cycles of MOPP and not to regard six cycles as a "magic" number. Once a complete remission has been well documented, treatment may be stopped since there is no evidence that maintenance therapy is of any clinical value.

   b. **Response to MOPP chemotherapy.** When MOPP has been administered in optimal fashion, 81 percent of patients achieved a complete remission. Of these patients, 66 percent (representing 53% of the total series) have remained in complete remission for 5 years, and an identical percentage have remained in complete remission for 10 years. Thus, 5-year disease-free survival is probably equivalent to cure. It should also be noted that the figure of 53 percent is a minimal estimate for the cure of advanced Hodgkin's disease since many patients who receive a complete remission and then relapse may still be cured with later salvage therapy.

   c. **Alternatives to MOPP induction therapy.** Many efforts have been made to develop combination regimens that are more effective and less toxic than the standard MOPP regimen. Some of these regimens represent minor variations of the MOPP regimen (Table 18-3) and other regimens are combinations of non-cross–resistant drugs (Table 18-4). These latter regimens may be used in MOPP failures, but may also be considered as initial therapy. While many of these regimens can produce remission rates similar to those rates achieved with MOPP therapy, there are no data that any of the regimens produce long-term results superior to MOPP. Two interesting alternatives to MOPP therapy have recently generated considerable interest. It is well known that patients with nodular sclerosing Hodgkin's disease, the most common type of Hodgkin's disease, tend to relapse at the site of prior nodal disease when treated with MOPP alone. For this reason, a number of programs combining MOPP or its variants with radiotherapy have been proposed for stage IV disease.

Another approach to treatment of advanced disease is to alternate 1 month of MOPP therapy with 1 month of non-cross–resistant therapy such as doxorubicin (Adriamycin™), bleomycin, vinblastine, and dacarbazine (ABVD regimen), and to administer a total of 12 cycles of

Table 18-3. Minor Variations of MOPP Chemotherapy

Regimen	Dosage
MOPP-Bleo	Mechlorethamine, 6 mg/m^2 IV days 1 and 8 Vincristine (Oncovin®), 1.4 mg/m^2 (not to exceed 2.0 mg) IV days 1 and 8 Procarbazine, 100 mg/m^2 PO days 1–10 Prednisone, 50 mg/m^2 PO days 1–10 (cycles 1 and 4 only) Bleomycin, 2 units/m^2 IV days 1 and 8 Repeat every 28 days
BVCPP	Carmustine, 100 mg/m^2 IV day 1 Vinblastine, 5 mg/m^2 IV day 1 Cyclophosphamide, 600 mg/m^2 PO day 1 Procarbazine, 100 mg/m^2 PO days 1–10 Prednisone, 60 mg/m^2 PO days 1–10 Repeat every 28 days
CVPP	Lomustine (CCNU), 75 mg/m^2 PO day 1 Vinblastine, 4 mg/m^2 IV days 1 and 8 Procarbazine, 100 mg/m^2 PO days 1–14 Prednisone, 30 mg/m^2 PO days 1–14 (cycles 1 and 4 only) Repeat every 28 days

Table 18-4. Alternatives to MOPP: Non-Cross–Resistant Regimens

Regimen	Dosage
ABVD	Doxorubicin (Adriamycin™), 25 mg/m^2 IV days 1 and 15 Bleomycin, 10 units/m^2 IV days 1 and 15 Vinblastine, 6 mg/m^2 IV days 1 and 15 Dacarbazine, 150 mg/m^2 days 1–5 Repeat every 28 days
BCAVe	Bleomycin, 2.5 units/m^2 days 1, 28, and 35 (IV or IM) Lomustine (CCNU), 100 mg/m^2 PO day 1 Doxorubicin (Adriamycin™), 60 mg/m^2 IV day 1 Vinblastine, 5 mg/m^2 IV day 1 Repeat every 42 days
ABDIC	Doxorubicin (Adriamycin™), 45 mg/m^2 IV day 1 Bleomycin, 5 units/m^2 IV or IM days 1 and 5 Dacarbazine, 200 mg/m^2 IV days 1–5 Lomustine (CCNU), 50 mg/m^2 PO day 1 Prednisone, 40 mg/m^2 PO days 1–5 Repeat every 28 days

chemotherapy. Preliminary results have suggested that this approach may be superior in stage IVB disease, but confirmatory studies are needed.

8. **Salvage therapy for treatment failures.** Relapse in Hodgkin's disease does not mean death, since salvage therapy is capable of producing cures. However, the chance of curing a patient with Hodgkin's disease who has relapsed is greater if the recurrence is nodal than if the recurrence is visceral. Also, the chance of salvaging a patient with Hodgkin's disease is greater when the initial stage of disease was limited than when the initial stage was relatively advanced.

For patients with limited nodal relapses following radiation therapy, additional radiation therapy may be considered. Alternatively, chemotherapy may be used in these patients and in patients who relapse following chemotherapy. It has long been appreciated that patients who relapse following initial radiotherapy may achieve a complete remission and may be potentially cured with combination chemotherapy. Recently, it has been shown that patients who achieve a complete remission with MOPP therapy and who remain in remission for more than 1 year may be reinduced with MOPP therapy at the time of relapse and may be cured by this salvage therapy. In past years, many of these patients, who are not truly MOPP resistant, were treated with one of the regimens listed in Table 18-4 as salvage therapy. Inclusion of these relatively favorable patients in studies of newer regimens as salvage therapy has led to overestimating the value of these regimens as salvage therapy in the patient who is truly MOPP resistant. When patients are truly resistant to MOPP, that is, when they relapse within 1 year of discontinuing MOPP therapy or even during MOPP therapy, the chance of cure is only between 15 and 30 percent.

II. Non-Hodgkin's lymphoma

A. Classification and natural history.
The non-Hodgkin's lymphomas (NHL) are a group of malignancies that involve lymphocytes. Although NHL is often considered as a single disorder with respect to incidence and staging, the disorders included in NHL differ in many basic characteristics. At the time of presentation, some types of lymphoma are almost always disseminated and have a high incidence of bone marrow and liver involvement (poorly differentiated lymphocytic lymphoma). Other lymphomas (diffuse histiocytic lymphoma) are limited to a single lymph node region, or to two adjacent areas in up to 30 percent of cases.

1. **Clinical course.** The most important clinical differences among the types of lymphoma, however, relate to clinical course. In some types of lymphoma, particularly those lymphomas included in the category diffuse histiocytic lymphoma, median survival is only 6 months unless combination chemotherapy induces a complete remission; these complete remissions are often equivalent to cures. By contrast, in other lymphomas, primarily nodular lymphomas, patients may survive many years with only minimal palliative therapy or with no therapy at all. Even when therapy produces a complete remission in these indolent lymphomas, the patients invariably relapse and eventually die.

2. **Classification.** Because of these biologic differences, it is important that an accurate classification system for the lymphomas define diseases that behave in a relatively uniform manner. Since lymphomas are disorders of the immune system, it would seem that a meaningful classification would have to consider immunologic variables and to attempt to define immunologically homogeneous entities. Unfortunately, the standard classification of lymphomas, the Rappaport classification, does not consider immunologic characteristics and instead classifies lymphomas on the basis of cytology (poorly differentiated, so-called histiocytic, or mixed cell) and pattern (nodular or diffuse). Table 18-5 presents the incidence of the various lymphomas defined

Table 18-5. Incidence of Histologic Types of Lymphoma (Rappaport Classification)

Cytology	Incidence (%)	
	Nodular	Diffuse
Well differentiated lymphocytic lymphoma (WDL)	—	2–5
Poorly differentiated lymphocytic lymphoma (PDL)	20–30	10–15
Mixed cell (lymphocytic–histiocytic) lymphoma (MC)	5–15	5–10
Histiocytic lymphoma (HL)	3–7	30–40
Undifferentiated lymphoma	—	3–5

by the Rappaport classification. Although most studies in the past decade have used the Rappaport classification, recent studies have suggested that two of the common disorders defined by the Rappaport classification (poorly differentiated lymphocytic lymphoma-diffuse and diffuse histiocytic lymphoma) are immunologically heterogenous entities within which more homogenous disorders may be defined. Thus, while the Rappaport classification provides the framework for this discussion, reference to immunologic findings will be made whenever pertinent to clinical care.

B. Staging

1. **Limited versus advanced disease.** The Ann Arbor staging system for Hodgkin's disease (section **I.B**) is also used in NHL. However, in contrast to Hodgkin's disease, which arises at an extranodal site in less than 1 percent of cases, approximately 10 to 20 percent of NHL cases arise at extranodal sites. Furthermore, the clinical applicability of the four stages of Hodgkin's disease to non-Hodgkin's lymphoma is limited. For practical purposes, there may be only two stages: limited disease (stage I and perhaps some stage II patients), which is treated with radiation therapy, and advanced disease (stages III and IV, and in some cases stage II), which is treated systemically. The incidence of the various stages of NHL, as related to histology, is presented in Table 18-6.

2. **Special considerations.** As in Hodgkin's disease, staging forms the basis for therapeutic planning. However, additional considerations must be added to the staging of patients with NHL. In performing a physical examination, special care must be given to sites such as Waldeyer's ring, epitrochlear nodes, femoral nodes, and popliteal nodes, which are rarely involved by Hodgkin's disease. Bone marrow biopsy is a key diagnostic procedure in NHL owing to the high incidence of involvement, especially in poorly differentiated lymphocytic lymphoma. Abdominal CT scanning is of greater value in NHL than in Hodgkin's disease; in Hodgkin's disease involved abdominal nodes are small and may be missed by CT scanning whereas lymphangiography can detect small nodes in which the internal architecture is disrupted. In NHL, retroperitoneal masses are often large and easily detected by CT scanning. In addition, while mesenteric nodes are rarely involved in Hodgkin's disease, these nodes are involved in approximately 70 percent of cases of nodular lymphomas and may be detected by CT scanning, but will not be opacified by lymphangiog-

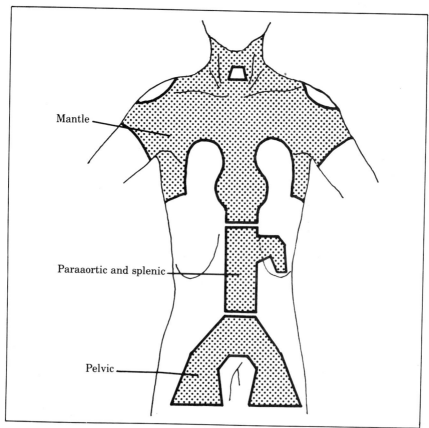

Fig. 18-1. Standard radiation therapy ports that are used in the treatment of Hodgkin's disease. For disease presenting above the diaphragm, the mantle plus paraaortic and splenic ports would be regarded as extended field therapy. The use of all three ports would be considered total nodal irradiation. (Reprinted by permission from J. R. Salzman and H. S. Kaplan, Effect of prior splenectomy on hematologic tolerance during total lymphoid radiotherapy of patients with Hodgkin's disease. *Cancer* 27:472, 1972.)

raphy. As in Hodgkin's disease, tests that are performed for purposes of staging establish a baseline so that patients can be evaluated for the occurrence of a complete remission when therapy has been given with curative intent.

C. Therapy of non-Hodgkin's lymphomas

1. **Radiation therapy; general considerations.** Since the majority of patients with NHL have disseminated disease, radiotherapy plays a more limited role in NHL than in Hodgkin's disease. However, the value of radiotherapy should not be overlooked. In most histologic types of nodular lymphoma, doses of 4400 rad can achieve control of local disease. Because disease occurs outside of treatment fields, such as bone marrow disease, radiation is rarely curative. However, when

Table 18-6. Stage at Completion of Staging Evaluation
as Related to Histology: Non-Hodgkin's Lymphomas

Histology	Stage (percent of patients)			
	I	II	III	IV
Nodular				
Poorly differentiated lymphocytic	4	0	27	69
Mixed cell (lymphocytic–histiocytic)	0	8	24	68
Diffuse				
Poorly differentiated lymphocytic*	7	14	0	79
Histiocytic	8	23	24	45

*For lymphoblastic lymphoma (convoluted cell lymphoma), the T-cell subset of diffuse poorly differentiated lymphocytic lymphoma, essentially all cases are stage IV.
Source: Modified from B. A. Chabner et al. *Cancer Treat. Rep.* 61:993–997, 1977.

patients with nodular lymphoma have large masses, local radiotherapy may be the most effective means of palliation. While a dose-response curve for histiocytic lymphoma is less well established, radiotherapy may also play a role in palliating patients with histiocytic lymphoma who have become refractory to chemotherapy. Although 30 percent of patients with histiocytic lymphoma may have stage I or II disease, the role of radiotherapy in these patients is not firmly established. Some authors feel that radiotherapy should be used only for histiocytic lymphoma patients in stage I, while chemotherapy should be used for patients in stage II or higher; other investigators have studied combination chemotherapy as the primary therapy even in stage I disease. Further studies will be needed to resolve these issues. Remember, however, that when radiotherapy of a histiocytic lymphoma requires use of a large port, as in the case of a large retroperitoneal mass, this therapy is likely to render impossible the later administration of curative combination chemotherapy.

Prior to initiating intensive chemotherapy, patients should be placed on allopurinol 300 mg/day to avert the hyperuricemia that may follow tumor lysis.

2. **Poorly differentiated lymphocytic lymphoma–Nodular (PDL–N).**
Patients with this type of lymphoma almost always have widespread disease at the time of presentation. However, despite this fact, median survival of patients with PDL–N has ranged from 4 to 8 years in most series. Therapy has had no impact on curability of PDL–N. Although combination chemotherapy regimens (Table 18-7) have produced complete remissions in up to 80 percent of patients with PDL–N, such remissions are never durable. Since the drugs included in combination regimens have considerable toxicity (myelotoxicity, nausea, vomiting, alopecia, and neurotoxicity), there appears to be no justification for the routine use of combination chemotherapy in these patients.

a. **Asymptomatic patients.** It has been shown that asymptomatic patients with PDL–N may do quite well in the absence of any initial therapy. Since one third to one half of patients with PDL–N may present without symptoms despite the presence of disseminated disease, it may well be that the best approach to PDL–N is no therapy or single agent therapy with chlorambucil, 2 to 4 mg/m^2

Table 18-7. Combination Chemotherapy for the Clinically Indolent Lymphomas

Regimen	Dosage
CVP*	Cyclophosphamide, 400 mg/m² PO days 1–5 Vincristine (Oncovin®), 1.4 mg/m² (not to exceed 2.0 mg) IV day 1 Prednisone, 100 mg/m² PO days 1–5 Repeat every 21 days
COPP*	Cyclophosphamide, 600 mg/m² IV days 1 and 8 Vincristine (Oncovin®), 1.4 mg/m² (not to exceed 2.5 mg) IV days 1 and 8 Procarbazine, 100 mg/m² PO days 1–10 Prednisone, 40 mg/m² days 1–14 Repeat every 28 days
CHOP*	Cyclophosphamide, 750 mg/m² IV day 1 Doxorubicin (Adriamycin™), 50 mg/m² IV day 1 Vincristine (Oncovin®), 1.4 mg/m² (not to exceed 2.0 mg) IV day 1 Prednisone, 100 mg PO days 1–5 Repeat every 21 days

*These regimens employ a sliding scale for myelotoxicity similar to that used for the MOPP regimen, Table 18-2. The alphabetical abbreviations used for these regimens consider doxorubicin (Adriamycin™) as hydroxyldaunomycin.

PO daily. If this minimal therapeutic approach is adopted, the more toxic combination regimens can be reserved for palliation of symptoms when the toxicity of therapy is more easily justified.

b. Symptomatic patients. Indications for the use of more aggressive therapy, such as the combination regimens in Table 18-7, in patients with PDL–N would include persistently enlarging nodes or spleen, development of cytopenias, development of fever, sweats, or weight loss, evidence of visceral involvement other than in bone marrow or of microscopic hepatic involvement, and evidence of autoimmune disease. In many patients, years may elapse before such therapy is required.

3. Poorly differentiated lymphocytic lymphoma–Diffuse (PDL–D). This type of lymphoma is generally regarded as an aggressive disease. However, during the past decade, research has shown that this disorder is actually composed of two diseases. One half of the patients have a disease that is similar to PDL–N, and, like PDL–N, the lymphoma is composed of small (cleaved) B-lymphocytes. These patients have a clinical course that is similar to PDL–N. Although survivals in patients with PDL–D have been shorter than survivals of patients with PDL–N, these differences have generally not been statistically significant. It is not known if the results of aggressive initial chemotherapy produces better results than watchful waiting in this group of patients.

PDL–D also includes a group of patients with T-cell lymphomas characterized by mediastinal masses and a high incidence of bone marrow involvement. Cytologically, this disease is indistinguishable from acute lymphocytic leukemia of T cells. This lymphoma is highly aggressive, and, in most series, median survivals have been less than 1 year. These patients are candidates for aggressive therapy but no established regimen for treatment exists. Experimental regimens in-

Table 18-8. Chemotherapy Regimens for Histiocytic Lymphoma

Regimen	Dosage
BACOP	Bleomycin, 5 units/m^2 IV days 15 and 22 Doxorubicin (Adriamycin™), 25 mg/m^2 IV days 1 and 8 Cyclophosphamide, 650 mg/m^2 IV days 1 and 8 Vincristine (Oncovin®), 1.4 mg/m^2 (not to exceed 2.0 mg) IV days 1 and 8 Prednisone, 60 mg/m^2 PO days 15–28 Repeat every 28 days
CHOP	Cyclophosphamide, 750 mg/m^2 IV day 1 Doxorubicin (Adriamycin™), 50 mg/m^2 IV day 1 Vincristine (Oncovin®), 1.4 mg/m^2 (not to exceed 2.0 mg) IV day 1 Prednisone, 100 mg PO days 1–5 Repeat every 21 days
COMLA	Cyclophosphamide, 1500 mg/m^2 IV day 1 Vincristine (Oncovin®), 1.4 mg/m^2 (not to exceed 2.5 mg) IV days 1, 8, and 15 Methotrexate, 120 mg/m^2 IV days 22, 29, 36, 43, 50, 57, 64, and 71 Leucovorin, 25 mg/m^2 PO q6h for 4 doses starting 24 hours after each methotrexate dose Cytarabine, 300 mg/m^2 IV days 22, 29, 36, 43, 50, 57, 64, and 71 Repeat every 91 days

cluding cytarabine and asparaginase have produced encouraging results in small preliminary studies.

4. **Mixed cell nodular lymphoma (MC–N).** Patients with this type of lymphoma have a course that is similar to that of PDL–N. However, when asymptomatic patients with MC–N have been followed with watchful waiting, the majority have required therapy in less than 1 year. For this reason, many physicians would treat these patients at presentation even though superior survival has not been established as occurring with this approach.

In one study of patients with MC–N, the cyclophosphamide, vincristine (Oncovin®), procarbazine, and prednisone (COPP) regimen (see Table 18-7) produced complete remissions in 77 percent of patients. Among these patients achieving a complete remission, 79 percent were still in remission at the time of publication of the study. Unfortunately, this finding has not been replicated.

5. **Diffuse histiocytic lymphoma (DHL)**

a. **Combination chemotherapy: COPP.** The remarkable clinical progress that has been made in treating DHL represents one of the brightest aspects of clinical cancer chemotherapy of the 1970s. In the age of single agent chemotherapy, DHL was a rapidly lethal neoplasm, with a median survival of 6 months and a 2-year survival of, at best, 5 percent. In 1974, workers at the National Cancer Institute published their findings concluding that the COPP regimen (see Table 18-7) produced complete remissions in approximately 40 percent of patients. More importantly, most of these remissions were durable. The 5-year disease-free survival was projected as 37 percent. These remissions have persisted with 10 years of follow-up.

b. **Alternative therapy.** Nevertheless, COPP has not become standard therapy for DHL. Shortly after the demonstration that histiocytic lymphoma was a curable neoplasm, other workers began publishing results using newer drugs as part of combination therapy. The best published results have used the regimens in Table 18-8. In the absence of a randomized trial, it is impossible to establish an optimal regimen. However, if attempts are made to compare the regimens, one point quickly emerges. Although complete remission in DHL is equivalent to cure in many cases, the percent of complete remissions that are reported for many drug combinations does not correspond to the 2-year disease-free survival. This discrepancy may represent inadequate evaluation by clinical investigators at the time that a complete remission appears to be present, or it may represent the fact that certain regimens produce remissions that are not durable. In any case, if regimens are compared in DHL, it seems more meaningful to compare the 2-year disease-free survival than to compare the "complete remission" rates that are reported. When this comparison is done, all of the regimens in Table 18-8 are associated with 2-year disease-free survivals of 45 to 62 percent.

c. **Immunologic subtypes.** The discussion in **II.C.5** considers DHL as a single disease entity. Immunologic studies have shown that this consideration is not correct. Specifically, approximately 85 percent of cases of so-called histiocytic lymphoma are B-cell lymphomas and the remainder are T-cell lymphomas. True histiocytic disorders are rare. Furthermore, among the B-cell disorders several different entities have been described: large cleaved cell lymphoma, large transformed cell lymphoma, small transformed cell lymphoma, and immunoblastic sarcoma. This distinction is not simply of academic importance. Although the data are only suggestive and not definitive, it appears that large cleaved cell lymphoma and large transformed cell lymphoma have a relatively favorable prognosis. Immunoblastic sarcoma of B cells and small transformed cell lymphoma appear to be relatively refractory to chemotherapy. Durable remissions are extremely rare in T-cell lymphomas included in so-called histiocytic lymphoma.

d. **Treatment of refractory disease.** Unfortunately, unlike Hodgkin's disease, patients with DHL who fail one induction regimen are generally refractory to all other regimens. Second-line approaches, such as high-dose methotrexate, one of the nitrosoureas, or one of the experimental epipodophyllotoxins, produce at best brief partial remissions in 20 percent of patients. It is to be hoped that identification of the subsets of histiocytic lymphoma that are resistant to present regimens will lead to these patients receiving the newer approaches as their initial therapy. It is unfortunate that these patients are identified merely as having histiocytic lymphoma and treated with ineffective regimens at the only time in their disease when a favorable response might be achieved.

Selected Reading

DeVita, V. T. et al. Curability of advanced Hodgkin's disease with chemotherapy. *Ann. Intern. Med.* 92:587, 1980.

Fisher, R. I. et al. Prolonged disease-free survival in Hodgkin's disease with MOPP reinduction after first relapse. *Ann. Intern. Med.* 90:761, 1979.

Portlock, C. S., and Rosenberg, S. A. No initial therapy for stages III and IV non-Hodgkin's lymphomas of favorable histologic types. *Ann. Intern. Med.* 90:10, 1979.

Rodgers, R. W. et al. ABDIC chemotherapy in MOPP-resistant Hodgkin's disease. *Cancer* 46:2349, 1980.

Stein, R. S. et al. Correlations between immunologic markers and histopathologic classifications. *Semin. Oncol.* 7:244, 1980.

Stein, R. S. et al. Anatomic substages of stage III-A Hodgkin's disease. *Ann. Intern. Med.* 92:159, 1980.

Sweet, D. L. et al. Cyclophosphamide, vincristine, methotrexate with leucovorin rescue, and cytosine arabinoside (COMLA) combination sequential chemotherapy in the treatment of advanced diffuse histiocytic lymphoma. *Ann. Intern. Med.* 92:785, 1980.

Sweet, D. L., Kinnealey, A., and Ultmann, J. E. Hodgkin's disease. Problems of staging. *Cancer* 42:957, 1978.

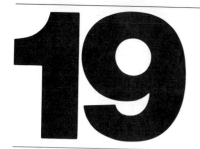

Multiple Myeloma and Other Plasma Cell Dyscrasias

Martin M. Oken

I. Introduction

A. Types of plasma cell dyscrasias.
Plasma cell dyscrasias or plasma cell neoplasms are a group of conditions characterized by unbalanced proliferation of cells that normally synthesize and secrete immunoglobulins. They range from malignant neoplasms, such as multiple myeloma, to monoclonal gammopathy of undetermined significance, a usually benign condition that is sometimes termed *benign monoclonal gammopathy*. Associated with the abnormal cellular proliferation in nearly all cases is the production of either a homogeneous monoclonal immunoglobulin, referred to either as *myeloma protein* or *M-protein*, or of excessive quantities of homogeneous polypeptide subunits of a monoclonal protein. The latter usually appear as monoclonal free light chains excreted into the urine. Frequently, both whole immunoglobulin M-protein and free light chain are produced. The plasma cell dyscrasias discussed in this chapter are multiple myeloma, macroglobulinemia (Waldenström's macroglobulinemia), heavy-chain diseases, amyloidosis, and monoclonal gammopathy of undetermined significance.

B. The M-protein.
Unlike most neoplastic diseases, which are followed objectively by serial evaluation of palpable or radiographically measurable tumor masses, most plasma cell dyscrasias are best followed by serial measurements of the monoclonal protein (M-protein) elaborated by the tumor. Effective use of this tumor marker is important to the proper evaluation of the disease course in most plasma cell dyscrasias and is, in most instances, essential to the determination of response to treatment. The basic immunoglobulin unit comprises two identical heavy chains with a molecular weight of 55,000 daltons linked to two identical light chains with a molecular weight of 22,500 daltons. The heavy chains are either γ, α, μ, δ, or ϵ corresponding to IgG, IgA, IgM, IgD, or IgE. The light chains exist as either κ or λ subtypes. Serum M-protein is a monoclonal whole immunoglobulin and will therefore possess only one heavy chain type and one light chain type. Urine M-protein consists of free light chain, or in the case of some heavy chain diseases, free heavy chain fragments of single specificity. Serum M-proteins may be quantitatively evaluated either by serum protein electrophoresis or by determining the concentration of the individual immunoglobulins (particularly IgG, IgA, and IgM) by radial immunodiffusion or by nephelometry. Urine M-protein, usually in the form of free light chain, should be characterized by immunoelectrophoresis as monoclonal κ or λ light chain and then followed sequentially expressed as urinary light chain excretion in g/24 hr. This characterization requires determination of 24-hour urine pro-

tein excretion, and scanning the urine protein electrophoresis to determine the percent of urine protein present as free monoclonal immunoglobulin light chain.

II. Multiple myeloma

A. General considerations and aims of therapy

1. **Diagnosis.** Multiple myeloma is a neoplasm of malignant plasma
   cells invading bone and bone marrow, causing widespread skeletal
   destruction, bone marrow failure, and problems related to quantitatively abnormal serum and/or urine M-proteins. The diagnosis of
   multiple myeloma requires histologic documentation by the demonstration of increased numbers (usually >10%) of abnormal, atypical,
   or immature plasma cells in the bone marrow, in addition to the
   finding of serum or urine M-protein or of characteristic osteolytic bone
   lesions. Some patients will have multiple plasmacytomas of bone with
   intervening normal areas of bone marrow. In these patients, a random bone-marrow aspirate and biopsy may fail to demonstrate the
   tumor, and biopsy of specific bone lesions may be necessary to establish the diagnosis.

2. **Incidence.** The annual incidence of multiple myeloma is 3 per
   100,000 population with a peak occurrence at age 50 to 70. While as
   many as 4 percent of myeloma patients may have indolent or smolder-
   ing disease at diagnosis, and an additional 5 percent may have an
   isolated plasmacytoma of bone, most multiple myeloma patients require chemotherapy of their disease soon after diagnosis.

3. **Effect of treatment.** The goal of therapy is to improve the duration of
   survival and to diminish or prevent the serious manifestations of this
   disease, such as bone pain, pathologic fractures, severe anemia, renal
   failure, or hypercalcemia. Treatment produces objective response in
   about 50 percent of patients as determined by a sustained 50 percent
   decline in the levels of serum or urine M-protein. Temporary, sometimes long-lasting, improvement in symptoms occurs in nearly all
   patients exhibiting objective response to treatment and in some additional patients with lesser degrees of objective improvement. The median survivals reported for treated patients range from 2 to 3 years
   and are strongly influenced by response to treatment and by initial
   tumor load.

4. **Prognostic factors.** Table 19-1 outlines a clinical staging system developed to estimate myeloma tumor cell mass utilizing readily obtained clinical findings. Severe anemia, hypercalcemia, advanced osteolytic lesions, and extremely high M-protein production rates are all
   associated with a high tumor burden and a poor survival prognosis.
   Renal failure, while not well correlated closely with tumor burden, is
   associated with poor prognosis. Advanced age, poor performance
   status, and λ light chain type have also been established as adverse
   prognostic signs.

B. Initial treatment

1. **General measures.** Complications of myeloma, such as infection, hypercalcemia, and renal failure, may be present at the time of diagnosis (section **II.D**). These complications should be promptly identified
   and treated before the start of chemotherapy. The small percentage of

Table 19-1. Myeloma Clinical Staging System

Stage	Criteria	Myeloma Cell Mass (cells/m²)
I	All of the following: 1. Hemoglobin >10 g/100 ml 2. Serum calcium value normal (≤12 mg/100 ml) 3. On x-ray film, normal bone structure or solitary bone plasmacytoma only 4. Low M-component production rates 　a. IgG value <5 g/100 ml 　b. IgA value <3 g/100 ml 　c. Urine light chain M-component on electrophoresis <4 g/24 hours	$<0.6 \times 10^{12}$ (low)
II	Fitting neither stage I nor stage III	$0.6–1.2 \times 10^{12}$ (intermediate)
III	One or more of the following: 1. Hemoglobin <8.5 g/100 ml 2. Serum calcium value >12 mg/100 ml 3. Advanced lytic bone lesions 4. High M-component production rates 　a. IgG value >7 g/100 ml 　b. IgA value >5 g/100 ml 　c. Urine light chain M-component on electrophoresis >12 g/24 hours	$>1.2 \times 10^{12}$ (high)
Subclass		
A	Serum creatinine ≤2 mg/100 ml	
B	Serum creatinine >2 mg/100 ml	

Source: Modified from B. G. M. Durie and S. E. Salmon, *Cancer* 36:842, 1975.

patients who present with stable or indolent, asymptomatic stage IA disease may be followed with observation alone until evidence of progression is obtained. Most patients will have more advanced or progressive disease at diagnosis and will require chemotherapy. Patients should be maintained on allopurinol, 300 mg/day PO through the first 2 months of chemotherapy to prevent urate nephropathy. A general supportive care regimen emphasizing ambulation and hydration should be maintained throughout.

2. **Standard induction chemotherapy** consists of the following:

   a. Melphalan, 8 mg/m² PO days 1 to 4 *and*

   b. Prednisone, 60 mg/m² PO days 1 to 4

   Repeat cycle every 28 days for at least 1 year.

   Because of erratic absorption of melphalan in a minority of patients, some recommend cautiously escalating the dose of melphalan on subsequent cycles of chemotherapy until a dose that produces moderate nadir leukocyte counts of 2000 to 3000 cells/μl is reached.

3. **Alternative induction chemotherapy.** A more intensive regimen termed the *M-2* or *VBMCP* represents an alternative approach to induction chemotherapy. In this program the prednisone schedule is frequently individualized so that slowly responding patients with persistent generalized bone pain or severe anemia receive low-dose pred-

nisone each day of the first 2 or 3 cycles in addition to the high scheduled dose on days 1 to 14. Furthermore, the second cycle may begin on day 29 if blood counts reflect complete recovery from the myelotoxic effects of the initial cycle of treatment. The VBMCP form of this regimen is the following:

   a. Vincristine, 1.2 mg/m^2 IV day 1 (dose not to exceed 2.0 mg)

   b. Carmustine (BCNU), 20 mg/m^2 IV day 1

   c. Melphalan, 8 mg/m^2 PO days 1 to 4

   d. Cyclophosphamide, 400 mg/m^2 IV day 1

   e. Prednisone, 40 mg/m^2 PO days 1 to 7 (all cycles) and 20 mg/m^2 PO days 8 to 14 (cycles 1–3 only)

Repeat cycle of VBMCP every 35 days for at least 1 year.

A prospective clinical trial is currently underway to determine which of these treatments is superior as primary therapy for myeloma patients. Survival in objectively responding multiple myeloma patients averages 3 years or more compared with a 1-year median survival in nonresponding patients.

   4. Role of radiotherapy. Solitary plasmacytoma of bone is best treated by local radiation therapy and may not require chemotherapy for months to years. Radiotherapy is also useful as palliative therapy for patients with extraskeletal plasmacytomas, large lytic lesions threatening fracture of long bones, spinal cord or nerve root compression by plasma cell tumor, and with certain pathologic fractures. Repeated local irradiation should be avoided where possible in patients with disseminated myeloma since chemotherapy is the only treatment demonstrated to improve survival while controlling systemic manifestations of the disease. Excessive use of radiation therapy can impair marrow reserves and render the patient less able to tolerate subsequent chemotherapy.

C. Maintenance therapy. Although no study has conclusively demonstrated benefit in continuing chemotherapy beyond 1 year in responding patients, several investigators have noted prompt reemergence of active myeloma shortly after cessation of therapy. Therefore, one acceptable approach is to continue the induction regimen beyond 1 year in responding patients, but to decrease its frequency to every 6 to 8 weeks while continuing to follow M-protein production carefully. It is probably safe to stop treatment at 1 year in those patients who started therapy with stage I disease and who maintain a 75 percent reduction in M-protein production. These patients should be observed carefully with reevaluation of serum and urine M-protein at least once every 3 months.

D. Complications of disease or therapy. Chemotherapy for multiple myeloma frequently causes moderate myelosuppression and packed red blood cell transfusions are often required, particularly during the early weeks of treatment and during the late refractory period. Toxicity of each chemotherapeutic agent is described in Chapter 4. In addition to these problems, several complications characteristic of multiple myeloma may occur.

   1. Hypercalcemia. This common complication of multiple myeloma is believed to result from the liberation of bone calcium stimulated by osteoclast activating factor released by the tumor cells. Presenting symptoms may include anorexia, nausea, vomiting, constipation, and polyuria progressing to lethargy, confusion, coma, and death. Dehydration and potentially reversible renal failure frequently occur during hypercalcemic crises. Control of hypercalcemic crises of multiple myeloma is usually accomplished with saline hydration, furosemide (40 mg q4–6h), and prednisone (40–80 mg PO daily for 3–7 days). When hypercalcemia occurs in previously untreated patients, prompt initiation of chemotherapy of the myeloma, in addition to these measures, will usually produce effective and durable control. In some patients, oral inorganic phosphates or mithramycin may be needed and can be used on the following schedule:

a. Inorganic phosphate as Neutra-Phos® or Fleet® Phospho-Soda at a dose equivalent to 0.5 g of phosphorus PO qid (diluted in water to reduce diarrhea).

b. Mithramycin, 25 µg/kg IV every 3 to 7 days. This agent is myelosuppressive and can cause hemostatic disorders and nausea. Its long-term or repeated use in myeloma should be avoided except in the most refractory instances of hypercalcemia.

2. Infection. Myeloma patients are highly susceptible to respiratory and urinary tract infections with common gram-positive and gram-negative bacterial pathogens. Deficiency of normal immunoglobulins, diminished bone marrow reserves, and immobilization owing to skeletal disease are important predisposing factors. The weeks immediately following initiation of chemotherapy represent a particularly high-risk period for infection. Prompt evaluation of fever or other manifestations of infection is essential. Antibiotic coverage for gram-positive and gram-negative organisms should be instituted while awaiting culture results in patients whose clinical picture suggests infection. Infection prophylaxis with gamma globulin injections or antibiotics has not been proven of value although further evaluation is needed.

3. Hyperviscosity. Hyperviscosity may present as CNS impairment, congestive heart failure, ischemia, or bleeding tendency. It is more characteristic of Waldenström's macroglobulinemia than of multiple myeloma, but it may be seen in patients with extremely high IgG or IgA concentrations or in patients whose M-protein tends to form aggregates. The treatment for symptomatic hyperviscosity is plasmapheresis.

4. Renal dysfunction. Renal dysfunction may be caused by myeloma kidney, amyloidosis, pyelonephritis, hypercalcemia with urate nephropathy, hyperviscosity syndrome, plasma cell infiltration of both kidneys (rare), and renal tubular acidosis. Most of these problems are at least partially reversible if recognized and treated promptly. Hypercalcemia and hyperuricemia are especially common potential causes of reversible renal failure and should be ruled out at the outset of the evaluation of a patient with myeloma. In patients with severe renal failure, hemodialysis should be considered as long as chemotherapy offers the potential for a prolonged remission.

5. Skeletal destruction is a major cause of disability and immobilization in multiple myeloma. Radiation therapy, surgery, or both may be needed to treat fractures or to prevent impending fractures to weight-bearing bones. The role of fluoride, calcium, and vitamin D in promoting skeletal repair during remission is under study.

6. **Leukemia.** Acute nonlymphocytic leukemia (ANLL) develops in about 4 percent of myeloma patients who receive chemotherapy. The incidence of ANLL is appreciably greater in patients surviving 4 years or more after the start of chemotherapy. Leukemia in this setting appears to represent the result of the interaction of a carcinogenic drug with a predisposed host. ANLL complicating multiple myeloma is frequently preceded by sideroblastic anemia.

E. **Recurrence and treatment of refractory disease.** Objective responses to chemotherapy that are accompanied by a 75 percent decrease in M-protein production have a median duration of about 2 years. Lesser degrees of response are usually under 1 year in duration. Patients with recurrent or refractory multiple myeloma pose a difficult clinical problem because of the small number of chemotherapeutic agents with proven activity in this disease. Patients relapsing months or years after last receiving melphalan can frequently be reinduced with the original regimen.

1. **Treatment of patients refractory to melphalan.** Patients refractory to melphalan or melphalan–prednisone regimens may still respond to other alkylating agents. The following are two suggested regimens:

   a. **CP**

      (1) Cyclophosphamide, 1000 mg/m^2 IV day 1

      (2) Prednisone, 60 mg/m^2 PO days 1 to 5

      Repeat every 3 weeks, *or*

   b. **BCP**

      (1) Carmustine (BCNU), 75 mg/m^2 IV day 1

      (2) Cyclophosphamide, 400 mg/m^2 IV day 1

      (3) Prednisone, 75 mg PO days 1 to 7

      Repeat every 4 weeks.

2. **Alternative regimens.** The effectiveness of the M-2, or VBMCP, regimen in patients refractory to melphalan–prednisone is currently under study. Alternative regimens include:

   a. Hexamethylmelamine, 280 mg/m^2 PO daily for 21 days *and* Prednisone, 75 mg PO daily for 7 days

   Repeat cycle every 28 days.

   b. Carmustine (BCNU), 30 mg/m^2 IV day 1 *and* Doxorubicin (Adriamycin™), 30 mg/m^2 IV day 1

   Repeat cycle every 21 days.

   c. Cyclophosphamide, 600 mg/m^2 IV days 1 to 4 repeated in 1 to 2 months, effectively produces pain relief of greater than 1 month duration and yields short-term objective responses in about 50 percent of patients refractory to prior treatments. Because this high-dose cyclophosphamide regimen is highly myelotoxic, its use should generally be limited to patients with clinically active, markedly symptomatic refractory disease in institutions equipped to render intensive support, including platelet and leukocyte transfusions and infectious disease consultation.

III. Waldenström's macroglobulinemia

A. General considerations and aims of therapy. This neoplasm is characterized by the proliferation of plasmacytoid lymphocytes that elaborate a monoclonal IgM. In contrast to multiple myeloma, skeletal destruction does not occur, but hepatosplenomegaly and lymphadenopathy are common. The major problems are hyperviscosity syndrome, severe anemia, and occasionally pancytopenia. The median survival is about 5 years from diagnosis, owing to, in part, the advanced age of most of these patients (60–75 years old) as well as to the common association with second neoplasms (20%) and chronic or recurrent infections (25%). The primary aims of therapy are to control complications and to decrease their incidence. Although response to chemotherapy has, not surprisingly, been associated with a more favorable median survival, the actual role of chemotherapy in prolonging survival in this disease has not been fully defined.

B. Treatment

1. Anemia. Most patients with macroglobulinemia are anemic; however, transfusions should generally be reserved for those with symptomatic anemia. Overtransfusion is dangerous because of the important contribution of red blood cells to whole blood viscosity.

2. Hyperviscosity. Hyperviscosity syndrome requires plasmapheresis for acute management and chemotherapy with alkylating agents for long-term control.

3. Chemotherapy. In general, chemotherapy is withheld until symptomatic disease or progressive cytopenias occur.

a. Standard chemotherapy

(1) Chlorambucil, 2 to 6 mg PO daily *or*

(2) Cyclophosphamide, 50 to 100 mg PO daily

(3) Prednisone, 40 to 60 mg PO days 1 to 4 every 4 weeks may be added

b. Alternatively, a high-dose intermittent chlorambucil–prednisone regimen may be used every 2 to 3 weeks.

(1) Chlorambucil, 30 mg/m^2 PO day 1

(2) Prednisone, 40 mg/m^2 PO days 1 to 4

4. Disease variants. Some patients with IgM monoclonal proteins have clinical CLL or lymphoma and should have their treatment directed at that disease. Rare patients with macroglobulinemia have prominent skeletal disease, and their disease should be approached as IgM myeloma and treated similarly to other multiple myelomas.

IV. Heavy chain diseases comprise a group of rare plasma cell dyscrasias in which the abnormal clone of plasma cells or B-lymphocytes elaborates a qualitatively abnormal polypeptide consisting of anomalous γ, α, or μ heavy chains from which segments have been deleted.

A. **Gamma heavy chain disease** presents as a lymphoma usually with lymphadenopathy, hepatosplenomegaly, and involvement of Waldeyer's ring. The latter may lead to characteristic palatal edema. Bone marrow involvement is the rule. Treatment by local radiotherapy or lymphoma-directed chemotherapy regimens is sometimes effective.

B. **Alpha heavy chain disease** appears to be the most common of the heavy chain diseases and occurs mainly in people under the age of 50. Its most common clinical presentation is in the enteric form with chronic diarrhea, malabsorption syndrome, and marked lymphoplasmacytic infiltration of the small bowel mucosa. Remissions have been reported using lymphoma chemotherapy regimens and occasionally with antibiotics alone.

C. **Mu heavy chain disease** is quite rare, usually presenting as chronic lymphocytic leukemia and should be managed as such.

V. **Amyloidosis.** Only primary amyloidosis with or without associated plasma cell or lymphoid neoplasms will be considered in this section. In these disorders the amyloid substance consists of fragments of immunoglobulin light chains and is therefore termed an AL-protein (amyloid L chain protein). This type of amyloid characteristically infiltrates the tongue, heart, skin, ligaments, muscle, and occasionally kidney, liver, and spleen. In patients with documented lymphomas or plasma cell neoplasms, treatment is of the underlying neoplasm but improvement in the amyloid is often minimal. In primary amyloidosis without a demonstrable underlying neoplasm, treatment with melphalan and prednisone has been shown to be of moderate benefit when tested in a randomized double-blind study, although the exact role of chemotherapy in this disease is not yet clear.

VI. **Monoclonal gammopathy of undetermined significance.** This disorder has been found in up to 3 percent of persons over 70 years of age. It had been termed *benign monoclonal gammopathy*, but since approximately 20 percent of patients with this finding progress, the term *monoclonal gammopathy of undetermined significance* has been introduced as more appropriate. In this condition, patients usually have an M-spike of less than 2.0 gm/100 ml, no bone lesions, no evidence of myeloma on bone marrow aspirate and biopsy, no anemia or bone marrow failure, and stability of the clinical picture and M-protein studies over a period of follow-up. Once initial stability in the amount of M-protein production is demonstrated, these patients should be followed at yearly intervals with evaluation of hemoglobin levels and M-protein status. No treatment is indicated unless progression to myeloma or symptomatic macroglobulinemia occurs.

Selected Reading

McIntyre, O. R. Current concepts in cancer multiple myeloma. *N. Engl. J. Med.* 301:193, 1979.

Durie, B. G. M., and Salmon, S. E. A clinical staging system for multiple myeloma. Correlation of measured myeloma cell mass with presenting clinical features, response to treatment and survival. *Cancer* 36:842, 1975.

Kyle, R. A., and Elveback, L. R. Management and prognosis of multiple myeloma. *Mayo Clin. Proc.* 51:751, 1976.

Kyle, R. A. Monoclonal gammopathy of undetermined significance. Natural history in 241 cases. *Am. J. Med.* 64:814, 1978.

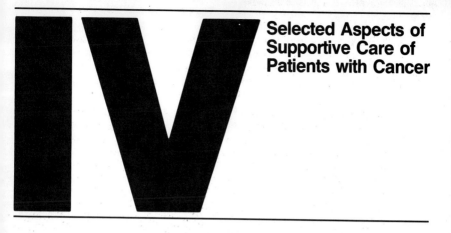

IV

Selected Aspects of Supportive Care of Patients with Cancer

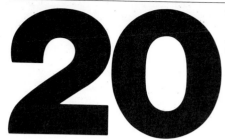

Treating Pain

Michael Weintraub

I. Goals and approach to therapy of cancer pain

A. Definition and significance.
Pain may be defined as an unpleasant sensory *and* emotional experience associated with actual or potential tissue damage or described in terms of such damage. The importance of both the sensory and emotional aspects of pain is particularly true in cancer pain. Whether or not specific therapy is available for the cancer, physicians always have the responsibility to attempt to achieve adequate analgesia for their patients. Cancer pain is not conceptually different from other chronic pain syndromes. However, the emotional overtones of pain in cancer make it even more important that it be adequately treated.

Initially, pain may be a signal for reassessment and diagnostic procedures. If specific therapy is possible, it should be undertaken as soon as the etiology of the pain has been discovered. However, physicians must prescribe analgesic drugs while attempting to establish the etiology of the pain and while waiting to begin specific treatment.

B. Goals of therapy.
The overall goal of analgesic therapy is to allow the patient to have as comfortable a life as possible at the highest level of daily activity commensurate with his or her physical status. The patient must be able to rest comfortably, to eat, and to perform self-care activities. Another goal of analgesic therapy is to enable the patient with cancer to maintain meaningful interactions with family members. Other ancillary goals are to allow the patient to maintain independence and live at home and be cared for in as normal a situation as possible. Some pain in patients with cancer may not be amenable to specific therapy. Nonetheless, analgesia should always be attempted.

C. General guidelines for analgesic use.
There are a number of general guidelines for analgesic use in patients with cancer. With the goal of therapy established and kept firmly in mind, the physician must next choose the agent.

1. **Choice of agent.** The choice of analgesic should be made not only on the basis of the analgesic goal and pain severity but also on a variety of other factors. These considerations include the etiology of the pain, the anatomic location of the pain, and the characteristics of the pain (e.g., sharp, paroxysmal pain or dull, constant pain).

2. **Dosage and schedule.** Once the agent has been chosen, the proper dose and dosing interval needed to achieve the therapeutic goal must next be decided. This decision is not the end of the therapeutic process,

however. Physicians must continually assess the response to the analgesic selected and modify the dose or the dose schedule based on the patient's response. In general, it is most often efficacious to begin treatment with higher doses when the pain is severe and taper medication as pain control is achieved. Regularly scheduled dosing is often more effective than "as needed" dosing. Patients suffering severe pain may benefit from a *pain-free period*—a period of intensive treatment allowing sleep and freedom from discomfort. Such a period often restores response to previously ineffective analgesics. The need for a pain-free period may occur whenever patients have escaped from previous analgesic therapy or if a new pain problem has arisen. When a previously effective chronic pain analgesic regimen fails, physicians should look for correctable new pain causes, such as infection, pathologic fractures, tumor extension, or neuritic involvement from radiation therapy or direct tumor extension.

3. **Adjunctive therapy.** Nonanalgesic adjunctive therapy such as muscle relaxants, sedatives, linaments, antiemetics, heat, cold, braces, and other appliances as well as other symptomatic therapy for cough, itching, or nausea can enhance the patient's response to analgesic medication and improve the overall quality of their life.

4. **Combinations of analgesics.** Quite often, rational combinations of different types of analgesics are beneficial for patients with cancer pain. Such combinations of analgesics may provide improved pain relief, delay the appearance of tolerance to narcotic medications, and avoid side effects from the medications in the combination. In some cases, combinations of narcotic analgesics and stimulants, such as amphetamines, may enhance narcotic effects, as will be discussed in section **IV.C.4.**

5. **Pain and suffering.** Physicians must always remember that chronic pain does not inure patients to pain; it makes them more sensitive to pain. Additionally, physicians and patients may share the puritanical belief that suffering builds character. Undertreatment with analgesic drugs may occur based on complicity between patient and the physician, nurse, or other health professional. Physicians may not prescribe analgesic treatment, a weak drug may be chosen, too low a dose may be given, or too long a dose interval may be utilized. Alternatively, patients may not ask for prescribed analgesics and will needlessly suffer.

II. Cancer pain type and etiology

A. **Visceral pain.** Cancer pain may arise from the pressure caused by the tumor growth in a tight tissue compartment. Occasionally, cancers may impede venous return causing engorgement and resulting in pain. Ischemia resulting from partial or complete arterial blockage causes severe pain. A hollow viscus may become obstructed as a consequence of tumor growth or of surgical intervention. Pain arising in solid or hollow visci related to these etiologies is often called *visceral pain*. Patients often describe the character of visceral pain as dull, constant, and aching. Visceral pain is often diffuse and poorly defined, except in the case of hollow viscus obstruction. The pain radiation may not be in the pattern usually associated with classic descriptions of somatic dermatomes. Visceral pain often responds best to narcotic and narcotic antagonist analgesics, particularly when it is severe.

B. **Inflammatory and somatic pain.** Cancer pain may also arise from tissue damage, such as that caused by necrosis, infection, or inflammation in pain-sensitive structures. Cancer patients may also complain of bone or musculoskeletal pain. This sort of pain may arise from periosteal irritation, fractures, or other causes. These two types of pain, plus dental and integumental pain, respond best to antipyretic or antiinflammatory analgesics such as aspirin, acetaminophen, or the new nonsteroidal antiinflammatory agents.

C. **Neuritic, neuropathic, and atypical pain.** *Neuritic pain* is pain arising from infiltration of nerves or nerve roots, as a distant effect caused by cancer, from extrinsic pressure on the nerves, or from postherpetic neuralgia. It often has burning, sharp, or "electric shooting" characteristics. Patients may complain of unpleasant distortions in their perception of normal stimuli. There may also be changes in anatomic function, such as blood flow changes or sweating, contemporaneous with the pain. *Neuropathic pain* occurs when the nervous system is damaged, or degeneration occurs in the part of the nervous system that normally transmits information about painful stimuli. Neuropathic pain may be caused by direct irritation, metabolic causes, immunologic effects on the nervous system, or late effects of radiation therapy, surgery, or chemotherapy. These types of pain often respond poorly to both narcotic analgesics and to antipyretic, antiinflammatory analgesics, but may respond well to socalled nonanalgesic analgesics, such as phenothiazines, tricyclic antidepressants, and antiepileptic agents.

III. Drug groups

A. **Narcotic and narcotic antagonist (partial agonist) analgesics.** Examples of drugs in this class of analgesic agents include the narcotic agonists morphine, methadone (Dolophine®), meperidine (Demerol®), and the narcotic antagonist or partial agonist analgesics, pentazocine (Talwin®), butorphenol (Stadol®), and nalbuphine (Nubain®). These drugs are most helpful in treating visceral pain as described in **II.A,** and should be used for severe pain of any type arising from any structure.

   1. **Mode of action.** These drugs are also called *centrally acting analgesics.* They work by interacting with specific receptors that are located in neuronal membranes and have their major effect within the central nervous system. These receptors are thought to be the same ones normally acted on by the "endogenous opioids"—primarily endorphins and enkephalins. The narcotic drugs presumably mimic the actions of these endogenous compounds. In addition to decreasing the patient's response to or processing of the pain stimulus at a central level, these drugs also directly decrease the severity of the pain.

   2. **Adverse effects.** Sedation may be a problem in the use of narcotic analgesics and narcotic antagonist analgesics. Other adverse effects, such as hypotension, may be seen with some of the agents in this class. Respiratory depression occurs with the narcotic agonists. *Tolerance* (the need to increase the dose to achieve the same therapeutic effect) and *physical dependence* (as manifested by a characteristic

withdrawal syndrome) have been described with these medications. True addiction arising from the medical use of narcotic analgesics is a *rare* phenomenon. Psychological and physical dependence may develop more or less rapidly based on various medication and patient characteristics. The medications that cause psychological and physical dependence more rapidly are those drugs that cross the blood-brain barrier quickly. Other effects of the medication, such as anticholinergic and euphoriant effects, increase drug abuse liability. Larger doses and more frequent doses of medication speed the development of tolerance. It has been said that tolerance and physical dependence may develop over a 48- to 72-hour period when the drug is administered in continuous IV infusions at a relatively high dose. The patient and the underlying physical problem also affect the rapidity and the development of tolerance and physical dependence. Some patients rarely develop this syndrome, others develop it more often.

Narcotic antagonist analgesics, which are, in reality partial agonists and partial antagonists, may induce or precipitate withdrawal syndrome in patients who have received chronic narcotic analgesic therapy. They thus should not be used in such patients.

3. **Effect of dose and route of administration.** There is a ceiling effect for some of the weaker narcotic analgesic agents such as codeine and propoxyphene (Darvon®). Thus, increasing the dose of codeine above 120 mg q4h may do nothing but increase adverse effects without concomitant increase in analgesia. However, morphine does not exhibit the ceiling effect, and in fact open-heart surgery has been conducted using morphine as the sole anesthetic agent. Many of the narcotic analgesics maintain some activity when administered orally. However, simply giving the same amount of drug orally as given parenterally will result in serious undertreatment with most narcotic analgesics. For example, an adequate IM dose of meperidine for an adult will be 75 to 100 mg. As much as 200 to 300 mg PO may be necessary to achieve the same analgesic response. Several narcotic analgesics are not completely metabolized in the gut wall or by hepatic cells and reach the systemic circulation with a good oral to IM potency ratio. These include levorphenol (Levo-Dromoran®), methadone, and oxycodone. Codeine, while less active, also has good oral to IM potency ratio. In Table 20-1, the starting doses of narcotic analgesics and narcotic antagonist-agonist analgesics are given.

4. **Duration of action.** Most narcotic analgesics have a duration of action of at least 3 hours. Medications found at this lower end of the scale include hydromorphone (Dilaudid®), oxycodone, pentazocine, and heroin, which is not available for medical use in the United States. Methadone has a longer duration of action (up to 6 hrs), particularly after chronic dosing, owing to drug accumulation. Meperidine and morphine are intermediate-acting with durations of action of approximately 4 hours. Physicians frequently over-estimate the duration of action of narcotic analgesics, which may result in undertreatment. Morphine and other narcotics may accumulate in patients with decreased renal function. Naloxone (Narcan®) reversal of excessive effects may thus be needed for long periods.

Table 20-1. Starting Doses and Duration of Action of Narcotic
Analgesics and Narcotic Antagonist–Agonist Analgesics

Drug	Initial Dose	Frequency (hr)	Duration of Action (hr)
PARENTERAL NARCOTICS			
Morphine	8–10 mg	q3–6	~ 4
Oxymorphone (Numorphan®)	1 mg	q3–6	~ 4
Hydromorphone (Dilaudid®)	1–2 mg	q4–6	~ 5
Levorphanol (Levo-Dromoran®)	2–3 mg	q4–6	~ 5
Methadone (Dolophine®)	8–10 mg	q5–8	~ 6
Meperidine (Demerol®)	75–100 mg	q3–4	2–4
PARENTERAL NARCOTIC ANTAGONIST–AGONISTS			
Pentazocine (Talwin®)	40–60 mg	q3–6	4–5
Butorphanol (Stadol®)	2–4 mg	q3–4	3–4
Nalbuphine (Nubain®)	10 mg	q3–4	3–4
ORAL NARCOTICS			
Meperidine (Demerol®)	200–300 mg	q4–6	4–5
Codeine	30–60 mg	q4–6	4–5
Propoxyphene (Darvon®)	130 mg	q4–6	4–5
Oxycodone (in mixtures)	20–30 mg	q3–4	~ 4
Methadone (Dolophine®)	10–20 mg	q6–8	~ 6
Levorphanol (Levo-Dromoran®)	2–4 mg	q4–6	~ 5
Hydromorphone (Dilaudid®)	4–6 mg	q3–5	3–4
ORAL NARCOTIC ANTAGONIST–AGONIST			
Pentazocine (Talwin®)	50–100 mg	q3–5	3–4
PHENOTHIAZINES (PARENTERAL)			
Methotrimeprazine (Levoprome®)	10–20 mg	q6–8	~ 6

5. **Formulation.** Some patients will prefer liquid oral formulations. These formulations are easy to take, have various flavors (limited only by the pharmacist's imagination), and are flexible in terms of dose titration. However, the excessive interest in liquid combination analgesics are not supported by objective data. Other patients will find tablets or capsules more convenient. Suppositories may also be useful in patients having swallowing difficulties or significant nausea. Patients must insert the suppository above the anal sphincter but not much further. This position may allow the absorbed drug to bypass the portal system and enter the systemic circulation since the inferior and middle hemorrhoidal veins enter the inferior vena cava system. Occasionally rectal administration of analgesics may irritate the mucosa or absorption may be irregular and slow. Patients also may not wish to use the suppositories. Most analgesics can be found in many formulations and the physician should prescribe one that the patient will find preferable and that best accomplishes the therapeutic goal.

6. **New developments**

   a. **Epidural narcotic analgesics.** A recent, exciting development in the use of opiate analgesics is the administration of these drugs into the extradural spaces. Potential advantages of this route of administration include lower drug doses than those used for systemic therapy and analgesia without autonomic changes, loss of motor power, or impairment of sensation other than pain reduction. Various medications with differing durations of action and routes of eliminations have been utilized in peridural or epidural analgesia. This method seems relatively safe, even if the material is inadvertantly injected into the subarachnoid space. If the medication is accidentally given IV or intrathecally, respiratory depression and other adverse effects can easily be antagonized by naloxone, a specific, safe, pure opiate antagonist. The use of epidural narcotic analgesics is based on the existence of spinal opiate receptors in the substantia gelantinosa. Recent studies involving large numbers of patients have concluded that the use of indwelling epidural catheters for narcotic analgesic administration has resulted in few adverse effects, rare development of tolerance (even over a 3-week period), need for low daily doses, and excellent analgesia. Respiratory depression may still occur following epidural morphine, however.

   b. Enkephalin Derivatives. Several enkephalin derivatives are currently under study as analgesic medications. Further understanding of the endogenous opiate system may result in clinically useful medications.

B. Antipyretic, antiinflammatory analgesics. The classic example of drugs in this class is aspirin. While acetaminophen is antipyretic, it is only weakly, if at all, antiinflammatory. Nonetheless, it remains a valuable analgesic replacing aspirin in patients who cannot tolerate the GI or platelet inhibitory side effects of aspirin. Acetaminophen does not affect uric acid excretion. The doses used for aspirin as an analgesic agent are less than those required for full antiinflammatory effect. Thus 650 mg (2 common tablets) of aspirin will provide analgesia for 2 to 4 hours. Other examples of the antipyretic, antiinflammatory analgesics include indomethacin and the new nonsteroidal, antiinflammatory agents such as ibuprofen (Motrin®), fenaprofen (Nalfon®), naproxen (Naprosyn®), sulindac (Clinoril®), and tolmetin sodium (Tolectin®).

   1. Use and mode of action. These drugs work peripherally rather than centrally. They are most effective in treatment of musculoskeletal, dental, or integumental pain of mild-to-moderate severity. They may also decrease inflammation. Data on precise mechanism of action of the antipyretic, antiinflammatory medications in decreasing pain are controversial. However, by blocking production of prostaglandins, these drugs may decrease sensitization of *nociceptors* (a receptor preferentially sensitive to a noxious or potentially noxious stimulus). Newer members of this analgesic class may also block other mediators of the inflammatory process. Sedation, of course, is not a problem with peripherally acting antipyretic, antiinflammatory analgesics.

   2. Adverse effects. Adverse effects are usually related to the GI system. Cardiovascular effects, respiratory depression, tolerance, and dependence do not accompany therapy with these agents. They do have a ceiling effect, however. All of these agents are orally active with a usual duration of action of approximately 4 hours. The rationale for the development of the newer nonsteroidal antiinflammatory agents has been to achieve similar antiinflammatory and analgesic effects compared to aspirin but with fewer side effects. Therefore, the possi-

Table 20-2. Starting Doses and Dose Ranges of Some Nonsteroidal Analgesic Agents

Drug	Starting Dose	Frequency (hr)	Dose Range
Aspirin	650 mg	q4–6	Up to 1300 mg q6h
Acetaminophen	650 mg	q4–6	Up to 975 mg q4–6h
Mefenamic acid (Ponstel®)	250 mg	6	Up to 375 mg q6h
Indomethacin (Indocin®)	50 mg	q6–8	Up to 100 mg q6–8h
Ibuprofen (Motrin®)	400 mg	q4–6	Up to 2400 mg daily
Fenaprofen (Nalfon®)	600 mg	6	Up to 3200 mg daily
Naproxen (Naprosyn®)	250 mg	q8–12	Up to 1250 mg daily
Naproxen sodium (Anaprox®)	550 mg	First dose	
	275 mg	q6–8	Up to 1375 mg daily
Zomepirac (Zomax®)	100 mg	q4–6	Up to 600 mg daily

bility of using these agents in patients who cannot tolerate the necessary doses of aspirin or acetaminophen always exists. Table 20-2 lists common starting doses of the nonsteroidal antiinflammatory drugs.) Antipyretic, antiinflammatory analgesics often form a logical component of rational combination analgesics either as manufactured by the pharmaceutical industry or as prepared individually for each patient by physicians.

3. **New developments.** Zomepirac sodium (Zomax®) is a recently introduced analgesic that has some attributes of narcotic analgesics and some of antipyretic, antiinflammatory analgesics. However, zomepirac is not a narcotic analgesic, does not induce tolerance, nor causes physical dependence or withdrawal syndrome. Its use does not result in respiratory depression. While it appears to be a valuable addition to our therapeutic armamentarium, zomepirac is a new agent that has not been widely used in the United States or abroad. Nonetheless, if our understanding of zomepirac's usefulness is substantiated over time, it will be a valuable agent.

C. **Nonanalgesic analgesics (phenothiazines, tricyclic antidepressants, and antiepileptic agents)**

1. **Agents and their use.** Examples of this class of medications include the standard analgesic drug methotrimeprazine (Levoprome®). This agent is a phenothiazine drug used in other parts of the world as an antipsychotic agent. It produces analgesia equivalent to that of morphine when given parenterally. The problems of its use include sedation (particularly after the first few doses) and postural hypotension. Tolerance and respiratory depression do not develop with methotrimeprazine.

Amitriptyline (Elavil® and others) given with or without a substituted phenothiazine such as perphenazine (Trilafon®) has been used in the treatment of atypical pain and a variety of painful syndromes involving nerves. Postherpetic neuralgia, phantom-limb pain, and other types of neuritic pain may respond dramatically and rapidly to these agents.

Amitriptyline plus perphenazine as well as other psychotropic drugs have been used with good success in the treatment of serious postherpetic neuralgia pain and in neuritic pain caused by direct or distant effects of cancer. Common starting doses include 50 mg of amitriptyline with 4 mg of perphenazine given before bed, followed by 25 mg of amitriptyline and 2 mg of perphenazine given in the morning. Patients with postherpetic neuralgia may report dramatic improvement in their pain after 1 or 2 days of such doses.

Carbamazepine (Tegretol®) has been used in the treatment of tic douloureux. It is, of course, an important antiepileptic agent.

Levodopa has been used to treat pain arising from bone metastases in patients with breast and other cancers. Along with a peripheral dopa-decarboxylase inhibitor, levodopa has also been successful in decreasing acute herpes zoster pain and perhaps preventing postherpetic neuralgia. The mechanism of levodopa's pain-decreasing effects is unclear.

These nonanalgesic analgesics may have both central and peripheral sites of action. Neuritic and atypical shooting paroxysmal pain respond best to these drugs. In fact, ablative neurosurgical procedures may be avoided by the appropriate use of these agents. They are efficacious in moderate to severe pain. Of course, methotrimeprazine may be used for any type of pain, particularly in bed-ridden patients or in patients needing the pain-free period discussed in section **I.C.2.** Methotrimeprazine is a standard analgesic available for use in postoperative or any serious pain.

2. **Side effects.** Sedation may occur with amitriptyline and phenothiazine drugs, but it is rarely a problem if they are prescribed on an appropriate schedule, such as before sleep. Postural hypotension occurs with methotrimeprazine and less often with the amitriptyline plus perphenazine combination. However, patients rapidly become tolerant to this effect without loss of analgesic effect. Respiratory depression, the need for dose escalation, and physical dependence do not occur. Except for methotrimeprazine, these drugs are orally active and have relatively long half-lives.

D. **Combination analgesics.** Rational combinations of antipyretic, antiinflammatory agents with mild narcotics, such as codeine, propoxyphene, or in some cases, the more euphoria-inducing agent oxycodone, are valuable therapeutic approaches to the treatment of cancer pain. The addition of nonsteroidal antiinflammatory agents to a narcotic regimen may delay the appearance of tolerance to the narcotic while maintaining adequate pain control. In the last several years, the pharmaceutical industry has altered the formulas of many of the combination analgesics. Therefore, it is important that each physician keep up-to-date and learn the exact ingredients of every combination drug. One important change has been to eliminate phenacetin from analgesic combinations. However, other ingredients have also been removed from some of the pharmaceutically produced analgesic combinations. Combination analgesics may, in the long run, save the patient money and produce the desired therapeutic effect more efficaciously than combinations created by the physician. Another valuable feature of pharmaceutically produced combination analgesics is assurance of compatibility, of both active ingredients and of the excipients. Pharmacists may charge separate fees for filling each of two prescriptions, thus increasing the cost of physician-created combinations. If physicians wish to create their own combinations, the drugs not requiring a prescription should be given to the patient on a separate paper and bought over-the-counter. To reduce drug costs, only the prescription medications should be written on a prescription blank.

IV. Analgesics: additional considerations on rational pain management

A. Saving patients money on analgesics.
Physicians must consider the cost of therapy, but they should not depend on price lists taken from wholesale catalogues, even with a standard markup added. The pharmacist, whose importance is often forgotten, is one of the major components of drug pricing. Many studies have shown that prices for the same amount of the same medication vary enormously among pharmacies and even within the same pharmacies over time. Prescriptions written generically to allow substitution usually do save patients some money. However, generic drugs may occasionally cost more than the brand-name product, depending on the pharmacy. Simplistic dependence on the prices in the "Red Book" often misleads prescribers. To achieve savings, patients must comparison-shop. Of course, the physician must prescribe the most effective medication for the patient since the medicine achieving the therapeutic goal represents the least expensive treatment.

B. Escalation of analgesic requirement

1. **Increase in symptoms may mean change in disease status.** If a patient who has been previously well-controlled on a therapeutic regimen of analgesics suddenly has increasingly severe pain, a diagnostic workup and perhaps new therapeutic approaches are required. Frequently the cause of the change in pain is a new disease process, which may be either related to or unrelated to the cancer. The search for correctable causes, such as infections, pathologic fractures, and new metastases (which may be sensitive to localized radiation therapy or alterations in chemotherapy) should be carried out immediately. If the etiology of the pain is an extension of the disease process (such as a new tumor mass) or is due to therapy (such as late effects of radiation therapy or surgery) this etiology must be diagnosed and treated appropriately.

2. **Increase in symptoms may mean insufficient drug or tolerance.** Another cause for the development of ineffective analgesia is that the patients have "fallen behind" in their therapy. Constant around-the-clock analgesic therapy is more effective than on-demand or as-needed therapy. Patients may omit analgesic doses either because they wish to avoid addiction or because they feel that the physician, nurse, and pharmacist may attribute their use of drugs to weakness. The development of tolerance to narcotic analgesics is another potential etiology for ineffective analgesia. Patients first notice a decrease in the duration of action of narcotic analgesics as tolerance develops. Later the peak effect decreases, and finally the onset of effect is delayed. Simply increasing the dose of medication can overcome this problem. Addition of nonsteroidal antiinflammatory agents may also help delay and overcome the development of tolerance.

C. Stepwise use of analgesic agents.
If the necessity occurs for the initiation of analgesics or therapeutic escalation to more powerful analgesics in cancer pain, a stepwise approach is often valuable. This approach assumes that non-drug therapy and other adjunctive therapies have all been attempted. Beginning with oral medication is a good idea unless the

patient needs either a pain-free period or high analgesic doses to achieve initial pain control. The first step is to begin with the milder drugs, later working toward combinations of mild drugs, and finally adding the more powerful agents.

1. **Mild drugs.** In step 1 the use of nonnarcotic oral analgesics, such as antipyretic, antiinflammatory agents, is often helpful. Acetaminophen has less GI toxicity than aspirin, although it may cause hepatic toxicity in overdose and in poorly nourished patients. It does not have antiinflammatory effects, however. Aspirin is a good alternative that not only has analgesic effects, but also has antiinflammatory effects. The nonsteroidal antiinflammatory agents, including indomethacin (Indocin®), the propionic acid derivatives, and newer agents such as zomepirac and the as yet unmarketed nefopam, may also be useful as first-step agents. This is particularly true if the pain is mild or if it involves the musculoskeletal system or the integument. Depending on the etiology of their pain and its severity, some patients may also respond to a mild narcotic given alone. These medications include codeine and propoxyphene, either as the hydrochloride or the napsylate salt (Darvon-N®). One of the milder mixed agonist antagonist analgesics, such as pentazocine, could also be used. Oxycodone, which is found only in combination drugs, such as Percodan® or Tylox,® may have a higher abuse potential than some of the other agents. Propoxyphene and its metabolite, norpropoxyphene, at least in high doses, may be associated with cardiac toxicity. There is also a small problem with abuse of propoxyphene.

2. **Adding mild narcotic to nonnarcotic analgesics.** Step 1A involves the combination of a nonnarcotic oral antipyretic, antiinflammatory analgesic with a mild narcotic. In manufactured combinations, they frequently include the mild stimulant caffeine and, more rarely, barbiturates. Other combinations that can be created by the physician include those using benezodiazepines.

3. **Using a stronger narcotic.** Step 2 involves the use of orally active, stronger narcotics. Some examples include hydromorphone. While 8 mg PO is equivalent to 10 mg of parenteral morphine, lower doses may also be useful for less severe pain. This drug is short acting and should be given approximately every 3 to 4 hours. Other examples include levorphenol, in which 4 mg is equivalent to 10 mg of morphine. Oxymorphone (Numorphan®) can be given as a suppository in patients who are nauseated. The oral dose equivalent to 10 mg of morphine is approximately 6 mg of oxymorphone. Methadone is the most useful of these orally active strong narcotics because of its long half-life and its tendency to accumulate with chronic dosing. While 20 mg of methadone has been said to be equal to 10 mg of parenteral morphine, patients frequently respond well to methadone in repeated doses of 10 mg PO. In fact, at the end of a 1-week period, many patients reduce their dose of methadone.

4. **Combining strong narcotics and nonsteroidal antiinflammatory agents.** Step 2A involves combining the strong narcotics and the nonsteroidal antiinflammatory agents. In some institutions, strong narcotics have been used in combination with stimulant drugs, such as amphetamine and, more rarely, cocaine. Patients sleep and eat

better even when receiving the stimulants because their pain has been decreased. Such combinations may be effective but their use has probably been over emphasized. At the Strong Memorial Hospital, University of Rochester, the frequent combination is methadone (1 mg) plus amphetamine (0.5 mg/cc of liquid preparation).

5. **Parenteral narcotics.** Step 3 involves the relief of serious pain necessitating hospitalization or placement in an institution where parenteral medications can be administered. Occasionally, family members can be taught to administer parenteral medications, and the patient can be kept comfortable and at home. Step 3 requires the use of parenteral strong narcotics or narcotic antagonist analgesics. This use includes parenteral meperidine, morphine, or if the patient has not already been on long-term narcotic treatment, the parenteral partial agonist–antagonists such as butorphenol and nalbuphine or pentazocine may be prescribed.

Step 3A is the use of a parenteral nonnarcotic such as methotrimeprazine. At each step, nonsteroidal antiinflammatory analgesics can also be added if appropriate.

6. **Adjunctive therapy** should be considered at every pain level. Physicians can now choose from among many forms of treatment, including transepidermal neurostimulation (TEN), neurosurgical ablative procedures, nerve blocks, hypnosis, heat, cold, and braces.

V. **New developments in pain control.** The exciting development of patient-controlled analgesia in hospital settings remains of interest. Patients can administer analgesic drugs to themselves, particularly drugs given IV through reliable drug administration systems equipped with fail-safe controls. Such systems may be valuable in achieving pain-free periods. Patients in studies of self-dosing, self-controlled analgesia have requested less total analgesics over a 3-day period after surgery. They decreased their demand for analgesic drugs after the first postoperative day. However, in the first 24 hours after abdominal surgery, for example, they administered on the average, 500 mg of parenteral meperidine. This dose is much higher than physicians usually prescribe. Other methods, such as controlled IM analgesia and patient-controlled epidural injection of narcotic analgesics, may also offer important benefits.

Continued research on endorphins and enkephalins may result in the achievement of orally active derivatives of these fascinating materials. Further definition of the specific opioid receptors may result in the development of medications that selectively stimulate analgesic receptors without any, or with minimal, euphoria, sedation, cardiovascular effects, and tolerance. The pharmaceutical industry is continually searching for more effective orally administered nonnarcotic analgesics. Physicians should keep in touch with the literature and use these drugs as soon as they become available and their efficacy for cancer pain is apparent. While we do not have the perfect drug nor do we have agents that accomplish all of our goals, we certainly can do a better job in using available drugs more effectively and more rationally.

Selected Reading

Beaumont, A., and Hughes, J. Biology of opioid peptides. *Annu. Rev. Pharmacol. Toxicol.* 19:245, 1979.

Epidermal opiates. *Lancet* 2:962, 1980.

Flower, R. J., Moncada, S., and Vane, J. R. Analgesic–Antipyretics and Anti-Inflammatory Agents. In A. G. Gilman, A. Goodman, and A. Gilman (Eds.), *The Pharmacologic Basis of Therapeutics* (6th ed.). New York: MacMillan, 1980. Pp. 682–728.

Houde, R. W. The Use and Misuse of Narcotics in the Treatment of Cancer Pain. In J. J. Bonica (Ed.), *Advances in Neurology* (4th ed.). New York: Raven, 1974.

Houde, R. W. Systemic Analgesics and Related Drugs: Narcotic Analgesics. In J. J. Bonica and V. Ventafredda (Eds.), *Advances in Pain Research and Therapy* (2nd ed.). New York: Raven, 1979.

Jaffe, J. H., and Martin, W. R. Opioid Analgesics and Antagonists. In A. G. Gilman, A. Goodman, and A. Gilman (Eds.), *The Pharmacologic Basis of Therapeutics* (6th ed.). New York: MacMillan, 1980. Pp. 494–534.

Sechzer, P. H. Studies in pain with analgesic demand system. *Anesth. Analg.* (Cleveland) 50:1, 1971.

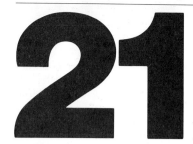

Bony Metastases

Gerald W. Marsa

Second in importance to maximizing a patient's chances for cure, perhaps, is the challenge the physician faces in minimizing the potential complications of cancer, which can markedly diminish the quality of remaining life for a patient with incurable disease. Metastatic involvement of the skeleton is the most commonly encountered problem; it has the potential to drastically change a patient's ability to continue living a relatively normal life. Thus, it is imperative that physicians and others caring for patients with cancer be continually alert to the possibility of skeletal metastases, so the devastating end result of pathologic fracture may be avoided. Accurate assessment of the patient's future course by knowledge of a tumor's natural history and realistic appraisal of chances for success of remaining therapy programs will assist the team of primary physician, orthopedic surgeon, radiation oncologist, and medical oncologist in deciding the correct approach in managing each patient with bony metastasis.

I. Clinical presentation

A. Pain. Bony metastases manifest themselves by producing pain or limiting function. Pain from skeletal metastases is usually of two separate and coexisting types. Patients with bone pain frequently complain first of constant *gnawing* pain in the affected bone, which usually is worse at night and may awaken the patient from sleep. This pain is due to pressure erosion of bone by an expanding metastatic deposit within the bone. A second component of pain, usually *sharp* in quality, is noticed by patients when stress (weight bearing etc.) is applied to the affected bone; classically, this is more prominent during the day while a patient is active and is relieved by resting. While the constant ache caused by bony erosion is frequently relieved within a few days of initiating radiotherapy or effective chemotherapy, the pain caused by structural weakening will persist until additional support is provided by external devices (brace, cast), internal orthopedic support (intramedullary rod, compression plate, methyl methacrylate cement, etc.), or by adequate bone reconstitution by the normal reparative process.

B. Radiologic studies

1. **Bone scans and radiography.** Radiographic evidence of bony metastasis may be lacking despite great pain, since nearly one half of the bone structure must be destroyed before the destruction will be apparent on a routine bone x-ray film; isotope bone scanning is much more sensitive and usually will show the increased bone turnover at a much earlier stage. It must be remembered, however, that the scan identifies only an area of increased osteoblastic activity that can be

the result of a variety of processes; radiographs of abnormal areas are a prerequisite to insure against a benign cause of the abnormality.

2. **Types of lesions.** Metastatic involvement may appear radiographically as a pure osteoblastic process (prostate carcinoma, osteosarcoma), a pure osteolytic process (multiple myeloma, oat-cell carcinoma of lung), or as a mixed process with varying amounts of each type (breast carcinoma, lung carcinoma, and most other malignancies, including those that can present as a pure process). Since bone scanning identifies areas of increased osteoblastic activity, lesions that are purely osteolytic may appear silent on bone scan in the presence of a large defect on x-ray.

3. **Sites of metastasis.** Malignancies that frequently metastasize to a solitary skeletal site include hypernephroma and gastrointestinal carcinomas. Breast carcinoma, lung cancer, and prostatic carcinoma nearly always involve multiple bones on initial metastasis. For this reason a systematic search for other, as yet asymptomatic, lesions should be undertaken as part of the overall reevaluation, which includes bone scan and x-rays of pelvis, proximal femurs, and any bones identified as abnormal on scan. Most metastases involve the axial skeleton and proximal extremities, but skull involvement is common in multiple myeloma and breast carcinoma; metastasis to distal extremity bones, although rare, is most frequently seen with hypernephroma, lung cancer, and neuroblastoma.

II. Surgical therapy

A. Pathologic fractures

1. **Long bones and ribs.** Since rapid return of the patient to as normal a life as possible is an overriding concern in treating patients with metastatic disease, surgical stabilization is most often the initial step in treating pathologic fractures of the long bones. If the fracture is the initial manifestation of tumor relapse, biopsy confirmation can also be obtained. Whereas fractures at sites of significant residual bony architecture can be satisfactorily stabilized with an intramedullary rod or pin, marked lytic destruction may necessitate additional structural support such as methyl methacrylate cement to fill the intramedullary canal and cortical defects. Casts are infrequently utilized owing to the long interval until restoration of normal bone strength through the healing process. In addition, a cast's bulkiness interferes with restoration of normal ambulation and makes the administration of adjuvant irradiation difficult. Pathologic fractures of non-weight-bearing bones can be managed by splinting (ribs) or sling immobilization (humerus or clavicle) while delivering radiotherapy to promote healing. Fixation may also be used in the upper extremities to speed recovery of function, particularly of the humerus.

2. **Compression fractures.** Compression fractures of the spine not only are a source of severe pain, but are also a potential source of spinal cord or nerve root compression. Adequate support to the weakened vertebral body can be provided with external supportive devices, ranging from a tight girdle in the least severe cases to a rigid spine brace in the most severe. In this manner, weight from the upper body can be partially transferred to the pelvic bones by way of the ribs and

soft tissues, preventing further deformity by reducing stress on the affected vertebral body. In many cases, this support must be maintained a number of months until adequate healing has occurred subsequent to intervening radiotherapy or systemic therapy.

3. **Prostheses.** Occasionally, severe destruction of the femoral head or acetabulum makes restoration to an ambulatory state impossible unless the bone is replaced by a prosthesis. Replacement is warranted when the prognosis would suggest a reasonable life expectancy of 6 months or more with continued stability of health following the procedure. An appropriate example is breast carcinoma in a patient without prior exposure to combination chemotherapy, and several systemic therapy programs exist with high probability of response. A prosthetic device would seldom be appropriate in lung carcinoma, a disease in which survival is short following the diagnosis of systemic metastasis, and responses to chemotherapy are less frequent and of shorter duration. With careful selection, total hip arthroplasty can give excellent palliation with marked improvement in the quality of life for the affected patient.

B. **Impending fractures.** Weight-bearing bones with marked cortical destruction are at high risk for subsequent fracture during the course of palliative radiotherapy or, following radiation, while awaiting restoration of adequate bone structure. Rather than consigning a patient to a prolonged interval of non-weight-bearing on the affected extremity with continued high risk of fracture with passive movement, better management is immediate "prophylactic" stabilization with an intramedullary rod or pin. Following stabilization, radiotherapy can be initiated without high risk of fracture and with the patient significantly more active. Prophylactic nailing is easy to perform and has less morbidity than fracture fixation.

III. Radiation therapy

A. **Indications.** Irradiation of weight-bearing bones with metastatic involvement is indicated early in the disease process before pathologic fracture can occur. Surgical stabilization does not obviate the need for irradiation to prevent further bony destruction by residual tumor. Symptomatic metastases to non-weight-bearing bones are also an indication for palliative irradiation. Relatively low doses of irradiation (1500–2000 rad) are frequently sufficient to afford dramatic pain relief, and 80 to 90 percent of patients with pain secondary to bone metastases will show significant improvement with intermediate doses (3000–4000 rad).

B. **Treatment schedules.** Treatment is structured to give therapy as rapidly as possible to afford relief of pain and promote bone healing for the remainder of the patient's life, while minimizing any concurrent radiation symptoms. In a patient in the terminal stage of illness with a life expectancy of a few weeks, a single fraction of 1000 rad if the portal is small, or 1500 to 2000 rad in 3 to 5 fractions will give the desired effect. Conversely, an occasional patient may have the potential for prolonged survival (i.e., early metastatic breast carcinoma) in which instance one might use high doses for longer control of disease and a large number of fractions to minimize late normal tissue effects (i.e., 5000 rad in 25 fractions). Most patients will receive optimal results from courses of 3000 rad in 10 fractions (2 weeks) or 4000 rad in 15 fractions (3 weeks). Should recurrent symptoms develop owing to reactivation of treated disease, a repeat course of radiotherapy can be undertaken with excellent prospects for another response, since patients with relapsing metastatic disease seldom survive long enough to develop the late radiation consequences of multiple radiotherapy courses.

C. **Treatment fields.** Radiotherapy fields should include the evident bone involvement as shown on x-ray film and bone scan with a sufficient extension to prevent relapse at the portal margin. It is seldom necessary to treat the entire bone unless the entire bone is involved, since encroachment on marrow reserve may compromise any systemic chemotherapy that may also be indicated. Supervoltage radiotherapy (cobalt or linear accelerator) is always preferrable to minimize acute skin reactions and late soft tissue fibrosis as a source of patient morbidity and to maximize the capacity to retreat the patient at a later date if required.

D. **Hemibody irradiation**

1. **Indications.** Sequential hemibody irradiation for palliation of widespread symptomatic bony metastases is an effective modality, recent experience has shown. It is indicated only in patients with diffuse symptomatic bony involvement for whom no effective systemic chemotherapy remains, since significant marrow depression can be expected.

2. **Technique.** The more symptomatic half of the body, divided at the umbilicus, is irradiated as a single large field through anterior and posterior portals, usually giving a single fraction of 1000 rad to the lower hemibody or 700 rad to the upper half-body. The other half is treated approximately 1 month later, following marrow recovery within the irradiated field.

3. **Side effects.** Despite the following side effects, hemibody irradiation should be considered in patients with diffuse symptoms who have exhausted conventional systemic therapies, because of the excellent transient responses which can be achieved.

   a. Nausea and vomiting in the first 12 hours subsequent to treatment, usually controlled with sedation and antiemetics

   b. Blood count depression at 7 to 10 days posttreatment, which rarely requires transfusion support in the patient previously heavily treated with chemotherapy

   c. Hypotension in the first 24 hours following upper hemibody irradiation in patients not pretreated with steroids

   d. Acute radiation pneumonitis at 4 to 6 weeks following upper hemibody irradiation, especially if the patient has had prior thoracic radiotherapy

IV. **Systemic therapy.** Patients developing bone metastasis have obvious need for effective systemic therapy of their disease if therapy is available. In diseases such as the lymphomas or breast carcinoma, there is a high probability of response to chemotherapy, and institution of systemic treatment alone can induce healing of the metastatic bony lesions. Even in such favorable instances, the physician must evaluate any involved weight-bearing bones regarding the potential for pathologic fracture, and maintain this close vigilance throughout the course of therapy. Any evidence of progressive bony involvement, especially in the proximal femurs, warrants immediate radiotherapy to reduce the risk of pathologic fracture and to avoid the need for surgical stabilization. Many neoplasms, such as gastrointestinal malignancies and non-oat-cell carcinomas of the lung, have a low probability of response to chemotherapeutic regimens, and in these, local irradiation to affected weight-bearing bones should be considered as part of the initial systemic program. With closely coordinated care among the primary physician, medical oncologist, and the radiotherapist, concurrent or sequential therapies can be given to minimize the risks of orthopedic catastrophe without compromise of systemic chemotherapy.

Selected Reading

Montague, E., and Delclos, L. Palliative Radiotherapy in the Management of Metastatic Disease. In G. H. Fletcher (Ed.), *Textbook of Radiotherapy* (3rd ed.). Philadelphia: Lea & Febiger, 1980. Pp. 943–948.

Turek, S. Secondary Tumors of Bone. In *Orthopaedics: Principles and Their Application* (3rd ed.). Philadelphia: Lippincott, 1977. Pp. 586–602.

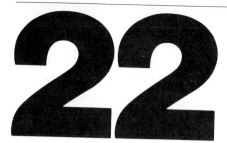

Superior Vena Cava Syndrome and Other Obstructive Syndromes

Gerald W. Marsa

Obstruction of blood vessels and other tubular passages is a common problem of untreated cancer, occurring as a presenting sign of localized tumor as well as a late manifestation of widespread disease. Irrespective of the extent of tumor involvement, it is a process that requires prompt recognition and appropriate treatment to avoid loss of organ function and to reduce the risk of abscess or other infection. While superior vena cava obstruction is among the most common of the obstructive syndromes encountered, a variety of different sites can become obstructed by neoplastic growths, and prompt treatment is important to relieve the patient's symptoms and reduce the likelihood of serious consequences.

I. Superior vena cava (SVC) syndrome

A. Clinical presentation. Symptoms of SVC obstruction include edema and cyanosis of the face, neck, and upper extremities (usually worse on arising in the morning and lessening during daytime activities), headache, and changes in sensorium. Examination reveals venous distention and elevated venous pressure in the neck and upper extremities, normal venous pressure of the lower extremities, and frequently visible superficial collateral circulation on the trunk with venous flow toward the groin.

B. Etiology

1. Malignant tumors. The high incidence of lung carcinoma today has made SVC obstruction increasingly common. It is nonetheless frequently overlooked in its earlier stages because of an insidious presentation. Although the majority of SVC obstructions are caused by bronchogenic carcinoma (usually metastatic to mediastinal lymph nodes), any neoplasm involving the upper right mediastinum in the vicinity of the SVC can obstruct it; other neoplasms frequently associated include undifferentiated carcinoma of the thyroid, diffuse non-Hodgkin's lymphomas, and mediastinal germinomas.

2. Nonmalignant disorders. The flagrant symptoms associated with SVC syndrome in cancer are caused by the rapid occlusion of the vena cava that occurs before sufficient collateral venous circulation can develop. The slow growth of benign mediastinal tumors allows more collaterals to develop and thus explains the much lower frequency of these symptoms with complete SVC compression by benign neoplasms. SVC syndrome from nonneoplastic conditions is extremely uncommon, and it is generally accurate to assume that the obstruction is caused by a neoplastic disorder.

3. **Intrinsic luminal occlusion.** Although obstruction usually is due to extrinsic compression, intrinsic venous involvement by tumor can also be seen. The syndrome can also develop from intraluminal thrombosis in the absence of neoplastic involvement.

C. **Diagnosis.** Superior venacavography can be useful in defining the site and extent of vena cava involvement. Because of the high risks of bleeding owing to elevated venous pressure, other invasive diagnostic studies (bronchoscopy, mediastinotomy) are generally not warranted until treatment has been initiated and signs of obstruction have subsided. If a surgical procedure is deemed necessary, meticulous attention must be paid to hemostasis to avoid severe uncontrolled bleeding.

D. **Treatment**

1. **General measures.** Since an element of tissue edema is usually associated with tumor obstruction, diuretics and high doses of corticosteroids can provide initial relief of symptoms and should be promptly prescribed. Dexamethasone, 8 to 16 mg daily in divided doses, or prednisone, 30 to 60 mg daily, will frequently give a partial response within 24 hours; additionally, it will help avoid further exacerbation of signs and symptoms at the initiation of antineoplastic therapy. Furosemide, 40 mg PO, is an effective diuretic with rapid action and can be repeated as symptoms require, providing cardiac output remains adequate.

2. **Surgery.** Since SVC obstruction is prima facie evidence of mediastinal involvement, surgical therapy is contraindicated, both because of tumor unresectability as well as the high risks of excessive bleeding.

3. **Radiotherapy.** Prompt irradiation of the site of vena cava obstruction is indicated as soon as SVC syndrome is recognized. Treatment need not be withheld pending histologic confirmation of malignancy, since benign conditions are so rare and the danger of waiting is high. Several daily high-dose fractions (400 rad daily for 2 or 3 days) is usually sufficient to provide temporary relief of symptoms. Additional diagnostic and staging procedures can then safely be undertaken to define the overall plan of therapy. For non-oat-cell lung carcinomas and other mediastinal neoplasms without evidence of systemic dissemination, definitive radiotherapy with high total radiation doses will be indicated. Therefore, emergency irradiation should be interrupted as soon as the desired response is seen, to avoid compromising definitive diagnosis and treatment.

4. **Chemotherapy.** In patients with previously diagnosed neoplasms that are highly responsive to systemic chemotherapy (lymphomas, small-cell undifferentiated lung carcinoma, etc.), chemotherapy can be initiated as primary treatment. Obviously, subsequent staging studies will be compromised after a course of systemic therapy; hence local irradiation will still be preferred in new patients presenting with cancer. Chemotherapy cannot be relied on to provide the desired rapid relief of SVC obstructive symptoms in neoplasms with low response rates to drug therapy and in neoplasms in which the chemotherapy response is achieved only following a prolonged interval. In these situations, local irradiation should precede planned chemotherapy.

II. Bronchial and tracheal obstruction

A. Etiology and diagnosis. One of the most common complications of uncontrolled bronchogenic carcinoma is loss of respiratory function secondary to airway obstruction. Symptoms can develop suddenly with increased dyspnea, or if obstruction is gradual, they can manifest as fevers caused by distal pneumonitis or abscess. Since obstruction can develop owing to causes other than neoplastic growth (especially mucous plugging), bronchoscopy should be performed if the etiology is uncertain, and it can be therapeutic if obstruction is due to nonneoplastic sources. Other neoplastic causes of bronchial obstruction include the lymphomas and a rare endobronchial metastasis from another site, such as breast or gastrointestinal (GI) carcinoma.

B. Surgery. In cases where only segmental atelectasis is present, a curative surgical resection is indicated if the neoplasm is localized and if the patient's medical condition will tolerate pulmonary resection. In cases that would otherwise be nonsurgical, palliative surgical resection may be necessary if significant localized pulmonary destruction owing to infection has occurred and can be resected in order to remove the nidus of an otherwise chronic infection.

C. Radiotherapy

1. General considerations. The most common therapy for major bronchial obstruction is localized irradiation. Because of the sensitivity of lung tissue to x-rays with risk for acute radiation pneumonitis and for late pulmonary fibrosis rising rapidly at doses above 1500 rad, it is important to achieve reexpansion of the collapsed normal lung as rapidly as possible to shield uninvolved lung from higher doses of irradiation. Intermittent positive-pressure breathing should be employed regularly during radiotherapy until reexpansion is achieved.

2. Potentially curative treatment. In newly diagnosed neoplasms where there is evidence of only localized or regional involvement, irradiation should be carried out with curative intent, delivering doses of 5000 rad or greater for attempted long-term control of the tumor.

3. Palliative treatment. More commonly, local obstruction owing to lung carcinoma is only a local manifestation of generalized disease; nevertheless, local irradiation is necessary to palliate what is or may progress to a most devastating complication of cancer—respiratory insufficiency. In such cases, a rapid course of lower total doses of radiation can be undertaken to the local area of tumor involvement to provide relief of obstructive symptoms, or at least to prevent further progression of lung collapse.

4. Prophylactic treatment. Anticipation of this potential complication with prophylactic treatment prior to onset of symptoms can be of marked value in maintaining a high quality of life in the patient with incurable disease, since it is often easier to avoid obstruction than to reverse the process once atelectasis has developed.

D. Chemotherapy. Systemic therapy should usually be reserved for the secondary management of disseminated carcinoma once the local problem of bronchial obstruction has been treated with local irradiation. Lymphomas and small-cell undifferentiated carcinoma of the lung have high response rates when treated with combination chemotherapy, and frequently obstruction can be relieved with systemic drug therapy alone. Even in these instances the response is seldom as rapid or complete as when local irradiation is also delivered.

E. **Tracheal obstruction.** Airway obstruction within the trachea is obviously acutely life threatening. It is caused most frequently by extrinsic compression by a mediastinal neoplasm. Since temporizing measures, such as tracheostomy, are impossible, recognition and treatment of pending obstruction before its development is vital.

1. **Endotracheal neoplasms** are rare. They are usually managed with bronchoscopic resection to temporarily enlarge the airway with corticosteroids followed by irradiation to the tracheal neoplasm and regional lymphatics. Tracheal resection with reanastomosis can seldom be accomplished, and utilization of prosthetic tracheal replacements has thus far proved unsatisfactory.

2. The more common **extrinsic tracheal obstruction** can be anticipated because tracheal narrowing can be observed on the chest x-ray film prior to development of obstruction. Since the trachea is composed of U-shaped rings of cartilage, it can withstand significant pressure before collapsing from extrinsic tumor compression. The collapse, usually complete, develops suddenly after the integral strength of the cartilage is exceeded. While emergency endotracheal intubation can be life sparing, it is seldom successful. It is, therefore, important that tracheal narrowing be noted early and be recognized for the potentially fatal complication it is, and that it be treated promptly with radiotherapy.

III. Biliary tract obstruction

A. **Etiology and diagnosis.** Obstruction of the biliary tract can develop owing to intrinsic blockade by a primary neoplasm or biliary stones, or owing to extrinsic compression by lymphadenopathy secondary to metastatic carcinoma. Identification of the site and probable cause of obstructive jaundice has been made easier with the advent of computed tomography (CT) body scanning, but other studies, including transhepatic cholangiography and endoscopic retrograde cholangiopancreatography (ERCP), may also be of benefit. Relief of obstructive jaundice is a legitimate goal even in patients having very limited survival.

B. **General measures.** Fever is a frequent symptom of biliary obstruction owing to a retrograde infection; and broad spectrum antibiotics that are concentrated in the bile (e.g., chloramphenicol or clindamycin) are the preferred treatment. Pruritus can be relieved in patients with partial biliary obstruction by cholestyramine resin, 4 g in water tid before meals, which chelates bile salts in the gut. Pruritus can also be lessened by such medicines as trimeprazine (Temaril®), 2.5 mg PO qid. Percutaneous biliary drainage through transhepatic catheter placement into the dilated proximal ducts can be utilized in instances where the obstruction is not amenable to surgical bypass procedures or in a patient whose medical condition makes surgery risky. Hypoprothrombinemia should be corrected with vitamin K, 5 to 10 mg IM or SC.

C. Surgery

1. **Curative resection.** Radical resection can provide both relief of obstructive symptoms and an opportunity for cure in some cases of ampullary carcinoma, an occasional carcinoma of the head of the pancreas, and rarely in carcinoma of the distal common biliary duct with radical pancreaticoduodenectomy (Whipple's operation).

2. **Palliative treatment.** The remaining cases will either have evidence of metastasis or will involve proximal biliary tracts not amenable to surgical resection for cure. In those instances with unresectable disease caused by intrahepatic or proximal obstruction, a permanent internal biliary drainage catheter can sometimes be passed through the obstructing tumor to act as a drain into the duodenum. In unresectable cases with more distal obstruction, bypass can be accomplished through choledochojejunostomy or external drainage by way of a T-tube from the dilated ducts proximal to the obstruction.

D. Radiotherapy

1. **Highly responsive tumors.** In patients with biliary blockage from highly radioresponsive neoplasms such as lymphomas or oat-cell carcinoma of the lung, local irradiation to the porta hepatis can provide rapid relief.

2. **Moderately responsive tumors.** Although radiotherapy will eventually cause sufficient tumor regression to reduce jaundice in most other neoplasms where only moderate radiosensitivity exists, the process may require several weeks or more; and, therefore, radiotherapy should be combined with a biliary drainage procedure whenever possible for best results. Irradiation following operative bypass or percutaneous transhepatic cholangial drainage can provide not only improved biliary drainage as the initial obstruction improves, but can also prevent reobstruction caused by progressive tumor growth. Palliative doses of irradiation (2000 to 4000 rad in 1 to 3 weeks depending on portal size) are indicated in cases of metastatic disease.

3. **Tumors with potential for long-term control.** In cases of primary carcinomas of the pancreas and biliary ducts without evidence of hepatic or distant spread, radical irradiation should be undertaken following surgical delineation of tumor extent and biliary bypass procedure. Radiation doses of 6000 rad or greater over 6 to 7 weeks, utilizing multiple shaped portals to minimize injury to surrounding normal tissues, can provide better local tumor control and occasionally improve long-term survival.

E. Chemotherapy.
Since response rates and regression intervals are poor in most tumors causing biliary obstruction, chemotherapy plays a secondary role of maintaining surgical and radiotherapeutic responses by preventing tumor extension with biliary reobstruction.

IV. Alimentary tract obstruction

A. **Clinical presentation and rationale of treatment.** Nausea, vomiting, and abdominal pain are common symptoms experienced by the patient with cancer. Obstruction of the GI tract must be constantly differentiated from other causes of these symptoms. Treatment of this complication is nearly always indicated, even in the patient with terminal disease, to relieve the undesirable alternatives of continued symptoms or continued suctioning of the alimentary tract. Even obstruction of the esophagus, which is not associated with the same symptoms, is best palliated by relief of the obstruction because of the unpleasantness associated with inability to handle salivary secretions.

B. General measures. Significant nutritional deficiencies are nearly always associated with GI obstruction, because of the longstanding condition that had existed subclinically before diagnosis of the blockage. Restoration of positive nutritional balance is vital to a good result. Usually nutritional balance should be initiated by IV hyperalimentation as a temporary supportive measure until GI tract integrity can be restored. In proximal obstructions (esophagus and stomach), feeding gastrostomy or jejunostomy can provide similar support and is to be preferred because of diminished expense and potential complications. Also continued hospitalization can be avoided. Intestinal dilatation associated with obstruction must be decompressed by nasogastric suction while preparing for surgery. Nonneoplastic causes of intestinal obstruction occasionally will be resolved by decompression of intestinal dilatation and subsidence of tissue edema.

C. Surgery. With few exceptions, surgical correction of GI obstruction is the treatment of choice.

1. **Tumors not helped by surgical resection** include carcinoma of the proximal esophagus and extensive carcinomas of the distal esophagus and stomach. In these cases the morbidity of the procedure overwhelms the palliative results. Feeding gastrostomy or jejunostomy can temporarily circumvent the obstruction while awaiting the results of radiotherapy. Placement of a semirigid plastic tube through an obstructive esophageal neoplasm into the proximal stomach can also be useful, although late displacement of the tube is common and local irradiation postoperatively is still indicated.

2. **Curative resections.** Resection is obviously indicated in other localized GI carcinomas causing obstruction, although it is often accomplished as a staged procedure following colostomy for colonic obstruction to reduce risk of infection and anastomotic leak.

3. **Palliative resection.** Palliative resection is also indicated in cases where metastases are evident and whenever this procedure can be accomplished without high risk. Palliative resection decreases the tumor burden for subsequent chemotherapy and removes the most likely site of future symptoms from the cancer. The recommendation for palliative resection includes obstructing rectal carcinomas with metastasis, in which abdominal perineal resection can prevent future pelvic and perineal pain, rectal bleeding and drainage, and rectal tenesmus. When an obstructing neoplasm cannot safely be removed, bypass of the obstructed viscus with side-to-side anastomosis should be performed.

D. Radiotherapy

1. **Potentially curative treatment.** Esophageal carcinoma is the only GI tract carcinoma commonly treated definitively with irradiation. In

the absence of evident systemic spread, radical irradiation is warranted to attempt long-term control of the local and regional disease, despite the dismal cure rates. Doses in the range of 6000 to 7000 rad are required, necessitating careful radiotherapy planning and multiple portals to avoid injury to lungs, spinal cord, and heart. Vigorous nutritional support is required during the treatment course.

2. **Palliative treatment.** Palliative irradiation of an unresectable GI neoplasm usually requires doses of 4000 to 5000 rad in 3 to 5 weeks. Restoration of esophageal and gastric patency can be accomplished in over one half of the cases with significant improvement in quality of life. Irradiation of unresected intestinal and rectal neoplasms following bypass or colostomy is frequently indicated to relieve pain and perineal discharge or bladder dysfunction.

E. **Chemotherapy.** Primary gastrointestinal carcinomas have low response rates to chemotherapeutic agents, and these should be considered only as an adjunct to surgery or radiotherapy in relieving obstructive symptoms. Responsive neoplasms such as lymphomas may be treated with drugs primarily in cases of incomplete obstruction, but usually they are best managed by relieving the obstruction surgically to improve nutrition before chemotherapy is begun.

V. Ureteral obstruction

A. **Etiology and diagnosis.** Because of the long abdominal and pelvic course of the ureter, it is subject to obstruction by a variety of cancers. The upper ureter can be compressed or invaded by carcinomas of the kidney or pancreas. The pelvic segment is most commonly compressed by extensive retroperitoneal lymph node metastasis from urinary bladder, prostate, uterus, cervix, or rectal carcinomas. Intraluminal obstruction by urothelial carcinoma must be distinguished from obstruction caused by clot or stone. Obstruction secondary to retroperitoneal fibrosis caused by previous surgery, by previous radiation therapy, or by primary disease should also be considered. Symptoms can be nonexistent until uremia develops, or they can develop acutely with flank pain, fever, or hematuria. Assessment of the site and extent of ureteral obstruction can be accomplished with an excretory urogram, cystoscopy with retrograde pyelography, and CT body scanning.

B. **General measures.** Preservation of remaining renal function requires prompt relief of ureteral back pressure. Indwelling retrograde catheters can be left in place until obstruction has been relieved or corrective surgery is undertaken. Ureteral stents can be utilized with lower obstructions to avoid the need for indwelling catheters. Where bilateral ureteral obstruction has occurred owing to uncontrolled neoplasm, one must assess the quality of remaining life before undertaking relief of ureteral obstruction. Since renal failure is one of the easiest modes of demise for patients with terminal cancer, it is inappropriate to prevent this in the patient with cancer who has significant pain and a minimal probability of future treatment response.

C. **Surgery.** In patients with localized recurrence of pelvic tumor following irradiation, exenterative surgery with ureteral implantation into an ileal or colonic conduit should be considered for possible salvage cure. If tumor resection is impossible, conduit diversion may still be the best palliation. Other diverting procedures such as ureterosigmoidostomy are less desirable. Occasionally, ureteral reimplantation into an unirradiated tumor-free bladder can be accomplished with excellent prognosis for success. Nephrectomy should be considered in the relatively healthy patient with unilateral nonfunctioning kidney caused by ureteral obstruction because of the high risk of future infection.

D. Radiotherapy. Ureteral obstruction caused by retroperitoneal lymphadenopathy or pelvic neoplasms not previously irradiated are usually best treated with radiotherapy. In instances of widespread metastases, palliative doses of 3000 to 4000 rad in 2 to 3 weeks are usually adequate (in conjunction with anticipated postirradiation systemic therapy). Objective response may take several weeks or more to be maximal. In cases of only localized or regional tumor involvement, higher doses are indicated in anticipation of longer potential survival or even cure.

E. Chemotherapy. With the exception of the lymphomas, most neoplasms causing ureteral obstruction have low chemotherapy-response rates. However, cisplatin alone or in combination may produce a satisfactory response in sensitive tumors. Since nephrotoxicity is markedly enhanced by poor renal function, chemotherapy with cisplatin is best withheld until ureteral obstruction has been relieved by surgery or irradiation. Ureteral obstruction due to disseminated lymphomas can be treated with combination chemotherapy in lieu of localized irradiation, but it should be recognized that the local response rate will be higher and the time to response shorter for patients receiving irradiation.

VI. Lymphatic obstruction. Lymphedema of an extremity in the patient with cancer can be discomforting and disabling; it can result from uncontrolled tumor growth within nodes blocking lymphatic pathways or from successful cancer therapy with surgery, irradiation, or both. Determination of the etiology of the edema in each patient, including separating lymphatic from venous obstruction, will maximize chances for successful therapy.

A. General measures. Reduction in total body fluids by salt restriction and diuretic therapy can somewhat reduce extremity lymphedema. Elevation of the affected extremity when possible and avoidance of strenuous muscular activities can also be of limited benefit. A fitted elastic stocking, encompassing the affected extremity and worn while nonrecumbent, can alleviate some of the aching and heaviness associated with this complication. A trial of intermittent elevated extremity pressures using a pneumatic pump occasionally may enhance development of collateral lymphatic channels.

B. Surgery. Patients without evidence of neoplasm and with lower extremity lymphedema owing to fibrotic obliteration of the lymphatic system have, on occasion, improved following placement of an omental graft across the area of prior high-dose irradiation to reestablish a lush lymphatic pathway.

C. Radiotherapy. Lymphatic blockage with distal lymphedema caused by metastatic lymphadenopathy usually responds best to local irradiation, although the probability of totally reversing the process is less than 50 percent except in highly radiosensitive tumors, such as the lymphomas. Since the local tumor burden is obviously great, relatively high doses of irradiation will be required. High-dose radiation carries with it higher risks of late radiation fibrosis and reexacerbation of initial symptoms, should the patient survive several years. The optimal radiation dose in the patient with reasonable life expectancy and regional metastatic carcinoma would be 6000 to 6500 rad in 6 to 7 weeks. Patients with poor prognosis can be treated with 3000 to 4000 rad in 2 to 3 weeks for optimal results.

D. Chemotherapy. Since lymphedema is not an emergency, systemic therapy with drugs or hormones can also be utilized in lieu of local irradiation for attempted relief of symptoms. Breast and prostate carcinomas and the lymphomas have higher expectations of response than many other neoplasms, where a lower probability of remission exists. In the latter cases, combined modality therapy with local irradiation and systemic therapy can provide maximal benefits.

Selected Reading

Davenport, D. et al. Radiation therapy in the treatment of superior vena caval obstruction. *Cancer* 42:2600, 1978.

Fielding, L. P., Stewart-Brown, S., and Blesovsky, L. Large bowel obstruction caused by cancer. A prospective study. *Br. Med. J.* 2:515, 1979.

Kanji, A. et al. Extrinsic compression of superior vena cava. An analysis of 41 patients. *Int. J. Radiat. Oncol. Biol. Phys.* 6:213, 1980.

MacCarthy, R. Nonsurgical management of obstructive jaundice in the patient with advanced cancer. *J.A.M.A.* 244:1976, 1980.

McNamara, T. E., and Butkus, D. E. Nephrostomy in patients with ureteral obstruction secondary to nonurologic malignancies. *Arch. Intern. Med.* 140:494, 1980.

Meyer, J. E. Palliative urinary diversion in patients with advanced pelvic malignancy. *Cancer* 45:2698, 1980.

Montague, E., and Delclos, L. Palliative Radiotherapy in the Management of Metastatic Disease. In G. H. Fletcher (Ed.), *Textbook of Radiotherapy* (3rd ed.). Philadelphia: Lea & Febiger, 1980. Pp. 943–948.

Osteen, R. T. et al. Malignant intestinal obstruction. *Surgery* 87:611, 1980.

Scarantino, C. et al. The optimum radiation schedule in treatment of superior vena caval obstruction. Importance of ^{99m}Tc scintiangiograms. *Int. J. Radiat. Oncol. Biol. Phys.* 5:1987, 1979.

Sharer, W. et al. Palliative urinary diversion for malignant ureteral obstruction. *J. Urol.* 120:162, 1978.

Singh, B. et al. Stent versus nephrostomy. Is there a choice? *J. Urol.* 121:268, 1979.

Sise, J. G., and Crichlow, R. W. Obstruction due to malignant tumors. *Semin. Oncol.* 5:213, 1978.

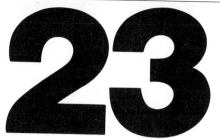

Malignant Pleural, Peritoneal, and Pericardial Effusions and Meningeal Infiltrates

Roland T. Skeel

Malignant pleural, peritoneal, and pericardial effusions and malignant meningeal infiltrates are uncommon early in the course of malignancy, but they occur frequently with disseminated disease. While pleural or peritoneal effusions may at times be of minor clinical importance, they, as well as pericardial effusions and meningeal infiltrates, may cause major disability and death. It is therefore important to be alert for signs and symptoms of these problems in patients with malignancy and to be prepared to take appropriate action to treat them effectively.

I. Pleural effusions

A. Causes. Malignant pleural effusions arise in association with malignant cells lining the pleura, exuded into the pleural space, or blocking veins or lymphatics. In females, the most common malignancy associated with pleural effusions is carcinoma of the breast, and in males, it is carcinoma of the lung. Other causes of malignant pleural effusions include lymphoma, mesothelioma, and carcinomas of the ovary, gastrointestinal (GI) tract, and uterus. Malignancy is not the only cause of effusions, even in patients with a known neoplastic disease, and therefore it is important to attempt to rule out other possible causes, such as congestive heart failure, infection, or pulmonary infarction.

B. Diagnosis

1. **Clinical.** Effusions are suggested by the symptoms of shortness of breath—particularly dyspnea on exertion—and occasionally cough. The patient may feel more comfortable when lying on one side when the effusion is unilateral. On physical examination decreased breath sounds, dullness to percussion, and egophony are the typical signs over the area of the effusion.

2. **A chest x-ray film** should be obtained to confirm the clinical impression. If fluid appears to be present, a lateral decubitus film must be obtained to help in the estimation of the volume of the effusion and how free it is within the pleural space.

3. **A diagnostic thoracentesis** should be performed to obtain fluid for bacterial culture, cytologic examination, protein, and cell count. The cytologic examination is most important and helpful, for if it is positive, as it is in 50 to 70 percent of cases with malignant effusion, the diagnosis is established. Other studies that may at times be helpful in the evaluation of pleural fluid include the lactic dehydrogenase (LDH) (which is > 0.6 times the serum LDH in most exudates) and the glucose, which is frequently low in malignancy and infections. A cy-

tologic examination of fluid from a newly discovered pleural effusion is wise, whether the patient is known to have malignancy or not, since in nearly one half of all malignant effusions, this finding is the first sign of malignancy.

4. **Pleural biopsy** may be helpful in establishing the diagnosis in up to 20 percent of cases in which the pleural fluid cytology is negative.

C. **Treatment.** As malignant pleural effusions are generally a sign of systemic rather than localized disease, the best therapy is treatment that effectively treats the malignancy systemically. Unfortunately effective systemic treatment is often not possible, particularly when the malignancy is commonly refractory to systemic treatment (such as in carcinoma of the lung) or in patients who have previously been heavily treated and systemic therapy is no longer effective. In these circumstances local–regional therapy is required for palliation of the patient's symptoms.

1. **Drainage.** Most malignant pleural effusions will recur in several days after a simple thoracentesis. Chest tube drainage (closed tube thoracostomy) will allow the pleural surfaces to oppose each other and, if maintained for several days, may result in obliteration of the space and improvement in the effusion for several weeks to months. It does not appear to be as effective when used alone as when a cytotoxic or sclerosing agent is added, and therefore one of these types of agents is commonly instilled into the space while the chest tube is in place.

2. **Cytotoxic and sclerosing agents.** A wide variety of agents including radioactive isotopes (gold, phosphorus, and yttrium), talc, tetracycline, quinacrine, mechlorethamine, thiotepa, fluorouracil, and bleomycin have been used in the treatment of pleural effusions. All are of similar effectiveness. All require the pleural fluid to be drained as completely as possible prior to instillation for maximal effectiveness.

a. **Method of administration.** The drug to be used is diluted in 50 ml of saline and instilled through the thoracostomy tube into the chest cavity after the effusion has been drained for at least 24 hours, and the rate of collection is less than 100 ml/24 hr. The thoracostomy tube is clamped, and the patient is positioned on his or her front, back, and sides for 15-minute periods over the next 2 hours. The tube is then reconnected to suction for at least 18 hours to assure that the pleural surfaces remain opposed and to prevent the rapid accumulation of any fluid in reaction to the instillation. If the drainage is less than 40 to 50 ml in the last 12 hours, the tube may be pulled and a chest x-ray film obtained to be certain that no pneumothorax has occurred during the removal of the tube. If the thoracostomy tube continues to drain more than 100 ml/24 hr after the instillation, then it may be necessary to leave it in place for an additional 48 to 72 hours to assure that a maximum amount of adhesion between the pleural surfaces has taken place.

b. **Recommended agents**

(1) Tetracycline, 500 to 1000 mg, has the advantage of being non-myelosuppressive.

(2) Mechlorethamine (nitrogen mustard), 8 to 16 mg/m². Systemic effects, including nausea, vomiting, and myelosuppression, are seen. Mechlorethamine may have an advantage because it is locally cytotoxic, particularly in the lymphomas.

(3) Thiotepa, 20 to 30 mg/m², causes less intense inflammation and therefore less pain than mechlorethamine. It also causes less nausea.

(4) Fluorouracil, 500 mg/m², may have a theoretical advantage in sensitive carcinomas, but whether that advantage is significant is not yet established.

c. Responses. A combination of chest tube drainage and instillation of one of the agents discussed in **I.C.2.b** will control pleural effusions more than 75 percent of the time. The duration of responses are short with a median between 3 and 6 months unless the patient's systemic disease comes under adequate control. In that circumstance, the effusion may not recur for years, at least until the systemic disease once more emerges.

II. Peritoneal effusions

A. Causes. Malignant peritoneal effusions usually occur in association with diffuse seeding of the peritoneal surface with small malignant deposits. In females, carcinoma of the ovary is the most commonly associated malignancy, and in males, GI carcinomas are most common. Other neoplasms that may cause peritoneal effusions include lymphoma, mesothelioma, and carcinomas of the uterus and breast. Peritoneal effusions may also result from impairment of lymphatic or venous flow. Liver metastasis by itself, unless it is far advanced, is not usually associated with symptomatic peritoneal effusions.

B. Diagnosis

1. Symptoms and signs. Patients may be completely asymptomatic or have so much fluid that they have severe abdominal discomfort and embarrassment of respiration. In the presence of peritoneal metastases, there may be abnormal bowel motility that at times resembles a paralytic ileus. On examination, the lower abdomen bulges when the patient stands, and the flanks bulge when the patient is supine. Confirmatory signs include shifting dullness, a fluid wave, or the "puddle sign." (Periumbilical dullness when the patient rests on his/her knees and elbows.)

2. Radiographic studies. Ascites may be suggested on recumbent film of the abdomen, although this is less sensitive than computerized tomography (CT) in detecting fluid. CT is also helpful in defining whether there are enlarged retroperitoneal nodes, tumor masses in the abdomen or pelvis, or liver metastases in association with the ascites.

3. A diagnostic paracentesis confirms the diagnosis by revealing malignant cells in about one half of patients. Other tests are not generally as reliable, and treatment decisions must often be based on incomplete data.

C. Therapy. As with malignant pleural effusions, malignant peritoneal effusions are optimally treated with effective systemic therapy. If the patient is resistant to all further systemic treatment, then regional treatment should be tried, but the likelihood of success is less and the complications are greater with peritoneal effusions than with pleural effusions. Success probably is less because of the greater likelihood of loculations to areas inaccessible to therapy and the impossibility of obliterating the peritoneal space in the same way that the pleural space can be obliterated. Complications are greater because of the increase in adhesions caused by instillational therapy and the resultant increase in obstructive bowel problems.

1. **Paracentesis** may be helpful in acutely relieving intraabdominal pressure. If the ascites has caused impairment of respiration, paracentesis may thus give temporary relief. Rapid withdrawal of large volumes of fluid (> 1 liter) can result in hypotension and shock, however, and if frequent paracenteses are performed, severe hypoalbuminemia may result. This procedure thus results in only temporary benefit.

2. **Diuretics** may be helpful in reducing ascites, but care must be taken not to be too vigorous in attempts at diuresis because of the possibility of dehydration and hypotension. A reasonable choice of diuretic is a combination of hydrochlorthiazide, 50 to 100 mg daily, together with spironolactone, 50 to 100 mg daily.

3. **Intracavitary therapy.** Radioisotopes, cytotoxic drugs, and sclerosing agents have all been used with some benefit in the treatment of malignant ascites, but overall, probably less than one half of patients will have a satisfactory response. The radioactive isotopes ^{198}AU or ^{32}P should be used only by those with experience and appropriate certification in their use. Thiotepa is associated with less risk for the person administering the therapy. It may be given in a dose of 20 to 30 mg/m^2. It is likely to cause myelosuppression, and therefore the dose should not be repeated until the blood counts have been observed to return to normal, and then only if there has been objective improvement in the ascites.

III. Pericardial effusions. Although 5 to 10 percent of patients dying with disseminated malignancy will have cardiac or pericardial metastases, far fewer will have symptomatic pericardial effusion. However, while malignant pericardial effusions are not particularly common, they are of great importance because of their potential to cause acute cardiac tamponade and death.

A. Causes. The most common neoplasms causing pericardial effusions are carcinomas of the breast and lung, leukemias, lymphomas, and melanoma.

B. Diagnosis

1. **Clinical.** Patients with developing cardiac tamponade may exhibit a variety of grave symptoms, including extreme anxiety, dyspnea, precordial chest pain, cough, and hoarseness. On examination they are likely to have engorged neck veins, generalized edema, a low systolic blood pressure, and a paradoxical pulse.

2. **ECG signs** include nonspecific low voltage, elevation of ST segments, and ventricular alternans or the more specific total electrical alternans.

3. **The chest x-ray film** typically shows an enlarged cardiac silhouette, often with a bulging appearance suggestive of an effusion.

4. **Echocardiography** can confirm the diagnosis and provide important information on the location of the effusion within the pericardium.

5. **Pericardiocentesis** will reveal neoplastic cells on cytologic examination in more than three-fourths of patients.

C. **Treatment consists of**

1. **General measures** to maintain blood volume (if that is necessary) and oxygenation.

2. **Pericardiocentesis** under ECG and blood pressure monitoring.

3. **Instillation of chemotherapeutic agents**

   a. **Fluorouracil,** 500 to 1000 mg in aqueous solution as supplied commercially *or*

   b. **Thiotepa,** 30 to 40 mg in 15 to 20 ml sterile water

4. **Radiotherapy** with radioisotopes or 2000 to 4000 rad external beam radiotherapy may help control effusions.

One of the chemotherapeutic agents or radiotherapy will control the effusion in about 50 percent of patients. If they are not effective, surgical intervention to create a pericardial window may be necessary and can be effective for several months. It is not recommended, however, unless simpler measures fail.

IV. Malignant subarachnoid infiltrates

A. **Causes.** Leptomeningeal involvement with non-CNS cancer is a very uncommon complication in most neoplasms, although in children with acute lymphocytic leukemia who have not received prophylactic treatment, the incidence approaches 50 percent. Of the nonleukemia diseases, breast carcinoma and lymphomas account for about 30 percent each in cases of malignant subarachnoid infiltrates. Carcinoma of the lung and melanoma account for 10 to 12 percent each.

B. **Diagnosis**

1. **Clinical.** Patients commonly present with headache, change in mental status, cranial nerve dysfunction, or spinal root derived pain, paresthesia, or weakness. Any onset of change in neurologic status, particularly of cerebral, cranial nerve, or spinal root origin should alert the clinician to the possibility of subarachnoid infiltrates.

2. **Lumbar puncture** is the most valuable test. Malignant cells will be found in nearly all cases, but two to four examinations may be performed before the cells are seen. Other CSF findings that suggest malignancy include an elevated pressure, low-grade leukocytosis (5–500 cells/m^3), elevated protein (70%), and depressed glucose (40%–70%).

3. Radiologic studies

   a. A myelogram may be helpful in finding larger infiltrates that may cause cord compression and identifying areas that may be benefitted by radiotherapy.

   b. Computed tomography can demonstrate tumor masses in the brain parenchyma or meninges and hydrocephalus.

C. Treatment. Malignant subarachnoid infiltrates may be treated with radiotherapy, intrathecal chemotherapy, or the combination.

   1. Radiotherapy. The radiation field is usually limited to the most involved field (frequently the brain), and intrathecal chemotherapy is used to control the infiltrates elsewhere. This is done although the entire neuroaxis is usually involved because total craniospinal radiation causes severe myelosuppression, which limits the patient's tolerance to concurrent or subsequent cytotoxic chemotherapy.

   2. Chemotherapy may be administered by lumbar puncture or into a surgically implanted reservoir that communicates with the ventricle. The latter has the advantages of (1) being easily accessible in patients who require repeated treatments and (2) giving a better distribution of drug than can be obtained through lumbar puncture.
   The most commonly used drugs are

   a. Methotrexate, 10 to 12 mg/m^2 twice weekly until the CSF clears of malignant cells, then monthly.

   b. Cytarabine, 45 to 50 mg/m^2 twice weekly until the CSF clears of malignant cells, then monthly.

   Thiotepa has been used, but experience with it is limited and it is not recommended. Other drugs used to treat effusions, such as fluorouracil, mechlorethamine, or radioisotopes should *not* be used to treat meningeal disease.

D. Response to treatment. Most patients with meningeal leukemia or lymphoma will respond to a combination of radiotherapy and intrathecal chemotherapy. Carcinomas are less likely to improve, but mild to moderate improvement may be seen in up to one half of the patients. Aseptic meningitis, seizures, acute encephalopathy, myelopathy, and radicular neuropathy may result from intrathecal chemotherapy with or without radiotherapy. Complications are infrequent, however, and in patients with advanced metastatic disease they are not a major problem.

Selected Reading

PLEURAL EFFUSIONS

Bayly, T. D. et al. Tetracycline and quinacrine in the control of malignant pleural effusions. A randomized trial. *Cancer* 41:1188, 1978.

Chernow, B., and Sahn, S. A. Carcinomatous involvement of the pleura. An analysis of 96 patients. *Am. J. Med.* 63:695, 1977.

Friedman, M. A., and Slater, E. Malignant pleural effusions. *Cancer Treat. Rev.* 5:49, 1978.

Von Hoff, D. D., and LiVolsi, V. Diagnostic reliability of needle biopsy of the parietal pleural. A review of 272 biopsies. *Am. J. Clin. Pathol.* 64:200, 1975.

PERITONEAL EFFUSIONS

Papac, R. J. Treatment of Malignant Disease in Closed Spaces. In F. F. Becker (Ed.), *Cancer, A Comprehensive Treatise,* Vol. 5. New York: Plenum Pr., 1977.

PERICARDIAL EFFUSIONS

Theologides, A. Neoplastic cardiac tamponade. *Semin. Oncol.* 5:181, 1978.

MALIGNANT SUBARACHNOID INFILTRATES

Olson, M. E., Chernik, N. L., and Posner, J. B. Infiltration of the leptomeninges by systemic cancer. *Arch. Neurol.* 30:122, 1974.

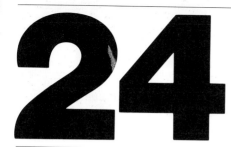

Endocrine Syndromes

Roberto Franco-Saenz

I. General considerations. The occurrence of endocrine syndromes secondary to the ectopic production of hormones by nonendocrine tumors has been recognized with increasing frequency over the past 20 years. Recognition of an endocrine or metabolic manifestation of cancer is most important since, in some patients, the effects of the endocrine syndrome are more deleterious to the patient than the neoplasm itself. Study of the responsible hormones and related products has further significance, for it is possible that they have the potential to be used clinically as tumor markers for early detection of tumors, an indication of the response to therapy, or an indication of recurrence of tumor.

A. Hormone production and clinical expression. Production of hormone precursors is a common occurrence in malignancy, but the clinical expression of an endocrine syndrome is less common, as it appears to depend on the capability of the neoplasm to release the active hormone from its precursor. Malignant tumors may also produce subunits of the parent hormone that under normal circumstances are not released by themselves. For example, the precursors of adrenocorticotropic hormone (ACTH), calcitonin, and other peptide hormones and their subunits are usually present in all lung tumors regardless of histologic type. However, only a minority of patients develop clinical or biochemical abnormalities related to ectopic hormone production. The so-called oncofetal proteins, such as α_1-fetoprotein and carcinoembryonic antigen, and the oncoplacental proteins represent another major category of ectopic production of proteins, and although they do not cause specific endocrine syndromes their production by tumors probably has similar pathogenetic significance.

B. Ectopic hormone production by nonendocrine tumors has been documented by several lines of evidence:

1. Arteriovenous differences in the hormone concentration across a tumor bed

2. High concentrations of hormone precursors in tumor extract

3. Incorporation of radiolabeled amino acids into the hormone by tumors

4. Production of the hormone by tumors grown in tissue culture

Furthermore, correction of the endocrine syndrome has followed total excision of the tumor with recurrence of the syndrome when metastases developed.

C. Mechanism of ectopic hormone production. Although the mechanism by which nonendocrine tumors synthesize hormones and hormone precursors is not known, several hypotheses have been advanced to explain this phenomenon.

1. **APUD hypothesis** postulates that tumors producing ectopic hormones derive from a single progenitor cell that is embryologically derived from the neural crest and capable of producing peptide hormones. (The *amine precursor uptake and decarboxylation* (APUD) hypothesis.) It is a possible explanation for some, but not all, of the ectopic hormone syndromes.

2. **Gene derepression hypothesis.** This concept implies that during the process of neoplastic transformation portions of DNA, which are inactive during normal cell differentiation, become activated, leading to the production of ectopic proteins.

3. **Dedifferentiation hypothesis.** This hypothesis postulates that neoplastic tissue regresses to a more primitive gene expression than that seen in the parent tissue.

4. **Sponge hypothesis.** This concept implies selective uptake of circulating hormones by tumor tissue. However, although there is evidence that tumor cells can bind specific peptides and steroids, the sponge hypothesis does not provide a satisfactory explanation for the majority of cases of ectopic hormone production.

II. Ectopic Cushing's syndrome (ectopic ACTH/β-LPH)

A. **Production of hormones.** ACTH-producing tumors have been shown to synthesize and release ACTH, β-lipotropin hormone (β-LPH), and β-endorphin, which are known to originate from a common precursor molecule, the *pro-opiomelanocortin*. Gamma-LPH, α- and β-melanocyte-stimulating hormone (MSH), and corticotropin-like intermediate lobe peptide (CLIP) have also been found in some tumors causing the ectopic ACTH syndrome. In view of these findings, the term *ectopic ACTH/β-LPH* is being used with increasing frequency. Simultaneous production of other unrelated peptide hormones, such as vasopressin (ADH) and calcitonin, has been reported. Furthermore, production of corticotropin-releasing factor (CRF) has been documented in several of these neoplasms.

The following tumors are most commonly associated with ectopic Cushing's syndrome:

1. Small-cell anaplastic (oat-cell) carcinoma of the lung

2. Thymoma

3. Carcinoid tumors in the lung and gastrointestinal (GI) tract

4. Medullary thyroid carcinoma

5. Pheochromocytoma

6. Ganglioneuroma

7. Melanoma

8. Prostatic carcinoma

B. **Symptoms and signs.** The ectopic ACTH syndrome is more common in males and has a higher frequency in patients over 50 years of age, probably because oat-cell carcinoma of the lung, which is the most common cause of the syndrome, is 10 times more common in males of this age group. The majority of patients with ectopic ACTH syndrome do not have the characteristic clinical appearance of Cushing's syndrome. The absence of this clinical picture is probably due to the catabolic effects of the neoplasm as well as to the sudden onset and rapidly deteriorating clinical course of patients with these malignant neoplasms. However, when the syndrome is caused by a less malignant or a benign tumor, such as bronchial carcinoid, classical cushingoid features may be found. Anorexia and weight loss, rather than obesity, are common. Hypertension and hyperpigmentation are more common than in other causes of Cushing's syndrome. Severe muscular weakness is one of the most common manifestations of the syndrome. Edema, polyuria, and polydipsia are often seen. The course of patients with ectopic ACTH syndrome is usually more rapid and the prognosis is worse than in patients with similar tumors without the ectopic ACTH syndrome. However, cures have been reported after successful removal of the bronchial carcinoid causing the ectopic ACTH syndrome.

C. Laboratory findings

1. **Hypokalemic alkalosis.** Severe, unexplained hypokalemia—with serum potassium levels usually below 3 mEq/liter and metabolic alkalosis with venous bicarbonate frequently greater than 30 mEq/liter—is one of the most common findings. *Hypokalemic alkalosis, when observed in a patient with cancer in the absence of diuretics, should alert the physician to the possibility of ectopic ACTH syndrome.* Severe muscle weakness, hyporeflexia, paresthesias, and muscle paralysis may occur. Cardiac arrhythmias, ECG findings of hypokalemia, and increased sensitivity to the effects of digitalis glycoside may occur.

2. **Hyperglycemia** or abnormal glucose tolerance is common.

3. **Hormone abnormalities.** Plasma cortisol is usually greatly elevated (> 40 µg/100 ml) and lacks diurnal variation. Plasma ACTH is also very high. Free urinary cortisol, 17-hydroxy, and 17-ketosteroids show marked increases. Typically, patients with ectopic ACTH syndrome caused by bronchogenic carcinoma show lack of suppression of the plasma cortisol, plasma ACTH, and urinary-free cortisol with high-dose dexamethasone (2 mg dexamethasone q6h for 2 days). In contrast, 20 to 50 percent of the patients with this syndrome owing to bronchial carcinoids show consistent suppression with 2 mg of dexamethasone.

D. Treatment

1. **Surgery.** The treatment of choice for ectopic ACTH syndrome is treatment of the primary tumor with surgery, radiotherapy, or chemotherapy. Unfortunately, as the most common cause of the syndrome is small-cell anaplastic carcinoma of the lung, complete removal or permanent eradication of this tumor is seldom possible. Complete removal of less aggressive tumors, such as bronchial carcinoids, may result in total cure of the syndrome.

2. **Correction of hypokalemia**

   a. **Oral therapy.** Owing to the concomitant alkalosis and hypochloremia, *only potassium chloride supplements should be employed.* Because of the severe potassium depletion, 40 to 100 mEq/day of potassium may be required to correct hypokalemia. Potassium chloride preparations are available in liquid, powder, and tablet forms. Liquid preparations of potassium chloride are available as 5%, 10%, and 20% solutions that contain 10, 20, and 40 mEq/15 ml (tablespoon). Nausea, vomiting, and GI irritation may be important deterrents for the use of oral potassium supplementation—especially in patients who may be receiving simultaneous chemotherapy. To minimize GI irritation, each 20 mEq of potassium chloride solution should be diluted with at least 3 ounces of water or fruit juice and taken after meals. The powder form of potassium chloride should be diluted in at least 4 ounces of water and taken after meals. The slow-release tablet forms of potassium chloride cause less irritation of the GI tract. However, some patients may develop intestinal or gastric ulcerations and bleeding. Furthermore, the concentration of potassium chloride in the tablets is too low for this to be an effective treatment.

b. **IV administration.** IV therapy is necessary for severe hypokalemia (serum potassium < 2 mEq/liter) if the patient cannot tolerate oral potassium or when cardiac arrhythmias, extreme muscle weakness, or paralysis are present. Under these conditions, the potassium chloride solution should be dissolved only in either *normal saline or half-normal saline solutions* and not in glucose-containing solutions, since the availability of glucose in nondiabetic patients may cause an intracellular shift of potassium and may aggravate hypokalemia. Potassium chloride solutions at concentrations no greater than 60 mEq/liter should be used and the rate of IV administration should never exceed 40 mEq/hr. However, if hypokalemia is not severe, more dilute solutions are advisable (20–30 mEq/liter), and slower infusion rates (10–20 mEq/hr) are recommended. The total daily dose of potassium chloride should not exceed 200 mEq/day. IV potassium therapy should be monitored by frequent determinations of serum potassium, venous bicarbonate, and pH. Also, at high infusion rates (30–40 mEq/hr), *continuous monitoring of the ECG is necessary.* Potassium chloride therapy should not be given to anuric or severely oliguric patients. In some patients with tumors producing multiple hormones (e.g., ACTH and ADH), correction of the hypokalemia may restore ADH sensitivity, and hyponatremia and water intoxication may develop.

c. **Spironolactone (Aldactone®)** is a specific pharmacologic antagonist of aldosterone that acts primarily through competitive binding of the mineralocorticoid receptors at the sodium-potassium exchange sites of the distal tubules. Doses of 100 to 400 mg daily may be necessary to correct hypokalemia. Spironolactone should not be used in conjunction with potassium supplements or other types of potassium-sparing drugs, since severe hyperkalemia may develop. Spironolactone is not always effective in preventing hypokalemia and metabolic alkalosis in patients with ectopic Cushing's syndrome, but it may be used temporarily until more effective measures are established. Spironolactone should not be used in the presence of severe impairment of renal function or oliguria. The most common side effects include gynecomastia, abdominal cramping, diarrhea, dizziness, lethargy, and confusion.

3. **Management of sodium and water retention.** In patients with severe hypertension and edema, moderate sodium restriction and diuretics are indicated.

   a. **Thiazides** are the most commonly used drugs for the treatment of sodium retention and hypertension in ectopic Cushing's syndrome. Hydrochlorothiazide, 50 mg bid or long-acting diuretics such as chlorthalidone, 50 to 100 mg daily, or metolazone (Zaroxolyn®), 2.5 to 5 mg/day are equally effective.

   b. **Other diuretics.** When severe hypertension with fluid overload and pulmonary congestion is present, more potent diuretics such as furosemide and ethacrynic acid are useful. Furosemide, 20 to 80 mg PO, may be used. If a good diuretic response is obtained, the dose may be repeated 6 hours later. If there is no significant response, the dose of furosemide may be increased by 20 to 40 mg q6h until the desired diuretic effect has been obtained. Furosemide is the diuretic of choice in patients with renal insufficiency. For more critical situations or for the treatment of pulmonary edema, furosemide should be administered IV (20–40 mg over 1–2 minutes) and, if necessary, increments of 20 mg can be given q2h. The maximum dose of furosemide should not exceed 600 mg/24 hr. Caution must be exerted with the use of diuretics in ectopic Cushing's syndrome since hypokalemia may be aggravated by their use. Careful monitoring of serum potassium and adequate potassium supplementation will prevent this complication.

4. **Treatment of metabolic alkalosis.** Metabolic alkalosis is of the chloride-resistant type and is caused by excess mineralocorticoids. This excess causes intracellular shifts of hydrogen ions and increased hydrogen ion secretion by the renal tubule and results in severe alkalosis. Characteristically, urinary chlorides are less than 15 mEq/liter. Treatment consists of potassium chloride supplement, spironolactone, and more importantly, correction of the mineralocorticoid excess by the use of inhibitors of adrenal steroid synthesis.

5. **Adrenal enzyme inhibitors**

   a. **Metyrapone (Metopirone®)**

      (1) **Mechanism of action.** Metyrapone is a synthetic compound that inhibits adrenal 11-β-hydroxylation causing a rapid reduction of cortisol production.

      (2) **Therapeutic use.** When used for therapeutic purposes metyrapone can be used at doses of 500 mg every 4 to 6 hours PO (2–3g/day), and according to the clinical response, the dose may be lowered.

      (3) **Effects of therapy.** Although metyrapone rapidly lowers plasma cortisol levels it does not lower the levels of desoxycorticosterone (DOC), which is a powerful mineralocorticoid. In patients with the ectopic ACTH syndrome, the plasma levels of DOC are usually 9- to 12-fold higher than normal. Therefore, rapid relief of symptoms caused by the excess cortisol is expected after metyrapone treatment, but hypokalemia and metabolic alkalosis may not improve by treatment with metyrapone alone. The most common adverse reactions have been

nausea, abdominal discomfort, dizziness, headache, sedation, and allergic reactions.

b. Aminoglutethimide (Cytadren®) is derived from the hypnotic drug glutethimide, which was formerly used for the treatment of epilepsy. Approximately two thirds of the patients with ectopic ACTH syndrome treated with aminoglutethimide show clinical, as well as biochemical, evidence of improvement.

(1) Mechanism of action. Aminoglutethimide is a competitive inhibitor of the mitochondrial enzyme cholesterol side-chain cleaving enzyme, and its primary effect is to inhibit the conversion of cholesterol to pregnenolone. By blocking the conversion of cholesterol to pregnenolone, aminoglutethimide causes a reversible medical adrenalectomy, with marked reduction in the production of adrenal glucocorticoids, mineralocorticoids, androgens, and estrogens.

(2) Dosage and administration. The recommended dose of aminoglutethimide for the treatment of Cushing's syndrome is 1 g/day in four divided doses. In some patients doses of 1.5 to 2 g/day may be necessary.

(3) Prevention of adrenal insufficiency. To prevent the development of adrenal insufficiency, glucocorticoids and mineralocorticoids should be replaced. Aminoglutethimide increases the rate of metabolism of hydrocortisone and dexamethasone, and it is necessary to use larger doses of dexamethasone or hydrocortisone than doses required for physiologic replacement. Adrenal replacement therapy can be done with either

(a) Hydrocortisone, 40 to 60 mg/day (10 mg at 8 AM, 10 mg at 5 PM, and 20 mg at bedtime), *or*

(b) Dexamethasone, 0.5 to 0.75 mg qid (2–3 mg/day). In patients receiving hydrocortisone replacement the response to aminoglutethimide therapy should be monitored by the plasma levels of dehydroepiandrosterone sulfate (DHEA-S). In patients receiving dexamethasone replacement, response to therapy can be monitored by the levels of plasma, or urinary cortisol, or both. If hypotension or hyperkalemia develops, the patient should also receive mineralocorticoid replacement therapy with fludrocortisone (Florinef®), 0.05 to 0.1 mg/day. Development of hyponatremia may be another indication of mineralocorticoid deficiency, but the possibility of concomitant production of ADH by the tumor has to be considered.

(4) Side effects. The most common side effects are related to CNS toxicity and include lethargy, sedation, dizziness, blurred vision, and depression. Morbilliform skin rashes with or without fever may also be seen 9 to 14 days after the initiation of aminoglutethimide therapy. These rashes may disappear spontaneously with continuation of therapy. CNS symptoms are usually transient and dose related and rarely occur in patients receiving 1 g/day. GI symptoms such as anorexia, nausea, and vomiting may also occur.

c. Mitotane (Lysodren®, o,p'-DDD)

(1) **Mechanism of action.** Mitotane is an oral chemotherapeutic agent best known by its trivial name o,p'-DDD. Mitotane is an adrenal cytotoxic agent, although it can also cause inhibition of steroidogenesis without cellular destruction.

(2) **Dosage and administration.** Treatment with mitotane should be instituted in the hospital until a stable regimen is achieved. *Signs and symptoms of adrenal insufficiency may develop in patients receiving mitotane.* Therefore, adrenal steroid replacement should be started (see p. 236) together with mitotane, although the effect of the drug on adrenal steroidogenesis is not immediate. Mitotane should be started at doses of 4 to 8 g/day in divided doses either qid or tid. If severe side effects appear, the dose should be reduced until maximum tolerated dose is achieved. If the patient can tolerate higher doses and if there is a possibility of further clinical improvement, the dose should be increased until adverse reactions interfere. Maximum tolerated doses vary from 2 to 16 g/day. Treatment should be continued as long as clinical benefits are observed. If no clinical benefits are observed after 3 months at the maximum tolerated dose, the drug should be discontinued. Doses as low as 4g/day, when combined with metyrapone (500 mg q4h), have been reported to cause complete remission of hypercorticism in patients with the ectopic ACTH syndrome.

(3) **Side effects.** A high percentage of patients treated with mitotane manifest at least one side effect. Approximately 80 percent of the patients develop GI disturbances such as anorexia, nausea, vomiting, and diarrhea. CNS side effects occur in approximately 40 percent of patients and consist primarily of depression, lethargy, and less frequently, dizziness, or vertigo. Dermatologic toxicity occurs in about 15 percent of cases, but the symptoms usually subside with continuation of treatment. A variety of other side effects have been reported but seem to occur only rarely. The combined administration of metyrapone, aminoglutethimide, and mitotane has been reported to be effective in some patients with ectopic Cushing's syndrome.

III. Hyponatremia and cancer

A. **The syndrome of inappropriate secretion of antidiuretic hormone (SIADH) and water intoxication.** Another endocrine syndrome that is frequently associated with cancer is *hyponatremia*. Hyponatremia in cancer patients can be caused by either inappropriate secretion of antidiuretic hormone (ADH) of central origin or ectopic production of ADH by the tumor. Also, hyponatremia can be caused by several drugs, including some drugs frequently used for cancer chemotherapy. A variety of tumors have been associated with ectopic production of ADH. The material synthesized by neoplasms has been characterized by bioassay, immunoassay, and chromatography and appears to be arginine vasopressin (AVP). Ectopic production of ADH has been reported in approximately 40 percent of patients with carcinoma of the lung and carcinoma of the colon without clinical evidence of this syndrome. The most common tumors associated with the SIADH syndrome are as follows:

Table 24-1. Drugs Associated with Hyponatremia

Drugs	Potentiates Renal Action of AVP*	Potentiates Release of AVP
Chlorpropamide (Diabinese®)	X	X
Tolbutamide (Orinase®)	X	
Clofibrate (Atromid-S®)		X
Carbamazepine (Tegretol®)		X
Vincristine (Oncovin®)		X
Vinblastine (Velban®)		X
Cyclophosphamide (Cytoxan®)		X
Opiates		X
Histamine		X
Phenformin	X	
Thiazides		X(?)
Nicotine		X
Barbiturates		X(?)
Isoproterenol		X
Thioridazine (Mellaril®)†		

*AVP = arginine vasopressin.
†Increases thirst.

1. Small-cell anaplastic (oat-cell) and squamous cell carcinoma of the lung
2. Carcinoid tumors
3. Pancreatic carcinoma
4. Esophageal carcinoma
5. Prostatic carcinoma
6. Adrenal cortical carcinoma
7. Bladder carcinoma
8. Hodgkin's disease
9. Acute myelogenous leukemia

B. **Other causes of SIADH and hyponatremia.** It is important to distinguish between ectopic production of ADH and other causes of SIADH. Also, it is important to discard the possibility that the syndrome may be caused by drugs that may affect water metabolism. The most common drugs that impair water metabolism and that are associated with hyponatremia are listed in Table 24-1.

C. **Spurious hyponatremia and hyperglycemia.** It must be recognized that the presence of lower than normal levels of serum sodium concentration does not always imply hypo-osmolarity.

1. **Spurious or artifactual hyponatremia** can occur in patients with marked elevation of *serum lipids* or *serum proteins.*

2. Severe **hyperglycemia** is another common situation that may lead to hyponatremia without hypo-osmolarity. In this condition, the increased osmolarity owing to hyperglycemia draws water from cells and results in dilution of plasma sodium.

D. Diagnosis of SIADH. In the absence of direct and clinically applicable measurements of ADH, the important criteria for the diagnosis of SIADH are

1. Hyponatremia with hypo-osmolarity of the serum

2. Inappropriate antidiuresis (urine osmolarity that is higher than that expected for the degree of hyponatremia and hypo-osmolarity of the serum)

3. Normal renal, adrenal, thyroid, and pituitary function

4. Evidence of sodium wasting in the urine (urine sodium is commonly greater than 20–40 mEq/liter)

5. Absence of clinical signs of hypovolemia and dehydration

6. Absence of generalized edema or ascites

7. Correction of the hyponatremia and hypo-osmolarity of the plasma by severe fluid restriction

Patients with mild SIADH may be asymptomatic. However, when the serum sodium levels fall to the range of 125 to 120 mEq/liter, loss of memory, apathy, and impairment of abstract thought may occur. When serum sodium levels fall below 115 mEq/liter, extrapyramidal signs, asterixis, convulsions, and coma may occur. Serum sodium levels below 115 mEq/liter indicate severe water intoxication and constitute a medical emergency.

E. Treatment of SIADH. Successful treatment of the tumor usually corrects SIADH, and reappearance of the syndrome is seen with recurrence of the tumor.

1. **Fluid restriction.** For mildly symptomatic patients or patients whose serum sodium has decreased below 125 mEq/liter, fluid restriction is necessary. In these patients, the major source of water loss is insensible. Therefore, to be effective in raising the serum sodium concentration, fluid restrictions to 500 ml/day or less may be necessary in some patients. Once the serum sodium returns to normal, fluid administration should be increased to replace sensible and insensible losses plus the urine output. Unfortunately, because of the continuous production of ADH by tumors, this approach alone is often impractical and unsuccessful.

2. **Demeclocycline (Declomycin®)** antagonizes the renal actions of AVP and therefore causes a reversible, dose-dependent nephrogenic diabetes insipidus. Demeclocycline, in divided doses of 600 to 1200 mg/day and combined with moderate water restriction, has been highly successful in treating chronic SIADH associated with tumors. The most common side effects of this drug have been anorexia, nausea, and vomiting. Skin rashes and hypersensitivity to ultraviolet light are also common. Because of the antianabolic effect of the tetracyclines, this drug may cause a rise in blood urea nitrogen (BUN). Also, when combined with fluid restriction, it may lead to sodium depletion and dehydration.

3. **Lithium carbonate** has also been used for the treatment of chronic tumor-associated SIADH, but it is more toxic and inferior to demeclocycline.

Table 24-2. Factors that May Be Responsible for
Hypercalcemia of Malignancy

1. Direct invasion of bone by tumor
2. Production of PTH or PTH-like substances by tumor
3. Production of PGE_2 or other substances by tumor
4. Production of osteoclast activating factor (OAF)
5. Coexistence of tumor with primary hyperparathyroidism
6. Coexistence with another cause of hypercalcemia (vitamin D intoxication, sarcoidosis, etc.)
7. Estrogen or androgen treatment of patients with carcinoma of the breast metastatic to bone

4. **Phenytoin** inhibits the release of ADH from the pituitary gland. At doses of 100 mg tid, phenytoin has been successful in the treatment of SIADH of CNS origin. However, this drug is not effective for the treatment of SIADH caused by ectopic production of ADH by tumor.

5. **Hypertonic sodium chloride.** For the treatment of severe hyponatremia and water intoxication (serum sodium below 115 mEq/liter associated with confusion, stupor, convulsions, and muscle twitching), therapy should be aimed at reversing the flow of water into the cells. This therapy may require the administration of small amounts of hypertonic sodium chloride, either 3% sodium chloride (513 mEq/liter) or 5% sodium chloride (855 mEq/liter). The quantity of hypertonic sodium chloride should not exceed the amount required to raise the concentration of serum sodium one half the distance to normality within 8 hours. It is unnecessary to correct serum sodium to normal levels within the initial 12 to 24 hours. The amount of sodium necessary to accomplish the desired correction can be estimated by the following formula:

[desired serum sodium (mEq/L) − observed serum sodium (mEq/L)] × [body weight (kg)] × .6 = sodium for replacement (mEq)

The use of hypertonic sodium chloride is a potentially dangerous mode of therapy that may result in fluid and circulatory overload, especially in elderly patients. To prevent these complications, IV furosemide can be added to the regimen. Alternatively, the IV use of furosemide (1 mg/kg) as initial therapy followed by the hourly replacement of the urinary losses of sodium and potassium with 3% sodium chloride with potassium chloride added to it is an effective way of correcting severe hyponatremia within 6 to 8 hours. However, this approach requires extremely careful monitoring of fluid and electrolyte balance as well as ready access to the laboratory, since hourly measurements of sodium and potassium in the urine are required.

IV. Hypercalcemia

A. **Causes.** The possible pathogenic mechanisms of tumor hypercalcemia are listed in Table 24-2.

1. **Associated tumors.** Hypercalcemia is relatively common in patients with malignancy. In fact, in a recent study it was shown that the most common cause of hypercalcemia in hospitalized patients is malignancy. Hypercalcemia of malignancy can be associated with bone metastasis, or it may occur in the absence of any direct bone involve-

ment by the tumor. Based on the findings of a recent study on 433 patients with hypercalcemia of cancer, 86 percent of the patients had identifiable bone metastasis. More than one half (225) of the cases were accounted for by patients with breast carcinoma, and cancer of the lung and kidneys accounted for a smaller proportion. Patients with hematologic malignancies accounted for approximately 15 percent of the cases. These patients usually had hypercalcemia in the presence of diffuse tumor involvement of bone, although in a small percentage evidence of bone involvement was absent.

2. **Humoral mediators.** In approximately 10 percent of the cases of malignancy, hypercalcemia develops in the absence of radiographic or scintigraphic evidence of bone involvement. In this group of patients, the pathogenesis of hypercalcemia appears to be secondary to humoral mediators.

   a. **Parathyroid hormone (PTH) production.** Evidence of synthesis and secretion of PTH by tumors have been obtained largely by immunoassay. By some radioimmunoassays, patients with hypercalcemia of malignancy show increased concentration of PTH in blood. However, the levels of PTH are substantially lower than those levels found in patients with primary hyperparathyroidism, although the values often overlap. Secretion of precursors of PTH or of smaller fragments of the molecule is a common occurrence. The tumors that have been associated with ectopic production of PTH are as follows:

      (1) Squamous cell carcinoma of the lung

      (2) Genitourinary: renal cell, bladder, testis, penis, adrenal, ovary, uterus, cervix, and vulva carcinomas

      (3) Breast carcinoma

      (4) Gastrointestinal: colon, esophagus, pancreas, liver, and biliary tract carcinomas

      (5) Adenocarcinoma of the parotid

      (6) Melanoma

      (7) Lymphoma

   b. **Prostaglandin (PG) production.** There is convincing experimental and clinical evidence indicating that PGs play a role in hypercalcemia of malignancy. PGs are potent stimulators of bone resorption. There are some reports of metastatic renal cell carcinomas in which high concentrations of PGE_2 have been found in the tumor or its metastasis and in which the hypercalcemia responded to treatment with indomethacin. Also, the urinary metabolite of PGE_2 has been found to be elevated in a number of patients with hypercalcemia associated with solid tumors, primarily bronchogenic carcinoma, and suppression of the PGE_2 metabolite levels and normalization of the serum calcium has been seen after treatment with indomethacin or aspirin in some patients. Therefore, solid tumors associated with hypercalcemia without evidence of bone involvement appear to produce hypercalcemia by synthesizing either a PTH-like material or PGE_2.

c. Osteoclast activating factor (OAF) production. A third hormonal mechanism for production of hypercalcemia is the elaboration of OAF. This material is a potent stimulator of osteoclast resorption and was initially found in the supernatant of human peripheral lymphocytes cultured with added antigens and phytohemagglutinin. OAF has been partially characterized and appears to be a polypeptide of 20,000 to 25,000 daltons. This material probably acts as a local hormone produced by the tumor. Besides increasing osteoclastic activity, it also inhibits bone collagen synthesis, thus leading to osteolytic lesions. It is thought that the hypercalcemia of multiple myeloma is probably associated with OAF production. Evidence of production of OAF has also been obtained in other hematologic neoplasms associated with hypercalcemia, such as Burkitt's and other malignant lymphomas. The release of OAF is macrophage dependent and may be affected through the synthesis and release of PGs by the macrophage. Also, the activity of OAF is sensitive to inhibition by glucocorticoids. Therefore, it appears that the hypercalcemia in some patients with hematologic malignancies may be explained by production of OAF rather than PTH or PGs.

3. Symptoms, signs, and laboratory findings. Hypercalcemia is often symptomatic in a patient with cancer and, in fact, may be the patient's major problem. Polyuria and nocturia, resulting from the impaired ability of the kidneys to concentrate the urine, occur early. Anorexia, nausea, constipation, muscle weakness, and fatigue are common. As the hypercalcemia progresses, severe dehydration, azotemia, mental obtundation, coma, and cardiovascular collapse may appear. In addition to hypercalcemia, the laboratory studies may show hypokalemia and increased levels of BUN and creatinine. Patients with hypercalcemia of malignancy frequently have hypochloremic metabolic alkalosis, whereas in primary hyperparathyroidism metabolic acidosis is more common. The concentration of serum phosphorus is variable. Parathyroid hormone levels may be normal, low, or high, but marked elevations are rarely seen. Bone involvement is best evaluated by a bone scan, which is often positive in the absence of x-ray evidence of bone involvement.

4. Treatment. The management of hypercalcemia of malignancy has two objectives: (a) reducing elevated levels of serum calcium and (b) treating the underlying cause. When hypercalcemia is mild to moderate (serum calcium < 12–13 mg/100 ml) and the patient is not symptomatic, adequate hydration and measures directed against the tumor (e.g., surgery, chemotherapy, or radiation therapy) may suffice. Severe hypercalcemia, on the other hand, is a life-threatening condition requiring emergency treatment. Therefore, for more severe degrees of hypercalcemia other measures must be taken, including enhancement of calcium excretion by the kidney in patients with adequate renal function.

a. Saline diuresis. Sodium competitively inhibits the tubular reabsorption of calcium. Therefore, the IV infusion of saline causes a significant increase in calcium clearance. Because of the large amounts of saline that may be required to correct hypercalcemia, it is advisable to continuously monitor the central venous pressure.

The infusion of normal saline (0.9% sodium chloride) at a rate of 250 to 500 ml/hr, accompanied by the IV administration of 20 to 80 mg of furosemide every 2 to 4 hours results in significant calcium diuresis and lowering of the serum calcium in the majority of patients. This type of therapy requires *strict* monitoring of cardiopulmonary status to avoid fluid overload and electrolyte imbalance. Also, it requires ready access to the laboratory since the urinary losses of sodium, potassium, magnesium, and water must be replaced in order to maintain metabolic balance.

b. **Glucocorticoids.** Large initial doses of hydrocortisone, 250 to 500 mg IV q8h (or its equivalent), can be effective in the treatment of hypercalcemia associated with lympho-proliferative diseases, such as non-Hodgkin's lymphoma and multiple myeloma, and in patients with breast cancer metastatic to bone. It may take several days for glucocorticoids to lower the serum calcium level. Maintenance therapy should be started with prednisone, 10 to 30 mg/day PO. The mechanisms by which glucocorticoids lower the serum calcium are multiple and involve (1) inhibition of OAF, (2) inhibition of phospholipase A_2, thereby blocking PG synthesis, (3) reduction of the rate of bone turnover, (4) reduction of the rate of intestinal absorption of calcium, and (5) reduction of the rate of renal tubular reabsorption of calcium.

c. **Calcitonin (Calcimar®)** is a peptide hormone that inhibits osteocytic and osteoclastic bone resorption. Salmon calcitonin, when given by infusion, will cause a modest reduction of serum calcium levels, usually by 1 to 3 mg/100 ml, which commonly reverses after discontinuation of therapy. To avoid anaphylactic reactions, skin testing should be performed prior to the administration of calcitonin. To avoid inconsistencies in the response, it is recommended that albumin (approximately 5 g) be added to the infusion to coat the infusion set and prevent absorption of the peptides to the walls of the set. The usual initial dose of calcitonin is 50 to 100 MRC units IV followed by 50 to 100 MRC units either SC or IM every 12 to 24 hours according to the serum calcium levels.

Nausea with or without vomiting has been noted in approximately 10 percent of patients treated with calcitonin. It is more common at the beginning of the treatment and usually subsides with continuous administration. Local inflammatory reactions at the site of SC or IM injection have been reported in about 10 percent of the patients. Skin rashes and flushing occur occasionally.

d. **Oral phosphate supplements (Neutra-Phos® or Fleet Phospho-Soda®).** Oral phosphate therapy is a useful adjunct for the treatment of hypercalcemia of malignancy. Oral phosphate decreases the intestinal absorption of calcium and enhances the deposition of insoluble calcium salts in bone and tissue. Oral phosphate supplements at doses of 1.5 to 3 g/day of elemental phosphorus can result in lowering of the serum calcium levels as well as a reduction in urinary calcium excretion. Diarrhea usually limits the amount of phosphate that can be given. Phosphate supplements should *never* be given to patients with renal failure or when hyperphosphatemia is present, since soft tissue calcification may occur. Monitoring of the level of calcium and phosphorus as well as the calcium × phosphorus ion product is important to prevent metastatic calcifications.

e. Mithramycin (Mithracin®) is a potent antineoplastic agent that was formerly used for the treatment of some malignant tumors of the testis. Mithramycin inhibits bone resorption and causes hypocalcemia. Mithramycin at doses of 15 to 25 μg/kg/body weight given by IV push as a single bolus usually causes a significant fall in serum calcium within 12 hours, and the effect may last for 3 to 7 days. Additional doses may be administered at intervals of 3 to 4 days in order to maintain the serum calcium below 12 to 13 mg/100 ml. Mithramycin should generally be used only for the treatment of hypercalcemia of malignancy that has been refractory to other modalities of therapy.

The most common side effects reported with the use of mithramycin consist of GI symptoms of anorexia, nausea, vomiting, diarrhea, and stomatitis. Other less frequent side effects include fever, drowsiness, weakness, lethargy, malaise, facial flushing, and skin rash. The most important form of toxicity associated with the use of mithramycin consists of a bleeding syndrome, which usually begins with an episode of epistaxis. The bleeding syndrome appears to be dose-related and is rarely seen at the doses used for the treatment of hypercalcemia.

f. PG inhibitors. Nonsteroidal antiinflammatory agents inhibit cyclo-oxygenase and thereby block PG synthesis. Inhibitors of PG synthesis have been clearly effective in selected cases of metastatic renal cell carcinoma and squamous cell carcinoma of the lung. Indomethacin, 50 mg tid, is the most potent inhibitor of prostaglandin synthesis. Aspirin, 1 g tid, has also been shown to be effective in selected cases.

V. Hypoglycemia and cancer. A wide variety of non-islet cell tumors may be associated with hypoglycemia. Hypoglycemia may occur months or even years before the recognition of the tumor, it may be present at the time of the diagnosis, or it may develop after the diagnosis of malignancy has been well established.

A. Most of the neoplasms associated with hypoglycemia are large and may present as masses in the mediastinum or retroperitoneal space. The most common non-β-cell tumors associated with hypoglycemia are as follows:

1. Mesenchymal or mesodermal: fibrosarcomas, mesotheliomas, neurofibromas, neurofibrosarcoma, spindle cell sarcoma, rhabdomyosarcomas, and leiomyosarcomas

2. Hepatocellular carcinoma

3. Adrenocortical carcinoma

4. Pancreatic and bile duct carcinomas

5. Lymphomas and leukemias

6. Miscellaneous: lung, ovary, neuroblastoma, Wilms' tumor, and hemangiopericytoma

B. The **pathogenesis of hypoglycemia** in patients with malignancy is not clear. The possible causes of hypoglycemia are

1. Production and secretion of insulin by the tumor
2. Production of NSILA-s or NSILA-p by the tumor
3. Excessive glucose utilization by the tumor
4. Production of metabolites that interfere with gluconeogenesis
5. Inhibition of glycogen breakdown
6. Destruction of liver by tumor
7. Suppression of counterregulatory hormones.

Secretion of insulin by tumors is rare. In only a few cases has an increased insulin concentration in the blood or in the tumors been reported. These tumors include teratoma of the mediastinum containing beta cells, bronchial carcinoid, carcinoma of the cervix, retroperitoneal fibrosarcoma, and in bronchogenic metastasis. At present, the best documented mechanism is the production of an insulinlike substance by the tumor. This substance has been named *non-suppressible-insulinlike activity* (*NSILA*) and has been found in approximately 40 percent of the non-islet cell tumors causing hypoglycemia. Two types of this material have been isolated: a low molecular weight NSILA-s and a high molecular weight NSILA-p, and both have been found to be elevated in some cases of tumor hypoglycemia. There is also evidence for a high rate of glycolysis of these large tumors associated with hypoglycemia, and this glycolysis could possibly contribute to excessive glucose utilization. It is likely that a variety of mechanisms may be responsible for the hypoglycemia in different tumors.

C. Symptoms, signs, and laboratory findings. The hypoglycemia that occurs with non-β-cell tumors usually occurs during fasting in the early morning or late afternoon, and its onset is usually insidious. In the majority of patients, symptoms of neuroglycopenia predominate. They usually develop when the plasma glucose falls below 45 to 50 mg/100 ml, and the patients may experience symptoms and signs that resemble a variety of neurologic or psychiatric disturbances. When the hypoglycemia is severe and protracted, generalized convulsions and coma may occur. Typically, the symptoms of hypoglycemia are relieved by the ingestion of food. The hypoglycemia caused by non-islet cell tumors cannot be differentiated clinically from that caused by insulinomas. However, they can be differentiated by measurement of fasting plasma insulin and glucose. Whereas, patients with insulinomas have fasting hyperinsulinemia in the presence of hypoglycemia, patients with non-islet cell tumors have hypoglycemia with low levels of insulin.

D. Treatment. Therapy of hypoglycemia associated with non-islet cell tumors is difficult because no specific agents are available. Amelioration of hypoglycemia may result from partial or complete resection of the tumor or by control of the tumor by either chemotherapy or radiation therapy.

1. **Diet.** The primary form of therapy is dietary. Frequent feedings between meals, at bedtime, and throughout the night may decrease the

frequency of hypoglycemic attacks. In severe cases it may be necessary to place an ileostomy tube for administration of continuous feeding, especially during the night. In some patients it is also necessary to administer continuous infusions of 10% to 20% glucose.

2. **Hyperglycemic hormones.** High doses of glucocorticoids (prednisone, 20–80 mg, or dexamethasone, 10–15 mg/day) may be used in patients that do not respond to diet therapy. Also, patients may benefit from the use of long-acting glucagon (zinc glucagon) and human growth hormone. In most cases, however, the effect of these agents is only temporary.

3. **Diazoxide (Hyperstat®)** is a nondiuretic derivative of the benzothiadiazine group that inhibits insulin secretion and thereby causes hyperglycemia. Diazoxide has been effective for the treatment of hypoglycemia associated with malignant insulinomas at doses of 300 to 600 mg/day IV given in conjunction with hydrochlorothiazide (100mg/day PO). However, in patients with hypoglycemia from non-islet cell tumors, diazoxide is frequently ineffective.

   Hypotension may occasionally result from the IV administration of diazoxide. Infrequently, severe hypotension and shock may be seen. Sodium and water retention after repeated injections are common, but may be obviated by the simultaneous use of hydrochlorothiazide or other diuretics.

4. **Phenytoin and somatostatin** are usually ineffective in patients with hypoglycemia owing to non-insulin producing tumors. Streptozocin and chlorozotocin, which may be effective in insulinomas, can be tried in refractory cases, but the results have been disappointing in non-islet cell tumors.

VI. Ectopic production of gonadotropins

A. **Causes and clinical observations.** Ectopic production of gonadotropin can result in gynecomastia in adults and in precocious puberty in children. Gynecomastia has been associated with carcinoma of the lung and is sometimes accompanied by hypertrophic pulmonary osteoarthropathy. Increased estrogen production has been reported in several patients with carcinoma of the lung and has been attributed to the production of gonadotropins by the tumor. Arteriovenous differences in follicle stimulating hormone (FSH) concentration have been found across the tumor from adenocarcinoma of the lung providing substantial evidence of hormone production by the tumor. Also, increased luteinizing hormone (LH) activity has been found in a hepatoblastoma from a patient with precocious puberty. In addition to carcinoma of the lung and hepatoblastoma, tumors of the testes, ovaries, pineal gland, mediastinum, adrenals, breast and bladder and melanomas may be associated with gonadotropin production. Assays not only for FSH, LH, and chorionic gonadotropin (HCG), but also for the alpha and beta subunits of these hormones have been developed and are used primarily for screening as tumor markers. HCG is closely related biochemically and biologically to LH and is generally produced by tumors that have trophoblastic characteristics. However, there is no specific syndrome that can be attributed to the ectopic production of HCG.

B. Treatment. There is no specific treatment for the ectopic production of gonadotropins other than therapy of the primary tumor.

VII. Ectopic thyrotropin secretion

A. Causes. Hyperthyroidism has been described primarily in patients with trophoblastic tumors, although a similar syndrome has been reported with epidermoid cancers of the lung and mesothelioma. The hyperthyroidism in these patients is usually mild, although severe cases have been reported in association with choriocarcinomas. The nature of the thyroid stimulator in chorionic tumors has been named *molar thyroid stimulating hormone* (*molar TSH*), and recent evidence suggests that thyrotropic activity cannot be separated from HCG.

B. Treatment. In patients with hydatidiform mole and hyperthyroidism, surgical removal is the treatment of choice and should be performed as soon as possible. If the hyperthyroidism is severe, administration of sodium iodide effectively reduces the concentrations of T_3 and T_4 in the plasma. Propranolol, 40 to 160 mg/day may be used for control of tachycardia. In patients with choriocarcinoma, symptomatic hyperthyroidism can be treated with propylthiouracil or methimazole as well as propranolol. Effective chemotherapy of the tumor will reduce the levels of HCG and thereby provide definitive treatment of the hyperthyroidism.

VIII. Osteomalacia and hypophosphatemia associated with tumors

A. Clinical observations. There are approximately 30 reports of patients displaying profound hypophosphatemia and osteomalacia associated with tumors. This condition has been called *oncogenic osteomalacia* and has been associated with a variety of mesenchymal tumors, including mesenchymomas, pleomorphic sarcomas, neurofibromas, sclerosing and cavernous hemangiomas, and hemangiopericytomas. Clinically, the patients may have profound muscle weakness and frequent fractures. Laboratory examinations reveal severe hypophosphatemia and phosphaturia. PTH levels are usually normal, and the levels of 1,25-dihydroxycholecalciferol are usually low. The pathogenesis of the syndrome appears to be abnormal vitamin D metabolism. It is thought that the tumor secretes a substance that inhibits the 25-hydroxycholecalciferol-1-hydroxylase activity resulting in a decreased synthesis of 1,25-dihydroxycholecalciferol, which causes the osteomalacia and the attendant biochemical abnormalities.

B. Treatment. Successful surgical removal of the tumor causes healing of the osteomalacia and restores the levels of serum phosphorus and 1,25-dihydroxycholecalciferol to normal. Treatment with 1,25-dihydroxycholecalciferol (Rocaltrol®), 3 μg/day for 2 weeks has been shown to correct the biochemical abnormalities and cause healing of the bone lesions. For severe hypophosphatemia, oral phosphate supplements (Neutra-Phos® or Fleet Phospho-Soda®) may be used (see section **V**).

Selected Reading

Bockman, R. S. Hypercalcemia in malignancy. *Clin. Endocrinol. Metab.* 9:317, 1980.

Bondy, P. D. Endocrine and Metabolic Effects of Cancer. In P. K. Bondy and L. E.

Rosenberg (Eds.), *Metabolic Control and Disease*. Philadelphia: Saunders, 1980. Pp. 1815–1841.

Imura, H. Ectopic hormone syndromes. *Clin. Endocrinol. Metab.* 9:235, 1980.

Kahn, C. R. The riddle of tumor, hypoglycemia revisited. *Clin. Endocrinol. Metab.* 9:335, 1980.

Myers, W. P. L. Hypercalcemia Associated with Malignant Diseases. In M. D. Anderson Hospital and Tumor Institute, *Endocrine and Nonendocrine Hormone Producing Tumors*. Chicago: Yearbook, 1973. Pp. 147–171.

Odell, W. D., and Wolfsen, A. R. Humoral syndromes associated with cancer. *Annu. Rev. Med.* 29:379, 1978.

Sherwood, L. M. Ectopic Hormone Syndromes. In S. H. Ingbar (Ed.), *Contemporary Endocrinology*. New York: Plenum Pr., 1980. Pp. 341–373.

Sherwood, L. M., and Gould, V. E. Ectopic Syndromes and Multiple Endocrine Neoplasia. In L. J. DeGroot (Ed.), *Endocrinology*. New York: Grune & Stratton, 1979. Pp. 1733–1766.

25

Infections and Bleeding

Mary R. Smith

I. Infections

A. Reasons for infection. Patients with cancer may be unduly susceptible to infections as a result of the disease process itself, direct complications of the therapy, or indirect complications of either the disease or the therapy.

1. **Underlying disease.** Infection related to the underlying disease process may occur as a result of one or more of several factors:

   a. **Granulocytopenia** remains the leading abnormality responsible for infection caused by the underlying disease.

      (1) **Causes.** Reduction in granulocytes may be due to bone marrow replacement, as in leukemia, or bone marrow invasion, as in carcinoma of the breast or prostate.

      (2) **Evaluation.** The peripheral blood smear is a very useful means of evaluating this form of leukopenia. If nucleated red-blood cells, "tear drop" red cells, or immature myeloid cells are noted on the smear, bone marrow invasion or replacement should be seriously considered, and a bone marrow aspiration and biopsy should be performed to further assess this possibility.

   b. **Reduction in immunoglobulins** (defective humoral immunity) results from several diseases of B-lymphocytes or plasma cells, including chronic lymphocytic leukemia, multiple myeloma, and Waldenström's macroglobulinemia. In each of these conditions, there is a particularly increased risk of bacterial illness.

   c. **Defective cellular immunity** may occur in lymphomas or other malignancies if the patient is severely debilitated. Such patients are at increased risk of viral and fungal illnesses.

   d. **Breakdown in normal skin or mucosal barriers** may occur, as in carcinoma of the colon.

   e. **Obstruction,** as in carcinoma of the bronchus, may lead to atelectasis and infection.

   f. **Defective leukocyte function** is a poorly documented but possible mechanism of increased susceptibility to infection in cancer.

2. **Direct complications of therapy.** As leukopenia (primarily granulocytopenia) also results from the effects of chemotherapy, radiotherapy, or both, treatment of the disease may make the patient more susceptible to infection. The effects of these two modes of therapy may

be more than additive, and great care must be taken when giving both radiotherapy and chemotherapy together. The nadir granulocyte count of various chemotherapeutic agents varies from a few days to many weeks, and knowledge of the expected time of the nadir is needed for safe planning of chemotherapy as well as radiotherapy.

Radiotherapy of 4500 rad or more to marrow-bearing bone may result in irreversible bone marrow damage. If such therapy is given to large areas of the bone marrow (e.g., pelvis or vertebral bodies), irreversible granulocytopenia or pancytopenia may develop.

3. **Indirect effects of either the disease process or treatment**

   a. **Malnutrition.** The risk of infection increases in patients who are in a catabolic state. In order to maintain nutrition, enteral tube feedings or IV hyperalimentation may be required.

   b. **Debility.** The bedridden patient has an increased risk of urinary tract and respiratory tract infections. Ambulation must be encouraged as much as can be tolerated. Decubitus ulcers, when they develop, may also act as portals for infection, and avoidance of these pressure-induced lesions is important.

B. **How to avoid infection**

1. Require **careful hand washing** of all staff who have contact with the patient.

2. **Change any IV site** every 48 hours if possible.

3. **Avoid use of plastic IV catheters** if possible. If such catheters are used, the tip must be sent for culture and sensitivity when catheter is removed.

4. **Avoid the use of urinary bladder catheters.**

5. **Minimize digital rectal exams** and rectal suppositories when possible.

6. **Minimize invasive procedures.**

7. **Minimize the number of hospitalizations** or other exposures to potentially infectious persons or places.

8. **Use vaccines or immune globulin** in selected patients.

   a. **Pneumococcal** vaccine may decrease the likelihood of pneumococcal infection.

   b. **Avoid the use of live vaccines** in severely immunosuppressed patients.

   c. **Gamma globulin injections** may be of value for certain patients with severe hypogammaglobulinemia.

   d. **Zoster immune globulin** can be effective in patients without herpes zoster antibodies who are at high risk when exposed to zoster infection.

9. Attempt to attain **optimal dental hygiene** for the patient.

   a. Optimal dental hygiene is particularly important for patients preparing for **head and neck radiation.**

b. In patients with acute leukemia or other tumors requiring urgent chemotherapy, defer invasive dental work until a remission or reasonable disease control (and granulocyte count) is achieved. Avoid vigorous brushing of teeth during periods of granulocytopenia.

C. Management of infection

1. Importance of fever and other signs of infection

a. Never assume that fever is due to the patient's underlying malignancy until a very diligent search for an infection has been made.

b. Fever is usually present when infection occurs in patients with cancer. However, when patients are severely debilitated, fever may not be seen.

c. Other clues that infection is present include

(1) Neutrophilic leukocytosis with or without increase in the number of band-form neutrophils

(2) Toxic granulation of neutrophils

(3) Vacuolation of neutrophils

(4) Unexplained hypotension (a manifestation of septicemia)

(5) Unexplained tachycardia

(6) Hypomotility of the bowel, including ileus (a rare manifestation of infection)

2. Steps to take if infection is suspected

a. In patients with a normal or elevated granulocyte count:

(1) Obtain a culture and sensitivity of all potential sites of infection as well as a gram stain where appropriate.

(a) Potential sites of infection include the following: urine, stool, sputum, any wound drainage, pharynx, vagina, rectum, CSF, and biopsy tissue.

(b) Send specimens for bacterial, viral, and fungal culture, and where appropriate, a search for parasites.

(c) Cultures should be done on patients in whom a marked fall in the white cell count is anticipated even if infection is not presently suspected (e.g., a patient with acute leukemia who is to begin chemotherapy).

(2) Attempt to quickly define site and type of infective process, and if possible choose one antibiotic that is most likely to deal with the suspected organism.

(3) Be prepared to change the antibiotic based on results of culture and sensitivity.

(4) Complete a "full course" of antibiotic or antifungal or other antimicrobial therapy.

(5) Repeat culture studies after therapy is completed.

Table 25-1. Guidelines for Granulocyte Transfusions

1. For any patient in whom profound granulocytopenia is anticipated as a part of the complications of therapy, alert the blood transfusion service of this potential problem, and put in motion action for HLA typing of the patient and appropriate family members.
2. Granulocytes should be begun only in patients who have <500 granulocytes/mm², and in whom 48 hours of appropriate antibiotics have failed to lead to reduction in fever.
3. Personnel must be available to handle any of the complications of granulocyte transfusions.
4. In general, plan to give granulocyte transfusions for at least 4 successive days before determining the effectiveness of this therapy.

   b. In patients with low white blood cell counts. A total granulocyte count of less than 500/mm² is accompanied by a severe risk of rapidly fatal infection. Such a situation should be viewed as an emergency, and therapy must be instituted as soon as possible.

   (1) Obtain all cultures as listed in **I.C.2.a.(1)**, page 251.

   (2) Immediately begin broad-spectrum IV antibiotic therapy if no site of infection is apparent (e.g., tobramycin, 3 mg/kg daily in divided doses q8h, and ticarcillin, 200-300 mg/kg daily in divided doses q3-6 h). If a specific site and infecting organism are known, choose appropriate IV antibiotic therapy.

   (3) Consider granulocyte transfusions using the guidelines in Table 25-1.

   (4) Ensure very careful hand washing of all personnel contacting the patient. (Protective isolation as done in most hospitals appears not to provide any greater protection than careful "routine" nursing care.)

   (5) Avoid taking rectal temperatures and using suppositories.

   (6) Do not permit fresh flowers or plants in the patient's room.

   (7) Allow no uncooked fruits or vegetables as part of the patient's diet.

   (8) Consider the use of oral trimethoprim, 160 mg, and sulfamethoxazole, 800 mg (Bactrim™ DS), bid, in the hospitalized granulocytopenic patient.

3. Problem areas in treating the granulocytopenic patient

   a. When no infectious source can be found, current data suggest that granulocytopenic patients with fever of unknown origin who become afebrile should be continued on broad-spectrum antibiotics until granulocytopenia is resolved.

   b. For the granulocytopenic patient who fails to respond to broad-spectrum antibiotic therapy, the following measures should be undertaken:

   (1) Granulocyte transfusions (see Table 25-1)

(2) Consider another type of infection (e.g., viral, fungal, or other opportunistic infection)

 (a) Check carefully for oral candida and if present, treat to prevent disseminated disease.

 (b) Consider open-lung biopsy when pulmonary infiltrates are progressing.

 (c) Consider tuberculosis as a cause of fever.

II. Bleeding in patients with cancer

A. Tumor invasion. It is well recognized that bleeding may be a warning sign of cancer: bloody sputum may indicate carcinoma of the lung; blood in the urine may be a sign of carcinoma of the bladder or kidney; blood in the stool may be due to carcinoma of the alimentary tract; and post-menopausal vaginal bleeding may be caused by endometrial carcinoma. In each of these instances, bleeding can be directly related to the invasive properties of cancer and a disruption of normal tissue integrity.

B. Hematologic abnormalities. Often, bleeding in patients with cancer is not due to direct effects of the neoplasm, but to indirect effects of the cancer or its therapy on one of the components of the hematologic system. Because of the frequency and the special management problems caused by abnormalities in the hematologic system in patients with cancer and the frequency with which these problems occur, it is important to consider the possible causes and corrective measures in detail.

 1. Increased vascular fragility may be due to chronic corticosteroid therapy, chronic malnutrition, or "senile purpura." Bleeding is usually not severe, but bruising, particularly around IV sites, is common.

 2. Thrombocytopenia may occur for a variety of reasons, each of which must be considered whenever the platelet count is low.

  a. Chemotherapy or radiotherapy regularly cause depression of platelets, and regular blood counts must be obtained while patients are being treated.

  b. Bone-marrow invasion or replacement is common only in leukemias or lymphomas, but it may cause thrombocytopenia.

  c. Splenomegaly is most common in leukemia or lymphoma.

  d. Poor nutrition causing **folate deficiency** is common in patients with cancer because of poor appetites. Dietary history should provide the clues to the diagnosis.

 3. Abnormalities of platelet function. The majority of cases will be secondary to drug effects, including (1) nonsteroidal antiinflammatory agents (e.g., aspirin), (2) antibiotics (e.g., carbenicillin), and (3) antidepressants (tricyclics) and tranquilizers. Consider any drug that the patient is taking as a possible offender until proven otherwise. Recall that from the platelet point of view, alcohol is considered a drug.

 4. Coagulation factor deficiencies may develop in patients with malignancy for several reasons:

a. Disseminated intravascular coagulation (DIC).

b. Liver failure causes deficiency of all clotting factors except factor VIII.

c. Malnutrition leads to deficiency of factors II, VII, IX, and X (the vitamin K-dependent factors).

d. Circulating anticoagulants, if present, are most commonly fibrin–fibrinogen split products. Specific anticoagulants may also be seen but are not common.

e. Functionally abnormal clotting factors are occasionally seen. The most commonly diagnosed abnormality is dysfibrinogenemia.

C. Laboratory diagnosis of bleeding. A patient with unexplained bleeding should have several tests to help determine what hematologic abnormalities, if any, are responsible for the bleeding. If all of the screening tests are normal, it is not likely that a hematologic cause exists for the bleeding, and local factors, such as an eroded blood vessel, should be considered.

1. Screening tests for bleeding. The following tests provide an adequate screening battery:

a. Platelet count

b. Bleeding time

c. Prothrombin time (PT)

d. Activated partial thromboplastin time (APTT)

e. Thrombin time

f. Fibrinogen level

2. Interpretation of screening laboratory studies. Abnormalities in the screening tests reflect hematologic problems caused by blood vessels, platelets, or coagulation factors. The following list provides clues to the interpretation of the screening tests that will help determine the most likely cause or causes, of the patient's bleeding.

a. Platelet count

(1) Normal is 150,000 to 450,000/mm^3

(2) If thrombocytopenia is less than 100,000/mm^3, consider the following:

(a) Bone marrow failure

(b) Increased consumption of platelets

(c) Splenic pooling of platelets

(3) Thrombocytosis greater than 500,000/mm^3 is

(a) Common in patients with neoplasms

(b) May be seen in association with iron-deficiency states

b. Bleeding time

(1) Normal bleeding time requires both adequate platelet number and function and adequate blood vessel function.

(2) Prolonged bleeding time may be due to thrombocytopenia, abnormal platelet function, or rarely, inadequate vessel wall function.

c. Prolonged PT is seen in the presence of the following:

(1) Deficiency of one or more of the following clotting factors: VII, X, V, II (prothrombin), or I (fibrinogen) (Oral anticoagulant therapy leads to a deficiency of II, VII, IX, and X)

(2) Circulating anticoagulant(s) against factors VII, X, V, or II

d. Prolonged APTT

(1) Deficiency of any of the following clotting factors: XII, XI, IX, VIII, X, V, II, or I. Factor XII deficiency is not associated with bleeding. Fletcher and Fitzgerald factor deficiencies (both rare) may also prolong APTT.

(2) Circulating anticoagulants against factors XII, XI, IX, VIII, X, V, or II.

(3) Anticoagulant therapy with

(a) Heparin

(b) Oral anticoagulants

e. Prolonged thrombin time. Prolongation of the thrombin time may be due to

(1) Hypofibrinogenemia

(2) Some forms of dysfibrinogenemia

(3) Fibrin–fibrinogen split products

(4) Heparin therapy

If the thrombin time is prolonged, further studies to clarify the cause may be required.

f. Low fibrinogen level. In evaluating the results of a fibrinogen assay, one must be familiar with the assay method used. Many laboratories use immunologic assays, which will measure both functionally normal and abnormal fibrinogens. If such an assay is in use, the thrombin time can be used to evaluate the functional integrity of the fibrinogen. A low functional fibrinogen level means that production is decreased or that consumption is increased.

D. Transfusion therapy

1. General guidelines

a. Avoid the use of whole blood if at all possible, as whole blood can cause further risk of bleeding by diluting clotting factors and platelets.

b. Use the specific blood component needed by the patient.

2. Blood component therapy

a. Platelet transfusions

(1) Available forms of platelets for transfusion are:

(a) Random donor platelets

(b) Single donor platelets

(c) HLA matched platelets

The latter two are reserved for use in patients who fail to respond to random donor platelets or who may be a candidate for bone marrow transplantation, or in patients expected to need many platelet transfusions.

(2) Check platelet count 4 hours and 24 hours after platelet transfusion to estimate survival of platelets in the patient.

(3) When to transfuse with platelets

(a) Prophylactic platelet transfusion should be considered when the platelet count is 20,000/mm^3 or less. This transfusion is particularly important in patients with acute leukemia.

(b) If surgery is contemplated (with the exception of intracranial surgery), the platelet count should be raised to 60,000/mm^3 (check bleeding time before surgery; results should be within 2 minutes of upper limits of normal).

(c) For intracranial surgery transfuse to a platelet count of 100,000/mm^3 (bleeding time must be checked before surgery and must be normal).

b. Coagulation factor support

(1) Fresh frozen plasma (FFP) contains all clotting factors (but not platelets) and should be used for multiple coagulation factor deficiencies. FFP requires 20 to 30 minutes to thaw, as it must be thawed at 37°C or lower.

(2) Cryoprecipitated factor VIII ("cryo") is a source of factor VIII, fibrinogen, and factor XIII. Each bag of cryo contains the factor VIII and fibrinogen harvested from 1 unit of fresh whole blood. Cryoprecipitate is stored in a frozen state and has the advantage of concentrating the clotting factors in a very small volume (≤10 cc/unit).

(3) Factor IX concentrates contain factors II, VII, IX, and X. Several precautions are worth noting.

(a) This concentrate is made from pooled plasma; therefore, the **risk of hepatitis** is high.

(b) There is a **small risk of disseminated intravascular coagulation (DIC)** resulting from the use of factor IX concentrates. Patients with liver dysfunction and newborns have an increased risk.

(c) Factor IX concentrates are stored in the lyophilized state. **Do not shake** when reconstituting.

E. Disseminated intravascular coagulation. DIC may occur with a broad range of signs and symptoms from an asymptomatic abnormality of laboratory tests to a rapidly fatal process characterized by diffuse organ damage. Because it is common, often complex, potentially life threatening, and may be difficult to diagnose with certainty, DIC will be considered in some detail.

1. **Common etiologies** of severe DIC include

   a. Gram-negative infections

   b. Obstetrical complications

   c. Acute promyelocytic leukemia and other neoplasms, especially mucin-producing lesions

   d. Liver failure

2. **Laboratory features** of DIC may be variable, depending on the severity and other underlying problems, such as liver disease, a poor nutritional status, and bone marrow function.

   a. Prolonged PT

   b. Prolonged APTT

   c. Thrombocytopenia

   d. Reduced fibrinogen

   e. Prolonged thrombin time

   f. Positive fibrinogen-fibrin split products

   g. Evidence of microangiopathic hemolytic anemia on peripheral smear

   h. Low factor V and VIII levels

   i. Shortened euglobulin lysis time

3. **Clinical features** of DIC

   a. DIC is often associated with hypotension.

   b. Renal, pulmonary, and/or CNS dysfunction may be present.

   c. Diffuse bleeding may occur, including petechiae, bruising, bleeding from mucous membranes, and bleeding from skin trauma sites.

   d. A disease process known to be associated with DIC may be present.

4. **Therapy** for DIC includes

   a. Urgently correct shock

   b. Treat underlying disease process

   c. Replacement therapy with blood components, for example, platelets and fresh frozen plasma

   d. Consider the use of heparin only when there is evidence of ongoing and organ damage to the brain, lungs, or kidneys owing to DIC in a patient who has been resuscitated from shock

e. There is no evidence that chronic warfarin therapy is of value in the treatment of chronic DIC that is seen in some patients with neoplasia

Selected Reading

Nauseef, W. M., and Maki, D. G. A study of the value of simple protective isolation in patients with granulocytopenia. *N. Engl. J. Med.* 304:448, 1981.

Parry, M. F., and Neu, H. C. A comparative study of ticarcillin plus tobramycin versus carbenicillin plus gentamicin for the treatment of serious infections due to gram-negative bacilli. *Am. J. Med.* 64:961, 1978.

Pizzo, P. A. et al. Duration of empiric antibiotic therapy in granulocytopenic patients with cancer. *Am. J. Med.* 67:194, 1979.

Ketchel, S. J., and Rodriguez, V. Acute infections in cancer patients. *Semin. Oncol.* 5:167, 1978.

Bick, R. L. Alterations of hemostasis associated with malignancy. Etiology, pathophysiology, diagnosis and management. *Semin. Thromb. Hemostas.* 5:1, 1978.

Note. The body surface area is given by the point of intersection with the middle scale of a straight line joining height and weight. (Reproduced from K. Diem and C. Lentner [Eds.], *Scientific Tables* [DOCUMENTA GEIGY, 7th ed.], 1970, with permission of CIBA-GEIGY Ltd., Basel, Switzerland.)

Height	Surface Area	Weight

Note. The body surface area is given by the point of intersection with the middle scale of a straight line joining height and weight. (Reproduced from K. Diem and C. Lentner [Eds.], *Scientific Tables* [DOCUMENTA GEIGY, 7th ed.], 1970, with permission of CIBA-GEIGY Ltd., Basel, Switzerland.)

Appendix II
Nomogram for Calculating the Body Surface Area of Children

Height	Surface Area	Weight

Height

cm 120 — 47 in
46
115 — 45
44
110 — 43
42
105 — 41
40
100 — 39
38
95 — 37
36
90 — 35
34
85 — 33
32
80 — 31
30
75 — 29
28
70 — 27
26
65 — 25
24
60 — 23
22
55 — 21
20
50 — 19
18
45 — 17
16
40 — 15
14
35 — 13
12
30 — 11
cm 25 — 10 in

Surface Area

1.10 m^2
1.05
1.00
0.95
0.90
0.85
0.80
0.75
0.70
0.65
0.60
0.55
0.50
0.45
0.40
0.35
0.30
0.25
0.20
0.19
0.18
0.17
0.16
0.15
0.14
0.13
0.12
0.11
0.10
0.09
0.08
0.074 m^2

Weight

kg 40.0 — 90 lb
85
80
35.0 — 75
70
30.0 — 65
60
25.0 — 55
50
20.0 — 45
40
15.0 — 35
30
25
10.0
9.0 — 20
8.0
7.0 — 15
6.0
5.0
4.5 — 10
4.0 — 9
3.5 — 8
7
3.0
6
2.5
5
2.0
4
1.5
3
kg 1.0 — 2.2 lb

Index

Index